Whole Person Healthcare

WHOLE PERSON HEALTHCARE

Volume 2

Psychology, Spirituality, and Health

Ilene A. Serlin, PhD, ADTR, General Editor

Kirwan Rockefeller, PhD, and
Stephen S. Brown, MA, Volume Editors

Praeger Perspectives

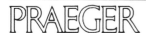

Westport, Connecticut
London

Library of Congress Cataloging-in-Publication Data

Whole person healthcare / Ilene A. Serlin, general editor
    p. ; cm.
  Includes bibliographical references and index.
  ISBN-13: 978–0–275–99231–6 (set : alk. paper)
  ISBN-13: 978–0–275–99232–3 (v. 1 : alk. paper)
  ISBN-13: 978–0–275–99233–0 (v. 2 : alk. paper)
  ISBN-13: 978–0–275–99234–7 (v. 3 : alk. paper)
  1. Integrative medicine. I. Serlin, Ilene A. [DNLM: 1. Mind-Body and Relaxation
Techniques. 2. Behavioral Medicine—methods. 3. Health Behavior. 4. Holistic
Health. WB 880 W628 2007]
  R733.W489 2007
  610—dc22   2007013444

British Library Cataloguing in Publication Data is available.

Library of Congress Catalog Card Number: 2007013444
ISBN-10: 0–275–99231–4 (set)   ISBN-13: 978–0–275–99231–6 (set)
          0–275–99232–2 (vol. 1)   978–0–275–99232–3 (vol. 1)
          0–275–99233–0 (vol. 2)   978–0–275–99233–0 (vol. 2)
          0–275–99234–9 (vol. 3)   978–0–275–99234–7 (vol. 3)

First published in 2007

Praeger Publishers, 88 Post Road West, Westport, CT 06881
An imprint of Greenwood Publishing Group, Inc.
www.praeger.com

Printed in the United States of America

The paper used in this book complies with the
Permanent Paper Standard issued by the National
Information Standards Organization (Z39.48–1984).

10 9 8 7 6 5 4 3 2 1

VOLUME 2:
PSYCHOLOGY, SPIRITUALITY, AND HEALTHCARE
CONTENTS

FOREWORD

When I was a senior resident in internal medicine, I was a little startled to hear one of the most respected senior physicians say to me one day, "You know, Dean, the mind doesn't really affect the body very much. I'm surprised that you believe that it does. And it can't be studied anyway."

This was not *that* long ago—in 1984. And it was at Harvard Medical School's Massachusetts General Hospital, which goes to show how much the field of behavioral medicine has evolved since then.

Because behavioral medicine is a relatively new field, it can be challenging to sort out what is most effective. This three-volume series does a lot of that work for you. It has assembled a group of accomplished experts in the field who can help guide you to understand better what works and what does not, for whom and under what circumstances.

We tend to think of advances in medicine as a new drug, laser, or other high-tech device. It can sometimes be hard for people to believe that relatively simple changes in behaviors, such as diet and lifestyle, can make such a powerful difference in our health and well-being, but they often do.

During the past 30 years, my colleagues and I at the nonprofit Preventive Medicine Research Institute and the School of Medicine, University of California, San Francisco (UCSF), have conducted a series of randomized controlled trials and demonstration projects demonstrating how powerful behavioral medicine approaches can be. We used the latest in high-tech, state-of-the-art diagnostic technology (including quantitative coronary arteriography and cardiac PET scans) to prove the power of low-tech, low-cost, and often ancient interventions.

At the time the conventional wisdom was that the progression of coronary heart disease could only get worse and worse. At best, you might be able to slow the rate at which the disease progressed, but that was about it. We were able to show, for the first time, that the progression of even severe coronary heart disease may begin to reverse using a multifactorial behavioral medicine program of comprehensive lifestyle changes. These included eating a whole-foods, low-fat diet rich in fruits, vegetables, whole grains, legumes, and soy products; getting moderate exercise; practicing stress management techniques, including yoga and meditation; and using support groups to build community and enhance love, intimacy, and healthier communication.

What did we find? Within a month, there was a 91 percent reduction in the frequency of angina, and most patients became essentially pain-free. These patients not only *felt* better, they *were* better; their hearts received more blood flow, and they pumped blood more efficiently. Within a year, we found that even severely blocked coronary arteries became measurably less occluded, and there was even more reversal of their coronary artery disease after five years than after one year. In contrast, coronary artery disease continued to worsen in patients in the usual-care control group. After five years, 99 percent of patients were able to stop or reverse the progression of their heart disease as measured by cardiac PET scans, and there were 2.5 times fewer cardiac events. These findings were published in the *Journal of the American Medical Association*.

Last year, we published the first randomized controlled trial (in collaboration with Dr. Peter Carroll at UCSF and Dr. William Fair at Memorial Sloan-Kettering Cancer Center) showing that the progression of prostate cancer may be affected by a similar behavioral medicine intervention. This study was published in the *Journal of Urology*.

After completing these randomized controlled trials showing how medically effective these behavioral medicine approaches could be, we conducted a series of three demonstration projects showing that these approaches are not only medically effective, but also cost-effective, in people with coronary heart disease. Through our nonprofit institute we began training hospitals throughout the country in our behavioral medicine program that integrates the best of traditional and complementary interventions. Mutual of Omaha found that almost 80 percent of people who went through this program and were eligible for coronary bypass surgery or angioplasty were able to safely avoid it, saving almost $30,000 per patient in the first year. In a second demonstration project, Highmark Blue Cross Blue Shield found that they were able to reduce their costs by 50 percent in the first year and by an additional 20 percent to 30 percent in subsequent years.

On the basis of these findings, Medicare conducted a demonstration project of our approach and another behavioral medicine program based on our work by Dr. Herbert Benson, a pioneer in behavioral medicine who conducted research documenting the power of meditation to elicit what he termed the "relaxation response." Our data were peer reviewed in an all-day hearing at the Centers for Medicare and Medicaid Services by 16 experts, who concluded in a national coverage determination that Medicare should now cover cardiac rehabilitation programs that include behavioral medicine interventions. Since reimbursement is a major determinant of medical practice, this Medicare coverage may help to increase the demand for behavioral medicine practitioners and thus help make the field more sustainable.

Also, medical care costs are reaching a tipping point. Many corporations are beginning to find that their employees' medical care costs are exceeding their entire net profits, which is clearly not sustainable. For example, Starbucks spends more for healthcare for their employees than for coffee beans, and General Motors spends more on healthcare than on steel. As a result, there is a growing receptivity for behavioral medicine programs that have been shown to reduce costs and improve health.

At a time when the power of behavioral medicine approaches is becoming increasingly well documented, the limitations of high-tech medicine are becoming more evident. For example, tens of billions of dollars each year are spent on angioplasty and cardiac stents, even though a recent meta-analysis of all the randomized controlled trials showed that these approaches do not prolong life, or even prevent heart attacks, in stable patients with coronary heart disease. Newer, more expensive technologies, such as coated stents, actually *increased* the risk of having a heart attack. There is a growing realization that it often makes more sense to pay for behavioral medicine interventions than for ones, such as angioplasty, that are dangerous, invasive, expensive, and largely ineffective.

In contrast, the landmark Interheart study examined almost 30,000 people in 52 different countries throughout the world. The investigators found that heart attacks can be prevented in more than 90 percent of people simply by changing nine easily measured risk factors (smoking, lipids, hypertension, diabetes, obesity, diet, physical activity, alcohol consumption, and psychosocial factors), all of which are the focus of behavioral medicine.

Ultimately, behavioral medicine is about transforming our lives, not just our behaviors. Meditation, for example, can be presented as a stress management technique, which it is, but it can be even more powerful if used to help people quiet down their minds and bodies enough to rediscover and experience an inner sense of peace, joy, and well-being.

In our studies, we found that it was not enough to focus on behaviors; we had to work at a deeper level. Many people smoke, overeat, drink too much, abuse other substances, and work too hard as a way of numbing their pain, depression, and loneliness. We found that when we work at that level, people are more likely to make and maintain comprehensive lifestyle changes that are life enhancing rather than self-destructive.

Dean Ornish, MD

Founder and President, Preventive Medicine Research
Institute Clinical Professor of Medicine, University of
California, San Francisco

PREFACE

Minding the body and embodying the mind are two challenges that face medicine, psychology, and related healthcare disciplines. The better we get—and we are indeed getting better—at treating life-threatening illness, the more we convert previously terminal diseases like cancer and heart disease into chronic illnesses. As life expectancy increases, we expect more from medical care and life itself. The technology that has brought us elegant noninvasive imaging, monoclonal antibodies in the treatment of cancer, statins to lower cholesterol, microsurgery, antidepressant and antipsychotic medication, and microarrays of gene expression, has, oddly enough, created a greater demand than ever for mental methods of controlling and understanding our bodies. It is as though the technological advances in medicine provide not just methods but processes that inspire us to find other ways to manage our bodies better from a psychosocial as well as a biotechnological perspective.

Indeed, the public appetite for integrative approaches to healthcare has grown remarkably. In the past decade the use of integrative services has grown by 1 percent of the population per year (Eisenberg et al., 1993, Eisenberg, Davis, & Ettner, 1997). Americans now spend more money on alternative and complementary medical care than they spend out of pocket on doctors or hospital care. They make more appointments with such practitioners than with primary care doctors. They are clearly seeking something they do not find in modern high-tech medicine. In the past, such contacts were something of a secret—two-thirds of patients did not tell their doctors they were availing themselves of herbal, meditative, or physical treatments such as acupuncture, yoga, and massage. But physicians are increasingly accepting of what is now being called integrative care, and more patients are open about their bimedicality, which is good for both kinds of care.

Another force driving those with medical illnesses to integrative care is the fact that, by and large, integrative services are outside the grasp of health insurers. This means that good old-fashioned market forces drive the development of services. People pay out of pocket for what they want, rather than running the thicket of regulations, approvals, copayments, limitations, and other artificial bureaucracy that plagues healthcare in the United States. People feel more in control of their integrative treatment than of their mainstream medical care. This is a crucial and helpful dimension, since the essence of serious stress is helplessness—the inability to do anything about the stressor. Feeling in charge of a treatment elicits cooperation and a sense of competence. In a classic study of the effect of patient involvement in treatment, Ralph Horwitz and colleagues (Horwitz et al., 1990) examined the effects of beta blockers in reducing risk of death after a heart attack. These widely used drugs, which block arousal of the sympathetic nervous system, are now standard care. Horwitz and colleagues' study demonstrated that these drugs were indeed effective in reducing mortality and that better adherence to the medication regimen was associated with lower mortality. But the surprise in this large randomized trial was that better adherence was also associated with reduced mortality among those receiving *placebo* medication. Apparently, it was their adherence that kept them alive, as much as the medication.

I was asked to see the CEO of a large corporation in the coronary care unit because he was suffering from intractable hiccups. He had suffered a myocardial infarction, and the heart injury may have been irritating his diaphragm. But he had been unresponsive to medication, so they asked me to try hypnosis with him. I saw this man, accustomed to controlling everything around him, flat on his back, wearing little, with tubes going in and out of every orifice. He felt demoralized and helpless. He turned out not to be hypnotizable, but I taught him a relaxation exercise to try to minimize his reactive muscle tension that accompanied the frustration he felt about his illness and annoying symptom. I returned the next day to see how he was doing, and his wife greeted me excitedly, saying he had felt much better after seeing me and was eager to have another visit. Surprised, I asked about his symptom. "Oh, he still has the hiccoughs but just felt so much better after talking to you," she said. When I asked him why, he said, "I have been flat on my back for a week having things done to me. You were the first person who told me there was something I could do for myself." So while objectively I didn't help him with the symptom, finding a way that he could participate in his recovery made a difference to him.

The average doctor spends some 7 minutes with a patient; the average practitioner of integrative medicine 30 minutes per patient. These numbers suggest what is missing in high-tech medical care: attention to the person with the disease. Sir William Osler said that it is more important to know the person who has the disease than the disease the person has. The twentieth century ushered in the era of scientific medicine with the Flexner report, which recommended that medicine be taught in organized curricula emphasizing two years of basic training in the fundamental sciences of medicine, including biochemistry, pathology, anatomy, immunology, and pharmacology. This was a departure from the apprenticeships that had dominated medical training until that time. The Flexner report promoted tremendous advances in healthcare, emphasizing more the science rather than the art of medicine, which was needed, since we were not far from the era of purgatives and blood-letting, which had often inflicted more harm than good. The oldest adage of medicine had been, "to cure rarely, to relieve suffering often, to comfort always." However, in the twentieth century we rewrote that job description to be, "to cure always, relieve suffering if you have the time, and let someone else do the comforting." This was a swing of the medical pendulum too far in the other direction. No matter how good we get at medical treatment, the death rate will always be one per person. Medicine and medical intervention will have to help us live with dying as well as cure diseases.

Whole Person Healthcare addresses this need, presenting in a lively and scholarly way a variety of approaches to helping the person with the disease learn to live better with it. Interventions ranging from essentials of mind-body medicine through psychological and spiritual approaches to art, music, dance, writing, and other applications of creative expression to healthcare are presented by experts in these areas. These experts provide a varied and authoritative review of methods to harness the human in the service of better health. We ignore what is most human in us at our peril. The science and art of psychologically, socially, emotionally, spiritually, and physically expressive intervention in healthcare is growing rapidly and is much needed. These volumes address that need, both for those with medical illnesses and for those who treat them. They are timely and timeless. Enjoy them.

David Spiegel, MD

Willson Professor and Associate Chair of Psychiatry & Behavioral Sciences
Medical Director, Center for Integrative Medicine
Stanford University School of Medicine
Stanford, California

REFERENCES

Eisenberg, D., Davis, R., & Ettner, S. (1997). Trends in alternative medicine use in the United States, 1990–1997. *Journal of the American Medical Association, 280,* 1569–1575.

Eisenberg, D. M., Kessler, R. C., Foster, C., Norlock, F. E., Calkins, D. R., & Delbanco, T. L. (1993). Unconventional medicine in the United States. Prevalence, costs, and patterns of use. *New England Journal of Medicine, 328,* 246–252.

Horwitz, R. I., Viscoli, C. M., Berkman, L., Donaldson, R. M., Horwitz, S. M., Murray, C. J., et al. (1990). Treatment adherence and risk of death after a myocardial infarction. *Lancet, 336*(8714), 542–545.

ACKNOWLEDGMENTS

Many people have served as inspiration, believed in this project, and read drafts of various sections. First, our editor at Praeger, Debora Caravalko, has encouraged and supported us through three years of gestation to give birth to these "triplets." Second, I want to thank my family, Florence, Barbara and Erica Serlin, and Jeff Saperstein for putting up with my preoccupation all these years. Friends and mentors, Kirk Schneider, Tobi Zausner, Stan Krippner, and Pat DeLeon were always there with wise advice. Fellow editors, with whom I have collaborated on projects over many years, Marie DiCowden, Kirwan Rockefeller, Stephen S. Brown, Jill Sonke-Henderson, Rusti Brandman, and John Graham-Pole, have been unflagging believers and collaborators in this work. Thanks to Dean Ornish and David Spiegel for supporting the work with their foreword and preface. Finally, all the editors and contributors, whose names appear in each volume, have given generously of themselves and shared their work and expertise.

Ilene A. Serlin, PhD, ADTR

INTRODUCTION

Mind-body therapies offer an exciting new healthcare frontier. This series introduces the public, healthcare professionals, and students to this future. Mind-body therapies address the complex interaction of mental, physical, and spiritual dimensions of health and illness. Because these therapies deal with the whole person in his or her setting, rather than in terms of isolated disease entities or body parts, this integrative approach is referred to as whole person healthcare. Each volume of this series demonstrates the application of mind-body therapies in a variety of contexts, showing their relevance across a wide range of settings and disciplines. Healthcare practices are expanding from traditional medical settings into new areas such as rehabilitation, wellness programs, and community education—offering practitioners new opportunities and challenges.

These developments are consistent with a variety of recent trends within psychology, such as the "Year of the Whole Person" (Serlin, 2001–2002; Serlin, Levant et al. 2001) and the addition of the word *health* into the mission statement of the American Psychological Association (APA) in 2001. An APA Health Care for the Whole Person Task Force in 2004, under the leadership of APA's president Ron Levant, began to gather evidence of the effectiveness and best practices of integrative collaborative care.

This series presents theory and clinical instruction for bringing a *whole person* perspective to healthcare. Each volume features chapters written by experts in various areas of mind-body healthcare, with case examples and a Tool Kit that lays out basic principles of clinical practice in this area. The afterword for each volume is by a renowned expert in the interface of psychology and healthcare, including the director of the APA Practice Directorate, the director of the APA Education Directorate, a member of the APA Board of Directors, and a former APA president. The preface is written by David Spiegel, Medical Director of the Center for Integrative Medicine at Stanford University Medical Center, and the foreword is by Dean Ornish, Founder and President of the Preventive Medicine Research Institute. This series has been blessed with contributions from some of the most inspired and creative leaders of the psychology and healthcare community.

What is whole person healthcare? Whole person healthcare integrates the best of medical and psychological practices into a biopsychosocialspiritual model. While traditional psychology has celebrated the Decade of Behavior and the Year of Cognition, it is now time for a psychology of the whole person, which integrates behavior, cognition, and consciousness—body, mind, and spirit. It takes into account the impact of life-style on health issues and educates patients to be informed consumers who practice prevention and make changes in their lives toward self-care and health. It relies on experiential as well as theoretical learning and utilizes symbolic and nonverbal as well as linear and verbal modes of expression, data gathering, and verification. Cynthia Belar, APA's Executive Director for Education, called for an integrative psychology:

> I have spent years educating physicians and other health professionals that psychology had a scientific knowledge base and practice relevant to both "mental" and "physical" health . . . the biopsychosocial model cannot be segmented into its component parts without attention to interactive efforts. (Belar, 2000, p. 49)

Russ Newman, Executive Director of the APA Practice Directorate, used the term "strategic resilience" to describe a new collaboration of psychology with healthcare in which lifestyle plays an important aspect of psychological and physical health.

The whole person approach considers the person in the context of his or her world. It seeks to understand the *meaning* of symptoms, as well as their biological and behavioral causes. Adapting a whole person model is becoming critical for healthcare professionals as an increasingly educated public demands integrative approaches. Growing numbers of people are turning to integrative practitioners for the treatment of a broad spectrum of medical conditions, as well as to reduce stress and enhance personal effectiveness through methods such as meditation, yoga, and acupuncture. These techniques are far less effective if applied mechanically and require a new way of thinking about integration. Psychologists and other healthcare practitioners who hold a whole person perspective are showing how to integrate them into the therapeutic process. The enormous popularity of Bill Moyers's television series "Healing and the Mind" and the revelation in the January 28, 1993, issue of the *New England Journal of Medicine* that over one-third of Americans utilize unconventional medicine, yet do not tell their doctors, signaled a major shift in public attitudes toward healing (Eisenberg et al., 1998). The trend is growing; a rigorous study done in 2004 shows that 80 percent of cancer patients use complementary, alternative, and integrative therapies (Dittman, 2004; Dossey, 1991, 1992). With its emphasis on prevention and education, integrative healthcare is also cost effective (DeLeon, Newman, Serlin, Di Cowden, et al., 1998; Gazella, 2004, p. 83). The National Institutes of Health (NIH) funded a National Center of Complementary and Alternative Medicine to support research into alternative approaches, and the center's budget and prominence have been growing yearly. NIH also issued a "Roadmap" with an emphasis on prevention and education. The Consortium of Academic Medical Centers for Integrative Medicine consists of 23 medical schools with programs in integrative medicine that include education, research, and clinical training.

Mind and body are interrelated (Rossi, 1986). Candace Pert's groundbreaking work on psychoneuroimmunology demonstrated that the processing of emotions often affects physical illnesses and the ability to heal. Research on healthy humans, as well cancer and HIV-positive patients, has shown that significant increases in immune function and positive health outcomes correlate with constructive emotional expression (Pert, 1997). Holistic perspectives on the self can be found in humanistic psychology, humanistic medicine, preventive medicine, health psychology, and wellness practices.

Integrative healthcare addresses a three-fold crisis in our medical systems: (1) the "completely disgruntled health care consumer," (2) the "disenfranchised, disillusioned physician," and (3) the growing perception that our approach to health care "is a broken model" (Gazella, 2004, p. 86). Combining whole person psychology with healthcare practices will revive the morale and effectiveness of healthcare practitioners while opening a wide range of opportunities. Since so many Americans already utilize integrative healthcare, but do so with little useful information for quality control or sound decision making, healthcare practitioners can make a large contribution simply by offering a systematic whole person evaluation and providing listings of available resources. This series goes beyond this, building upon state-of-the-art practices and existing literature to describe how a whole person model can be applied in a wide range of settings and areas of practice.

Beyond making sound theoretical sense, an integrative whole person approach is urgent as we face ever-more complex health issues. For example, one-third of California's 2 million teens are very overweight or obese and are at risk for life-threatening illnesses by the time they reach age 30. The highest rates of these at-risk teens are among Latin Americans and African

Americans. In a study carried out by the U.S. Department of Agriculture, over one-half of all American adults are considered overweight or obese, spending about $33 billion each year on diet books, diet pills, and weight loss programs (Squires, 2001). Both losing weight and keeping weight off are psychological issues that require understanding of motivation, stress factors, coping mechanisms, and social support. An encouraging study at the University of California, San Francisco, suggests positive results from an approach to weight loss (PRNewswire, 2000) in which sustained weight loss resulted from training people in two basic internal skills of self-nurturing and limit setting. Psychological interventions give people more conscious control over their lives while improving their self-esteem and sense of meaning (Yalom, 1980). Integrative therapies are also cross-cultural, opening healthcare to diverse, disabled, and marginalized populations.

Psychosocial support groups have proven to be a significant whole person intervention in healthcare. They have increased quality of life and survival time in cancer patients (Fawzy, Fawzy, et al., 1993; Spiegel, Bloom, et al., 1989). Supportive-expressive group therapies are existentially based and aim to help patients live their lives more fully in the face of a life-threatening illness. A wellness model would focus on how to help ordinary individuals cope with such extraordinary circumstances, while support groups address questions of meaning, mortality, and expression.

A NEW INTEGRATIVE PARADIGM

A new healthcare approach must move away from the culture's "scientific materialism"—with its fragmentation of mind, body, and spirit—to a new integrative paradigm. Nobel laureate Roger Sperry described the coming paradigm shift as moving from this scientific materialism to an integrative, holistic, nonmechanistic, bidirectional model. Scientific materialism is based on the Cartesian dualism of mind and body. The new paradigm would provide "a more realistic realm of knowledge and truth, consistent with science and empiric verification" (Sperry, 1991, p. 255), while including the "ultimate moral basis" (Sperry, 1995, p. 9) of environmental and population sustainability. In Sperry's interactionist, nondualistic model of mental and physical states, causation is determined upward from physical states as well as downward from mental states. In this model, the mind affects the body, just as the body affects the mind.

Consciousness, which brings together the physical and mental aspects of experience, comprises the area of meaning, beliefs, and existential choice. An illness such as breast cancer, for example, might involve the symbolic aspects of a woman's body, her attitudes and sensibilities about her life's meaning, and her understanding of the spiritual dimensions of her existence, as well as a confrontation with her mortality. Out of such confrontations can come a renewed will to live, hardiness, and optimism (Maddi & Hightower, 1999).

Stories of death and rebirth descend into sadness and ascend to joy. Disconnection and reconnection are ancient themes reflected in the myths common to all humankind. With the courage to create (May, 1975), new narratives move the self from deconstruction to reconstruction (Feinstein & Krippner, 1988; Gergen, 1991; May, 1989; Sarbin, 1986). These healing narratives are experienced as coherent and meaningful and have been gaining attention in many areas of clinical practice, including family therapy (Epstein, White, & Murray, 1992; Howard, 1991; Omer & Alon, 1997; Polkinghorne, 1988; Rotenberg, 1987). The act of telling stories has always helped humans deal with the threat of nonbeing, and sometimes the expressive act itself has a healing effect (Pennebaker, 1990). Not all expressive acts are verbal, however. Whole person healthcare embraces diversity of technique and approaches that include nonverbal and multimodal modalities such as the expressive therapies and mindfulness meditation (Kabat-Zinn, 1994). The arts are a particularly effective way to bring symbolic expression and coping mechanisms to people who cannot express trauma verbally or cognitively. From a humanistic whole person perspective, the creative act is a courageous affirmation of life in face of the void of death. Art comes from the basic human need to create, communicate, create coherence, and symbolize. The arts are also transcultural, expressing archetypal symbols that are universal throughout history and across cultures. By bringing the body, ritual, and community back into healthcare, diversity is served by countering the dominance of a white, individualistic European male verbal psychological and medical tradition. Whole person healthcare goals include achieving a gender and culture balance of emotional empathy, self-awareness, assertiveness, instrumental problem solving, and expressiveness (Levant, 2001).

The religious and spiritual dimensions of human nature and human fate are ultimate questions that are integrally related to whole person healthcare. Although long banished by Western medicine, spiritual concerns are proving vital in whole person healthcare. One of the three major themes the National Multicultural Conference and Summit sponsored by the APA in 1999, for example, was "spirituality as a basic dimension of the human condition." It recommended that

> psychology must break away from being a unidimensional science, that it must recognize the multifaceted layers of existence, that spirituality and meaning in the life context are important, and that psychology must balance its reductionistic tendencies with the knowledge that the whole is greater than the sum of its parts. Understanding that people are cultural and spiritual beings is a necessary condition for a psychology of human existence. (Sue, Bingham, Porche-Burke, & Vasquez, 1999, p. 1065)

A healthcare system that separates science from spirit is culturally narrow and "may not be shared by three quarters of the world nor by the emerging culturally diverse groups in the United States" (Sue et al., 1999, p. 1065). Spiritually based rituals have been shown to be effective coping strategies for dealing with life stresses (Pargament, 1997) and serious trauma (Frankl, 1959). However, while a national survey showed that 92 percent of all American reported that "my religious faith is the most important influence in my life" (Bergin & Jensen, 1990, p. 5), most healthcare professionals are unprepared to deal with these issues (Shafranske & Malony, 1990). Learning to deal professionally and objectively with these issues is, in fact, an ethical concern (APA, 2003).

STRUCTURE OF THE SERIES

Each volume of this series is designed to guide readers into a different area of whole person healthcare, and each provides a coherent overview of the field. The contributions are transdisciplinary, from practitioners and programs in psychology, medicine, clergy, public policy, and the arts.

- **Volume 1: Humanizing Healthcare,** edited by Marie Di Cowden, lays a foundation of definitions and practices of integrative healthcare for the twenty-first century. It helps practitioners develop protocols and assess efficacy of alternative practices, emphasizes the relevance of integrative healthcare for marginalized populations, and discusses risk prevention, policy, and issues of patient protection.
- **Volume 2: Psychology, Spirituality, and Healthcare,** edited by Kirwan Rockefeller and Stephen S. Brown, focuses on issues of meaning in illness; the role of spirituality; health and mental health; chaplaincy and pastoral care; and research and practice in yoga, meditation, imagery, QiGong, prayer, ritual, and death and dying.
- **Volume 3: The Art of Health,** edited by Jill Sonke-Henderson, Rusti Brandman, Ilene Serlin, and John Graham-Pole, introduces readers to the history and practices of art and healthcare throughout the ages. It presents the history of art and health in ancient healing rituals; shows the relevance of rituals in the growing number of international contemporary art-in-health programs; and discusses applications of art, music, dance, drama, and poetry therapy programs at the bedside, in groups, and in cross-cultural conflict.

SUMMARY

The Year of the Whole Person provides a timely focus for a much-needed collaboration among healthcare professionals. This collaboration can bring together the best practices from psychology and medicine for a comprehensive treatment approach. The current unsustainable U.S. healthcare system urgently needs a more efficient utilization of services; the underserved patients are demanding that their healthcare professionals talk to each other and combine quality traditional and complementary practices—an experience through which healthcare professionals can rediscover their modern yet ancient roles as healers of the mind, body, and spirit.

REFERENCES

American Psychological Association. (2003). Guidelines for multicultural education, training, research, practice and organizational change for psychologists. *American Psychologist, 58*(5), 377–402.

Belar, C. (2000, September). Learning about APA. *APA Monitor, 31*(8), 49.

Bergin, A. E., & Jensen, J. P. (1990) Religiosity of psychotherapists: A national survey. *Psychotherapy, 27*(1), 3–7.

De Leon, P., Newman, R., Serlin, I., Di Cowden, M., et al. (1998, August). *Integrated health care.* Town Hall symposium conducted at the meeting of the American Psychological Association, San Francisco, CA.

Dittman, M. (2004). Alternative health care gains steam. *American Psychological Association Monitor, 35*(6), 42.

Dossey, L. (1991). *Meaning and medicine.* New York: Bantam.

Dossey, L. (1992). Era III medicine: The next frontier. *ReVision: A Journal of Consciousness and Transformation, 14*(3), 128–139.

Eisenberg, D., Davis R., Ettner, S., Appel S., Wilkey S., Van Rompay, M., & Kessler, R. (1998). Trends in alternative medicine use in the United States, 1990–1997; Results of a follow-up national survey. *Journal of the American Medical Association, 280*(18), 1569–1575.

Epstein, D., White, M., & Murray, K. (1992). A proposal for the authoring therapy. In S. McNamee & K. J. Gergen (Eds.), *Therapy as social construction.* London: Sage.

Fawzy, F. I., Fawzy, N. W., et al. (1993). Malignant melanoma: Effects of an early structured psychiatric intervention, coping, and affective state on recurrence and survival 6 years later. *Archives of General Psychiatry, 50*(9): 681–689.

Feinstein, D., & Krippner, S. (1988). *Personal mythology.* Los Angeles: Tarcher.

Frankl, V. (1959). *Man's search for meaning.* New York: Praeger.

Gazella, K. (2004, July/August). Mark Hyman, MD. Practicing medicine for the future. *Alternative Therapies, 10*(4), 83–89.

Gergen, K. (1991) *The saturated self.* New York: Basic Books.

Howard, G. (1991). Culture tales: A narrative approach to thinking, cross-cultural psychology, and psychotherapy. *American Psychologist, 46,* 187–197.

Kabat-Zinn, J. (1994). Foreword. In M. Lerner, *Choices in healing* (pp. xi–xvii). Cambridge, MA: MIT Press.

Levant, R. (2001). *We are not from Mars and Venus!* Paper presented to the American Psychological Association, San Francisco, CA.

Maddi, S., and Hightower, M. (1999). Hardiness and optimism as expressed in coping patterns. *Consulting Psychology Journal: Practice and Research, 51*(2), 95–105.

May, R. (1975). *The courage to create.* New York: Bantam Books.

May, R. (1989). *The art of counseling.* New York: Gardner Press.

Omer, H., & Alon, N. (1997). *Constructing therapeutic narratives.* Northvale, NJ: Aronson.

Pargament, K. I.(1997). *The psychology of religion and coping.* New York: Guilford Press.

Pennebaker, J. W. (1990). *Opening up: The healing power of expressing emotions.* New York: Guilford Press.

Pert, C. B.(1997). *Molecules of emotion.* New York: Scribner.

Polkinghorne, D. E. (1988). *Narrative knowing and the human sciences.* Albany: State University of New York Press.

PRNewswire. (2000, October 18). First obesity treatment to report sustained weight loss-skill training vs. drugs and diets.

Rossi, E. L. (1986). *The psychobiology of mind-body healing.* New York: Norton.

Rotenberg, M. (1987). Re-biographing and deviance: Psychotherapeutic narrativism and the Midrash. New York: Praeger.

Sarbin, T. (Ed.). (1986). *Narrative psychology: The storied nature of human conduct.* New York: Praeger.

Serlin, I. A. (2001–2002). Year of the whole person. *Somatics,* Fall/Winter, 4–7.

Serlin, I., Levant, R., Kaslow, N., Patterson, T., Criswell, E., & Schmitt, R. (2001). *Healthy families: A dialogue between holistic and systemic-contextual approaches.* Paper presented to the American Psychology Association, San Francisco, CA.

Shafranske, E. P., & Maloney, H. N. (1990). Clinical psychologists' religious and spiritual orientations and their practice of psychotherapy. *Psychotherapy, 27,* 72–78.

Sperry, R. W. (1991). Search for beliefs to live by consistent with science. *Zygon, Journal of Religion and Science, 26,* 237–258.

Sperry, R. W. (1995). The riddle of consciousness and the changing scientific worldview. *Journal of Humanistic Psychology, 35*(2), 7–34.

Spiegel, D., Bloom, J. R., et al. (1989). Effect of psychosocial treatment on survival of patients with metastatic breast cancer. *Lancet, 2*(8668): 888–891.

Squires, S. (2001, 10 January). Only high-carb, modest-fat diets work for long. *San Francisco Chronicle,* A2.

Sue, D. W., Bingham, R. P., Porche-Burke, L., &Vasquez, M. (1999). The diversification of psychology: A multicultural revolution. *American Psychologist, 54*(12), 1061–1069.

Yalom, I. D. (1980). *Existential psychotherapy.* New York: Basic Books.

VOLUME EDITORS' NOTES

Kirwan Rockefeller, PhD and Stephen S. Brown, MA

To stay healthy, we all know what we need to do: eat right, get plenty of exercise, rest or sleep when we're tired, and avoid bad habits. When our health suffers, we also know what to do: go to the doctor. At the doctor's office, we're examined with diagnostic instruments that aid our physician in determining what is happening to our bodies and assist with providing treatment to alleviate or cure our ailments.

Yet as we leave the doctor's office we may feel deeply unsatisfied, as our spirits lag, our hearts tremble, and our minds are overcome with negative thoughts. While the physical symptoms we experience may have been addressed, there's no magic pill for our deepest fears and concerns. And, as we all know, we humans are much more than just our bodies. We are our heart, soul, longings, memories, traits, and we're imbued with the inevitable human quality of wanting to make sense out of what we're experiencing. We may wonder why it is that our bodies fail us, why our health falters, why disease is a part of the human condition, and eventually even why someday we will die.

The chapters in this volume, Psychology, Spirituality and Healthcare, speak to the myriad ways in which people attempt to make meaning of an illness or diagnosis, and explore modalities that people use to answer the existential questions that arise with illness or disease. The authors of this volume, who are at the forefront of their respective fields, invoke the common knowledge that mind and body are indeed integrally connected. This connection is bound by psychology on the one side and spirituality on the other. Spirituality encompasses the many and diverse ways that people find meaning in suffering or pain and in their life's journey. When combined with psychology, spirituality brings peace of mind, resolution, and safety to soothe the ravages of disease or illness.

For hundreds of years, physicians who have carried on the tradition of Western, allopathic medicine have not been comfortable with the presence of spirituality in healthcare. Historically under the influence of Cartesian mind-body dualism, spirit and meaning have been relegated to the domains of theology and philosophy, and far removed from the examining or surgery room.

However, over the course of the past 30 years, people from all walks of life have increasingly been turning to age-old methods of healthcare: spas, meditation, yoga, qi gong, prayer, imagery, and ritual to bring aid in times of uncertainty and pain. The authors in this volume speak to the current shift occurring in the conventional paradigm of Western medicine that addresses the psychological, emotional, imaginal, metaphorical, and symbolic elements of being human. While this volume does not cover all the topics that pertain to the holistic trends in medical care and the healing arts in psychology, spirituality, and healthcare, it nonetheless provides good evidence for the growing need of attending to the whole person with a humanistic approach.

Chapter One

CLINICAL HEALTH PSYCHOLOGY: FROM HOSPITAL PRACTICE INTO THE COMMUNITY

Ronald H. Rozensky, PhD, ABPP, Lauren Vazquez, MS, and Samuel F. Sears, PhD

Professional psychology in hospitals and medical settings emerged in the past decade with increased accomplishments, value, and potential to impact overall healthcare outcomes (Tovian, Rozensky, & Sweet, 2003). Among the numerous accomplishments of those practicing and conducting research in these venues, authors have noted (1) the significant increase in the number of psychologists on medical school faculties and on hospital professional staffs; (2) the decision by the American Psychological Association (APA, 2001) to amend its bylaws to state that psychology is a health profession not just a mental health profession; (3) the political successes that allowed the inclusion of psychology as an independent healthcare profession for internship funding by the federal government's Graduate Medical Education Program and the funding by the Bureau of Health Professions for the Graduate Psychology Education Program; (4) the establishment of new current procedural terminology (CPT) codes specifically for psychological assessment and interventions associated with physical health problems and traditional medical interventions and diagnosis; and (5) the further expansion of recognized professional practice specialties—that is, "board-certified" specialties, as granted by the American Board of Professional Psychology that include those practicing clinical health psychology, clinical neuropsychology, and rehabilitation psychology (specialties and specialists associated with healthcare and hospital practice; Tovian, 2006). Further, Rozensky (2006a) details how psychologists are currently, de facto, important members of the healthcare team with indispensable roles and responsibilities in patient care ranging from prevention and primary care through tertiary care.

The clinical utility of health psychology was founded on the diverse set of skills that are reflected in the scientist-practitioner tradition. The scientist-practitioner model of professional psychology has been described as a generative model (Papas, Belar, & Rozensky, 2004) and has resulted in both the advancement of scientific knowledge in medical settings and the expansion of practice opportunities in such specialties as clinical health psychology, clinical neuropsychology, pediatric psychology, geropsychology, primary care psychology, and rehabilitation psychology. Rozensky (1994, p. 2) noted that "there is a growing recognition, both within clinical psychology and in medicine in general, that psychological services are essential in both the treatment of 'the whole person,' as well as in helping to contain spiraling health care costs." Rozensky (2004) argued that the autonomy of psychological services in medical settings and psychology's wide scope of practice in healthcare assures the continued growth and success of these clinical programs.

The role of consultant in the medical and surgical hospital setting has been part and parcel of those activities, and it has been psychology's commitment to the hand-in-hand blending of the scientific basis of psychological practice and clinical interventions in hospital settings with medically ill patients that is key to its successful adoption and expansion within healthcare (Barron, Fennell, & Voeller, 1995; Belar & Deardorf, 1995; Blechman & Brownell, 1998; Camic & Knight, 2004; Frank, Baum, & Wallender, 2004; Frank & Elliot, 2000; Freidman and Silver, 2007; Gatchel & Blanchard, 1993; Johnson, Perry, & Rozensky, 2002; Nezu, Maguth, & Geller, 2003; Nicassio & Smith, 1995; Resnick & Rozensky, 1996; Rozensky, Sweet, & Tovian, 1997; Sweet, Rozensky, & Tovian, 1991; Sweet, Tovian, & Suchy, 2003; Tartar, Butters, & Beers, 2001). Evidence-based research demonstrates that the application of behavioral principles to the treatment of the broadest range of medical problems improves health outcomes, and the literature illustrates that the ongoing collaborative endeavors between psychology and various medical and surgical specialties and subspecialties in tertiary care medicine also improve health outcomes. Among many available texts, Sweet, Rozensky, and Tovian (1991) and Johnson, Perry, and Rozensky (2002) offer chapter after chapter of assessment, diagnostic, and psychotherapeutic approaches to the full range of medical disorders and diseases found in the International Classification of Diseases (Ninth Revision)—or ICD-9—classification system. Johnson and colleagues (2002) recognize that the ICD-9 approach to classification of illness "suffers from the mind-body dualism so common to Western medicine's approach to disease and its management" (p. 4) but that health psychology, on a day-to-day basis, clearly relies on the integrative biopsychosocial model that "underlies health psychology as a science and as a profession" (Johnson et al., 2002, p. 4). Rey (2004) punctuates this by noting that illness and cure are related to the interaction of psychological, social, cultural, biochemical, and physiological processes within the human condition.

Psychological services have been established as reliable interventions that offset medical costs (Chiles, Lambert, & Hatch, 1999; Mumford, Schlesinger, Glass, Patrick, & Cuerdon, 1984; Prigatano & Pliskin, 2003; Sobel, 1995). Chiles and colleagues (1999), carrying out a meta-analysis of 91 studies between 1967 and 1997, noted about a 20 percent *decrease* in medical costs after the implementation of psychological interventions. Beyond the hospital setting, psychology successfully has taken its clinical work from the consulting room and hospital into the community in both prevention and treatment (Frank, Baum, & Wallender, 2004; Rozensky, Johnson, Goodheart, & Hammond, 2004). Thus, for both clinical and economic reasons, psychologists are no longer outsiders in medical settings and function as well-recognized members of the modern-day healthcare alliance and important partners in quality continuity of care.

Given the diverse roles that psychologists can now play in healthcare (Brown et al., 2002; Levant et al., 2001; Newman & Rozensky, 1995), this chapter focuses on the clinical responsibilities taken by psychologists in general medical and surgical hospital settings. It focuses on issues germane to that practice environment, including expectations of clinical competency needed to work with patients with medical disorders, surviving as a successful practitioner in the complicated environment of hospital practice, and treatment approaches and continuity of care from bedside practice to follow-up in the community. Clinical examples are provided to illustrate these issues.

COMPETENCY TO PRACTICE

The first thing practicing health psychologists must assure themselves is that they are competently prepared to consult with and treat medically ill patients referred to them in the hospital. This includes a true understanding of the medical diagnoses they will encounter and the utility and side effects of various medications and medical procedures the patient might have to undergo. Equally important in the traditional hospital setting is the ability to communicate clearly with the medical team and physicians. Rozensky, Sweet, and Tovian (1997) provide a list of recommendations to enhance clear communication in the hospital setting. They specifically entreat behavioral health clinicians to be concise, avoid jargon, and "avoid use of theory-bound concepts" (p. 27) so that clinical input is more likely to be integrated into the overall patient care plan. Even more critical today with shortened hospital stays is Wright's (1982, p. 3) statement that "physicians respect critical thinking more than exotic intuition…[and] this serves to make a more natural union of psychology with…medicine." The science of health psychology and the literature supporting treatment must be readily in the toolkit of hospital practicing clinicians and should form the basis of parsimonious, data-driven clinical services and communications.

The American Psychological Association's (2002) Ethical Principles of Psychologists and Code of Conduct states that psychologists should only practice within the boundaries of their competency (p. 4). To assure that this ethical responsibility is met when working with medically ill patients, Belar and colleagues (2001) offer a model for self-assessment and continuing education that facilitates the ethical expansion of practice into the domain of clinical health psychology. These authors suggest that, before traditionally trained, mental-health focused psychologists (who might have had only minimal training in health psychology during graduate school) seek to work clinically with medically ill patients, they should "develop the necessary expertise to provide quality services across a broader range of health problems" (p. 136). To prepare for diagnosing and treating medically ill patients, these authors suggest that clinicians ask themselves 13 questions to self-assess their readiness to deliver services to patients with medical-surgical problems. The content of this self-assessment routinely should be built into graduate education for clinical health psychologists or should be used by clinicians in a hospital-based practice or those who want to expand their clinical work and begin seeing patients with a diagnosis new to their practice. The self-study questions recommended by Belar et al. (2001, p. 137) are as follows:

1. Do I have knowledge of the biological bases of health and disease as related to this problem? How is this related to the biological bases of behavior?
2. Do I have knowledge of the cognitive-affective bases of health and disease as related to this problem? How is this related to the cognitive-affective bases of behavior?
3. Do I have knowledge of the social bases of health and disease as related to this problem? How is this related to the social bases of behavior?
4. Do I have knowledge of the developmental and individual bases of health and disease as related to this problem? How is this related to developmental and individual bases of behavior?
5. Do I have knowledge of the interactions among biological, affective, cognitive, social, and developmental components (e.g., psychophysiological aspects)? Do I understand the relationships between this problem and the patient and his or her environment (including family, healthcare system, and sociocultural environment)?
6. Do I have knowledge and skills of the empirically supported clinical assessment methods for this problem and how assessment might be affected by information in areas described by Questions 1–5?
7. Do I have knowledge of, and skill in implementing, the empirically supported interventions relevant to this problem? Do I have knowledge of how the proposed psychological intervention might impact physiological processes and vice versa?
8. Do I have knowledge of the roles and functions of other healthcare professionals relevant to this patient's problem? Do I have skills to communicate and collaborate with them?
9. Do I understand the sociopolitical features of the healthcare delivery system that can impact this problem?
10. Do I understand the health policy issues relevant to this problem?

11. Am I aware of the distinctive ethical issues related to practice with this problem?
12. Am I aware of the distinctive legal issues related to practice with this problem?
13. Am I aware of the special professional issues associated with this practice with this problem?

This list of questions first and foremost challenges clinicians to not only understand the interplay of all aspects of the biopsychosocial dimensions of the disease at hand but to have a working knowledge of the empirically supported assessments and treatments for the management of the disorder and its contributing psychological factors or sequelae. By focusing on the biopsychosocial paradigm, psychologists, physicians, and other healthcare professionals can readily conceptualize problems in a truly integrative manner, enhancing dialogue and encouraging successful collaboration in primary healthcare (Gatchel & Oordt, 2003; McDaniel, 1995) as well as in secondary and tertiary healthcare settings (Belar & Deardorff, 1995). This model, an antidote to potential reductionistic tendencies in medicine, rejects the long outdated premise of mind-body dualism (Engel, 1977) by highlighting and connecting the biological, psychological, interpersonal, and social factors as a larger framework of multiple systems interacting with each other. This paradigm serves as more than a conceptual framework in building an understanding of illness and disease processes and thus demands that clinicians and healthcare teams integrate patients' experiences in a more comprehensive manner (Tovian, 2006). This, then, enhances patient care, providing the efficient use of resources and removing barriers (i.e., stigma) to access of care (Gunn, Seaburn, Lorenz, Gawinski, & Maukush, 1997). It is this model that assures that physicians will include the mind in their medical/body diagnostic and treatment recommendations, thus assuring the place for psychological services to be a key component in all patient care.

HEALTH PSYCHOLOGY AND EVIDENCE-BASED PRACTICE

Sackett, Straus, Richardson, Rosenberg, and Haynes' (2000) original definition of evidence-based practice was adapted by the Institute of Medicine (2001) to read "Evidence-based practice is the integration of best research evidence with clinical expertise and patient values" (p. 147). The American Psychological Association's policy statement on evidenced-based practice closely parallels the institute's definition: "Evidenced-based practice in psychology is the integration of the best available research with clinical expertise in the context of patient characteristics, culture, and preferences" (APA, 2005a, p. 5). The APA's Report of the 2005 Presidential Task Force on Evidence-Based Practice notes that "there is broad consensus that psychological practice needs to be based on evidence, and that research needs to balance internal and external validity" (APA, 2005b, p. 6). That report goes on to list issues that must be addressed in order to adequately integrate research into everyday practice.

These include evaluating different research methods; assuring representative research samples, including minority and marginalized populations, are part of research being evaluated; and assessing the generalizability and transportability of both efficacy- and effectiveness-controlled studies to treatment. Further, the task force report noted specifically that "clinical expertise is essential for identifying and integrating the best research with clinical data" (p. 9) and crafted a review of what is referred to as "multiple types of research evidence" (p. 7). It is beyond the scope of this chapter to discuss what Davison (2006) has called for vis-à-vis the current working model of evidence-based practice—that is, "a thoroughgoing analysis and passionate discussion...[and] to study [this] complex issue from all possible angles" (p. 1). Suffice it to say, clinical health psychologists should be cognizant of the issues surrounding evidence-based medicine and evidenced-based psychology and practice. This is essential for the assurance of quality patient care and for the continued enhancement of the viability of scientifically based health psychology in the hospital.

LOCAL STANDARDS OF PRACTICE

An important component of successful practice in medical settings is the knowledge of currently supported treatments in the literature, an understanding of the scope of practice allowed for psychologists within the given medical setting in which one practices, and the local standards of practice used by psychologist in that particular setting. The Joint Commission on Accreditation of Healthcare Organizations (JCAHO; 2000) states that "the exercise of clinical privileges within any department is subject to the rules and regulations of that department and the authority of the department's director" (p. 271). Further, the JCAHO states that clinicians practice in the hospital setting within the scope of their own competences as "indicated by the score of their delineated privileges" (p. 271). Thus, the hospital practice setting can be experienced very differently than the relative freedom that is explicit in an independent office practice. While psychologists in independent practice are free to practice as trained and competent, the hospital setting contains a peer group of colleagues and director of psychology who has the ultimate responsibility to oversee all clinicians' work within the walls of the hospital . This scrutiny can include routine chart reviews, audit committees, and quality improvement activities as mandated by external review agencies and explicated in the hospital's bylaws and policies and procedures. This local standard of practice should not hamper anyone's work, but it must be clear that local standards of practice might well dictate common, acceptable clinical work with patients. Rozensky (2006a) notes,

> For example, a psychologist might come from a cognitive behavioral approach to working with patients with difficulties adhering to medical regimes. A patient with

diabetes, for example, does not follow her diet nor take her medications as prescribed by her physician and the psychologist has been working on that problem with her when she is hospitalized for an insulin reaction. Now, for sake of argument, the local hospital where the psychologist has privileges takes a psychodynamic approach to adherence problems. The psychologist might have to assure his or her peers, both when seeking professional staff appointment initially, and when providing care once on staff, that his approach is indeed acceptable practice and effective. (p. 262)

Practicing according to acceptable, routine, local practice patterns is important for continuity of care to assure that, for example, unit nursing staff that have to implement the patient care recommendations and treatment plans understand and can follow up around the clock with the patient. "Hospital-based psychologists cannot avoid external scrutiny of their practices given the requirements of quality improvement and assurance within the hospital milieu" (Rozensky, 1997, p. 33). Similarly, clinician who wish to practice in the hospital environment do not simply walk into the facility to see their medically hospitalized patient. They *must* have the appropriate credentials and privileges that assure them that they can legitimately attend their patient and have rights to put clinical notes in the patient's medical chart as a recognized member of the hospital's professional or medical staff. Psychologists wishing to practice in the hospital setting should consult with the department head of the psychology service and review the hospital's bylaws and policy and procedure manual to understand how to properly seek formal credentialing (Rozensky, 2006a) and what the expectations of practice are for staff members.

HOSPITAL CONSULTATION

Access to referrals may also be influenced by models of psychological consultation (Gatchel & Oordt, 2003). Pace, Chaney, Mullins, and Olson (1995) describe two approaches that characterize psychological consultation: the problem-oriented approaches that rely heavily on psychological expertise in the assessment and treatment of the patient and the process-oriented approach that focuses on collaboration with medical expertise and an integrated understanding of the biopsychosocial context. Roberts and Wright (1982) discuss three consultation models based on the problem-oriented approach: the direct-consultation model in which the psychologist may be asked by the attending physician to assess affective or neuropsychological functioning; the informal consultation model in which the psychologist never actually sees the patient but the physician seeks the psychologist's input; and the collaborative consultation model in which the psychologist assumes a more active role in the direct delivery of healthcare services, such as psychotherapy or behavior modification (Tovian, 2006). The process-oriented approach, on the other hand, is a more comprehensive model that involves multiple phases of frequent direct contact between psychologist and physician to review goals, objectives, and progress and to build a greater understanding of the patient and his or her relation to the entire biopsychosocial system with the psychologist often taking on more of the direct patient care responsibilities.

SURVIVING IN HOSPITAL PRACTICE

Psychologists in hospital practice encounter challenges that are unique to the setting, including patient and family psychological responses to acute, life-threatening illness as well as chronic disease exacerbations. Today, inpatient care is marked by increased attention and involvement with implantable medical technologies, such as drug-eluting devices and defibrillators and increasingly complicated multiple medication regimens. The psychological impact of these various technologies has only begun to be examined fully (Sears, Kovacs, Azzarello, Larsen, & Conti, 2004). Professional competency and comfort to practice in such settings for health psychologists can be daunting. Nonetheless, the needs of hospitalized patients for psychological care are greater than ever before. Biomedical technology, for example, requires patients to accommodate and ultimately to accept the technology as a part of themselves. Patients and healthcare professionals alike need to recognize that technology alone may never be able to mend the gap between a patient's premorbid functioning (what has been lost) and his or her postmorbid functioning (what has been gained). However, psychological adjustment remains a critical aspect of recovery throughout the treatment regime. Technology without patient acceptance can only provide short-term benefit of survival but not long-term quality of life.

CASE 1: HOSPITAL CONSULTATION AND POLYDEVICE THERAPY—PSYCHOLOGICAL INTERVENTION BEYOND MIND-BODY

The following case illustrates a cardiac patient whose cardiovascular treatment largely consisted of what we have coined "polydevice therapy." In the course of one year, he underwent implantable cardioverter defibrillator (ICD) implantation, left ventricular assist device (LVAD) implantation, and subsequent heart transplantation. An ICD is a surgically implanted biomedical device designed to contravene potentially lethal arrhythmias by the automatic delivery of an electrical cardioverting shock to defibrillate the heart and restore normal sinus rhythm. An LVAD is a surgically implanted mechanical device that helps maintain the pumping ability of a heart that cannot effectively work on its own.

Patients sometimes must wait long periods of time for a hearttransplant; LVADs can be used as a "bridge" to transplantation—as a means of improving deteriorating heart function until a donor heart is procured. The case of Mr. G is an example of what future hospital-based clinical health psychologists will have to be prepared to manage as the technology of cardiac device therapies continues to advance.

Mr. G, a 40-year-old Caucasian male, was admitted to the cardiovascular unit of the hospital with a prior history of nonischemic cardiomyopathy, status post-biventricular ICD implantation and subsequent LVAD within the last year, and recent placement on the list as Status 1-B for orthotopic heart transplant. Notably, his LVAD was found to be operating with caution monitoring, and he was admitted for purposes of surveillance of his cardiac device. Mr. G presented with a significant ICD shock history, self-reported fatigue, depressive symptoms, and recent weight gain, not secondary to fluid retention. After an extensive medical workup, Mr. G's LVAD was found to be in eminent cardiac failure, warranting his immediate placement as Status 1-A for transplant. Referral for psychological consultation was made by his cardiologist on the second day of hospitalization. A routine cardiac psychology assessment was conducted, and, based on this consultation, individual therapy was recommended; Mr. G was amenable to this suggestion. Suchday, Tucker, and Krantz (2002) reviewed the research-supported treatments for patients with cardiac disease, and these treatments and other references listed provided the evidenced-based foundation for the approaches to this patient's care.

While Mr. G was an inpatient, a course of individual psychotherapy consisting of six, 60-minute sessions was completed. Because depression has been determined to be an important predictor of mortality in cardiac populations (Ziegelstein et al., 2000), we were particularly motivated to deal immediately with his depressive symptoms and did so through cognitive and behavioral-focused techniques, including journaling, identifying automatic thoughts, and challenging cognitive distortions. Cognitive and behavioral strategies such as these have repeatedly demonstrated effectiveness in the treatment of both anxiety (Barlow, 1997) and depression (Dobson, 1989). Because research from a variety of sources and patient populations has yielded support for the beneficial effects of training in relaxation techniques (Burish, Carey, Krozely, & Greco, 1994; Taylor, 1995), relaxation techniques such as diaphragmatic breathing and progressive muscle relaxation were also introduced as strategies for decreasing Mr. G's depression and encouraging a sense of mastery over his psychological symptoms and bodily sensations. The

(Continues)

(Continued)

focus of therapy also included exploration of Mr. G's self-reported guilt over possibly accepting an organ from someone deceased, future planning of post-transplant functioning, and addressing his self-reported anxiety over the upcoming transplant operation. As links between anxiety and quality of life outcomes have been established in prior research in which pre–cardiac transplantation trait anxiety was associated with increased symptom frequency and decreased mental health at long-term post-transplantation follow-up (Sears, Rodrigue, Greene, & Mills, 1995), alleviating his anxiety over the transplantation was an essential part of therapy. After four sessions of therapy, an appropriate heart was procured for Mr. G, and he underwent orthotopic heart transplant and removal of his ICD and LVAD.

Following his time in the intensive care unit and transfer back to the cardiovascular unit, we again initiated psychotherapy. We met for two additional sessions focusing exclusively on future planning surrounding issues of quality of life. Mr. G was highly motivated for change and optimistic about his "second chance at life," having addressed and let go his feelings of guilt over receiving his new heart (at discharge he was seeking information about the donor so that he could thank the family). He was discharged from the hospital in stable condition and returned to his home over 300 miles from the hospital. Follow-up with Mr. G consisted of two 30-minute phone sessions, during both of which Mr. G reported desirable psychosocial functioning and described strengthened relationships with his wife and daughter, specifically referencing the cognitive and behavioral solutions for coping that he learned during his hospital stay.

CASE 2: INPATIENT PAIN MANAGEMENT

The case of Mr. S is one that exemplifies several challenges for hospital-based clinical health psychologists, including the assessment and treatment of pain patients, as well as interaction with a patient distrustful of the medical environment and its practitioners. The concept of pain is a widely subjective phenomenon. Pain is generally composed of two parts: affective-emotional factors and sensory-discriminative factors (Merskey & Bogduk, 1994). Pain results from the interaction of nociception, pain perception, pain appraisal, pain behavior, and social roles for chronic pain and illness over time (Dworkin, Von Korff, & LeResche,

1992). Regardless of definition or origin, the assessment and treatment of pain patients can be challenging because this population often exhibits accompanying psychological sequelae, including depression, anxiety, and hypervigilance (Doleys, 2000). Robinson and James (2005) state that psychologists who practice in general medical facilities should be able to make the distinction between physical illnesses that may have a psychological component and those that are entirely psychological in nature. This is particularly important when working with patients who present with complaints of pain. Clinical health psychology has a long history of evidenced-based approaches to the assessment and successful treatment of acute and chronic pain (Chapman, 1991; Jensen, Turner, & Romano, 2001).

Mr. S was a 65-year-old white male who was transferred to our hospital from his local community hospital for evaluation of atypical chest pain of undetermined etiology. He had a long history of cardiac problems, including a myocardial infarction approximately 15 years prior to admission and coronary artery bypass graft 1 year prior to the current admission. Current management of his chest pain included taking a nitroglyceride tablet when he experienced angina, and if the pain did not resolve within 15 minutes, he would travel to the emergency room; as a result, he had had multiple hospitalizations over the past several years. His angina had no clear pattern of precipitants or temporal factors. Mr. S had a history of problematic interaction with his healthcare providers and repeatedly expressed his concern that he was not receiving the care that he deserved. A referral for psychological consultation was made by his attending cardiologist.

Mr. S was forthcoming about his distrust of our intentions during the assessment and commented several times that we were there to determine whether his pain was "real" or "in his head." He presented with a dramatic interpersonal style and reported current dysphoria, fatigue, agitation, tension, and excessive worrying. Following our assessment, we recommended that Mr. S engage in individual psychotherapy while he was an inpatient; he was amenable to this recommendation.

Our treatment plan for Mr. S included cognitive-behavioral strategies that emphasized increasing his knowledge of chest pain etiology, effective communication with healthcare providers, and pain management techniques such as relaxation training and stress relief. Both behavioral and cognitive-behavioral strategies have repeatedly demonstrated benefit in pain populations (Compas, Haaga, Keefe, Leitenberg, & Williams,

(Continues)

(Continued)

1998; Turner & Romano, 1990). We also provided psychoeducation about the relationships between anticipatory anxiety and hypervigilance and the prophylactic benefit that alleviating stress and anxiety can have on pain. One of the mechanisms thought most effective in the treatment of pain is the prevention of future pain episodes (Linton & Bradley, 1996). We acknowledged the existence of Mr. S's pain and utilized supportive therapeutic techniques to increase his comfort level in discussing his frustration with his current health status as well as with his treating physicians, who he felt were dismissive of his repeated pain complaints.

Upon discharge, Mr. S had completed six sessions of therapy, reported an understanding of the relationship between anxiety, tension, and pain and the benefit of alleviating stress to prevent future pain. He learned deep muscle relaxation skills well and utilized them twice daily, noting the reinforcing nature of decreased tension. He also described more effective communication with his physicians that resulted in his perception of better care by his healthcare team. He appeared hopeful for an improved quality of life precipitated by more effective management of his pain.

CONTINUITY OF CARE FROM BEDSIDE PRACTICE TO FOLLOW-UP IN THE COMMUNITY

Due to healthcare cost concerns, a greater degree of recovery and rehabilitation from illness and injury has shifted from inpatient recovery to the outpatient setting. The impact of this strategy involves greater responsibility and burden on families to extend previously hospital-based care to home-based care. The primary benefits include lower healthcare costs and more patient comfort due to returning home sooner. This continuum of care also can stress and strain families into new roles that can impact family functioning. The importance of social support and its impact on decreasing anxiety and depression in times of stress has been detailed (Taylor, 2006). McDaniel, Johnson, and Sears (2004) focused on the family as a social network and its central role in successfully managing medical illness; while Berkman and Syme (1979) looked more broadly and found that the larger one's social network—including spouse, friends, relatives, church and other group membership—the lower one's chances of mortality over a nine-year period. Taylor (2006) concludes her review of the scientific literature in social support and health by stating that, "across the life span, nurturant, supportive contact with others, a sense of belonging or mattering to others, and participation in social groups have been tied to a broad array of mental health and health benefits" (p. 163). Collectively, successfully extending the continuity of care via family can be partially reliant on the strength of the relationships that predate the current healthcare needs. Psychologists can provide specific evaluation, recommendations, and treatments to determine and address the viability of this health trend for individual patients and families.

CASE 3: PALLIATIVE DECISION MAKING AND HOME FOLLOW-UP

The following case study exemplifies a focus on quality of life and psychosocial functioning in the context of a life-threatening disease and palliative decision making. Health-related quality of life reflects a patient's ability to function in a variety of life's domains and may be embodied in the biopsychosocial model of health (Engel, 1977) in which biological, psychological, and social functioning are interdependent. Quality-of-life issues are highly relevant to the practice of palliative care and should be considered when patients are faced with palliative decision making. According to the World Health Organization (2005), palliative care improves the quality of life of patients and their families facing problems associated with life-threatening illness, through the prevention and relief of suffering. The American Board of Hospice and Palliative Medicine (2000) adds that such relief requires the comprehensive assessment and interdisciplinary team management of the multidimensional needs of patients *and* their families or social network. This definition emphasizes the necessity of the added expertise of hospital-based clinical health psychologists to the healthcare team and the ability to optimize physical, psychosocial, and spiritual care of patients.

Ms. M, a 35-year-old white female, was admitted to the oncology floor of the hospital with a remote history of breast cancer that had recently metastasized to her liver. She was treated by a neighboring hospital with radiofrequency ablation for the liver metastases and subsequently developed a right-sided bronchobiliary fistula. The fistula progressively impaired Ms. M's ability to lie flat and to sleep comfortably and also created a chronic cough, greatly decreasing her health-related quality of life. She became debilitated by the fistula and was unable to work or perform most activities of daily living. After medical consultation, she elected to undergo operative treatment for the fistula. The operation was noted to be strictly palliative and not curative, as the liver metastases were significant and notably life threatening. Ms. M tolerated the surgery well but later developed complications from her

(Continues)

(Continued)

surgical wound. As a result of these complications, Ms. M was required to remain an inpatient for an extended period of time. After her third week of hospitalization, she began to report depressive symptoms, anorexia, sleep disturbances, and a strong desire to return home to her husband and three young children, all of whom lived over 200 miles from the hospital and were only able to visit her occasionally. Referral for psychological consultation was then made by her hepatologist, and a routine inpatient psychological evaluation was completed. Henderson and Baum (2002) detailed the range of evidence-based psychological treatments for patients with cancer and its medical and psychological sequelae.

Following the assessment, individual psychotherapy was initiated. Ms. M largely needed supportive therapy, as she reported feeling extremely isolated being away from her family. Helgeson and Cohen (1996) determined that perceptions of greater social support were consistent with more positive psychological adjustment to cancer. Research has also suggested that the presence of social support can improve medical outcomes (Maunsell, Brisson, & Deschenes, 1995). Several therapy sessions were arranged that included her husband and children and focused on helping them understand and accept her limitations and support her when she expressed frustration over the changes and limitations in her ability to be an active mother and wife. Despite her prognosis, Ms. M exhibited intense optimism over her condition given the support of her family. She reportedly was "not ready to give up" and was appropriately motivated to achieve better health. While Ms. M was depressed, lonely, and ill, she possessed a unique positive outlook on her life, which motivated her during her long stay in the hospital. Individual coping strategies such as active acceptance of one's cancer, positive appraisal, and seeking social support have been suggested to protect many women from adverse psychological effects (Stanton, 1998). Her optimism was also a key component of time spent in therapy and aided her in rapidly achieving better psychological resilience. We recommended that, as soon as medically appropriate, she be discharged to home. Soon after our fourth individual session of therapy and three sessions with her family, Ms. M was discharged from the hospital, in stable condition.

Following her discharge, we engaged in one 30-minute telephone follow-up session. Ms. M reported that she was experiencing great comfort in being home with her family, an increased appetite, and improved sleep. She also described a greatly increased quality of life, as the fistula no longer impaired her from lying supine or carrying out a limited range of activities of daily living. Although she chose not to return to work due to her medical condition, she expressed satisfaction in this decision, because she was able to spend more time with her family whose support she labeled as key to her positive psychological adjustment.

CASE 4: PEDIATRIC HEALTH PSYCHOLOGY—FROM BEDSIDE TO HOME TO SCHOOL

Miss D was a 14-year-old Caucasian child who had experienced a potentially deadly congenital heart condition for her entire life. This case illustrates the many difficulties that childhood chronic illness can create, including the psychosocial effects on the family and potential isolation from typical childhood activities. Research suggests that family functioning impacts pediatric patients' psychosocial functioning. Family cohesion and parental adjustment are two variables that tend to mediate the relationship between pediatric disease and psychosocial adjustment (Wallander & Thompson, 1995). Parents of children with chronic illnesses are thought to encounter stressors at the time of diagnosis, through ongoing medical care (including hospitalizations), and during childhood and adolescent developmental transitions (Melnyk, Feinstein, Moldenhouer, & Small, 2001). For this reason, Kazak (1989) recommends considering pediatric patients with chronic illnesses within the context of the family.

Miss D had been admitted to our facility on numerous occasions. As a neonate, she was diagnosed with congenital cardiac dysrrhythmia and remained in the hospital for the first six months of her life. Throughout early childhood, Miss D experienced frequent Torsades de pointes (a type of heart dysrrhythmia) with accompanying neurological sequelae and was status post three ICD implantations over the course of five years. Miss D had been most recently hospitalized after multiple shock therapies due to her dysrrhythmias. During this hospitalization, Miss D reportedly began expressing her dissatisfaction with her health status, making statements such as "I don't want this heart" and "just let me die," as well as refusing to adhere to her medical regimen. Her parents reported to physicians that she had become increasingly fearful and

(Continues)

(Continued)

anxious and increasingly attached to her mother; a referral for psychological consultation was made.

We conducted an assessment with both Miss D and her parents and recommended cognitive-behavioral psychotherapy while she was an inpatient and that she continue as an outpatient after discharge. We also recommended that Miss D's parents consider participating in marital therapy to help them cope with the stressor of having a child with a chronic illness. Miss D's family was receptive to both individual and marital therapy. We saw Miss D and her family for a period of three months, beginning in the hospital and then transitioning to outpatient status. Therapy with Miss D focused on cognitive-behavioral techniques that included psychoeducation about her health condition and implementing techniques to help manage worry and reduce anxiety-provoking thoughts. Engaging in individual psychotherapy with Miss D without the presence of her parents gave her an opportunity to speak freely about her fears as well as her frustrations with her medical regimen. Nonadherence to treatment regimens has been well documented in pediatric samples with prevalence rates of roughly 50 percent (Lemanek, Kamps, & Chung, 2001). Because the consequences of nonadherence include increased morbidity, exacerbation of symptoms, medical complications, and greater mortality, we also focused on aiding Miss D in accepting her medical condition and taking an active role in maintaining her medical regimen. Marital therapy with Miss D's parents focused on developing good communication skills to buffer each other's stress and address their fears and concerns about their daughter. We also emphasized the importance of allowing Miss D to develop independence in some areas, including becoming an active participant in the administration and monitoring of her treatment regimen.

By the end of our course of therapy, Miss D reported greater satisfaction and knowledge of her health status, as well as better relationships with her family and friends. Miss D's parents reported similar benefits, and described specific improvement in their marital relationship. Giving further attention to continuity of care within the Miss D's broader community, we met with her teacher, the school nurse, and the principal and observed her behaviors in the classroom. We instituted a behavioral protocol in her classroom that reinforced her spending more time in the classroom without seeking the nurse, her timely taking of prescribed medications, and increasing intervals of not asking to contact her mother. This protocol was phased out as she spent more independent time and she experienced the innate rewards of increased social interactions with peers. Although she continues to be at high risk for medical complications and life-threatening health changes, addressing her personal issues as well as her social milieu has done much to bring about as normal a daily functioning as can be expected of a child facing ongoing challenges to her physical well-being.

CONCLUSION

Psychologists' medical colleagues increasingly understand that psychological assessment and treatment complete the care of patients with medical conditions that are exacerbated by psychosocial stressors and preexisting anxiety or depression (Robinson & Baker, 2006). Friedman and Adler (2007) highlight this understanding by describing the growth of health psychology over the past 25 years and how it "has rapidly moved to center stage" (p. 15) in modern psychology. These authors argue that health psychology's historical roots and current definition are based on interactions of the fields of medical psychology and clinical psychology as well as epidemiology and public health, medical sociology and medical anthropology, psychosomatic medicine, and the biopsychosocial model. They point out that Matarazzo helped define the field as a combination of specialty training and research and brought together "research psychology, clinical psychology, and health care" in the founding of the field (p. 13). "Health psychology is more than clinical psychology applied to medical settings and more than traditional psychiatric approaches to mental health," argue Baum, Perry, and Tarbell (2004, p. 15). Those authors, like many others, highlight the scientific roots of health psychology and its application "through prevention and early intervention in primary, secondary, and tertiary care" (p. 16). Rey (2004) asserts that the newest approach to health "says loudly and clearly that the causes, development, and outcomes of an illness are determined by the interaction of psychology, social, and cultural factors with biochemistry and physiology." He goes on to say that "our physiology and biochemistry are not separate and district from the rest of our life and our experiences. The mind—a manifest functioning of the brain—and the other body systems interact in ways critical for health, illness, and well-being" (p. 29).

Baum and colleagues (2004) focus on the holistic approach to healthcare and the role of health psychology in the "unification of persistent elements of Cartesian dualism" (p. 25). And, along with authors such as Freidman and Silver (2007) and others, they emphasize the importance of the scientific underpinnings of health psychology and its implication for quality patient care. Rozensky (2006b) highlights the wide range of major causes of mortality and morbidity in the human condition that clinical health psychologists have studied scientifically and have provided clinical services for those needing to manage those diseases and disabilities. As stated in that review, and given the present chapter's illustration of the success of psychological interventions with medically ill patients, the future of clinical health psychology in medical settings is bright.

TOOL KIT FOR CHANGE

Role and Perspective of the Healthcare Professional

1. Healthcare professionals should make sure they have the requisite knowledge and skills—either through graduate education or continuing education and self-study—to ethically and competently treat patients with the range of medical diagnoses they are called upon to assess or treat.
2. Healthcare professionals should remain up to date on the most effective evidenced-based practices in psychology used within the medical hospital setting.
3. Healthcare professionals should seek appropriate privileges by presenting their credentials according to the policy and procedures of the organized healthcare setting or hospital in which they wish to practice and attend their patients.
4. Healthcare professionals should be aware of the local standards of practice and work within the organized professional staff and their discipline-specific clinical department.

Role and Perspective of the Participant

1. Patients, family, and significant others should expect to be educated about the interplay of the biopsychosocial aspects of their presenting complaints.
2. Patients should expect to be included in the preparation of their treatment plan and understand the implications of their psychological diagnoses and treatment plan.
3. Patients should expect that their mental and behavioral health professional is utilizing the most current evidenced-based clinical approach to their presenting complaint and should be encouraged to ask about both the research supporting those techniques and the experience and training of their mental and behavioral health professional.

Interconnection: The Global Perspective

1. Health psychological approaches to hospitalized patients should be based on the most current evidenced-based research approach to presenting problems.
2. The psychological responses and symptoms of medically ill patients are as important as other medical symptoms.
3. Psychological interventions with medically ill patients are an important part of healthcare, and mental health professionals should be an active part of the multi-disciplinary team.

REFERENCES

American Board of Hospice and Palliative Medicine. (2000). Definition of palliative medicine. Retrieved [September 1, 2006, from http://www.abhpm.org.

American Psychological Association. (2001). *Revised mission statement.* Washington, DC: Author.

American Psychological Association (2002). Ethical principles of psychologists and code of conduct. *American Psychologist, 57,* 1060–1073.

American Psychological Association. (2005a). *American Psychological Association statement: Policy statement on evidence-based practice.* Retrieved September 15, 2006], from http://www2.apa.org/practice/ebpstatement.pdf.

American Psychological Association. (2005b). *Report of the 2005 task force on evidence-based practice.* Retrieved September 15, 2006, from http://www.apa.org/practice/ebpreport.pdf.

Barlow, D. H. (1997). Cognitive-behavioral therapy for panic disorder: Current status. *Journal of Clinical Psychiatry, 58,* 27–32.

Barron, I., Fennell, E., & Voeller, K. (1995). *Pediatric neuropsychology in medical settings.* New York: Oxford University Press.

Baum, A., Perry, N. W., & Tarbell, S. (2004). The development of psychology as a health science. In R. G. Frank, A. Baum, & J. L. Wallander (Eds.), *Handbook of clinical and health psychology: Models and perspectives in health psychology* (pp. 9–27). Washington, DC: American Psychological Association.

Belar, C. D., Brown, R. A., Hersch, L. E., Hornyak, L. M., Rozensky, R. H., Sheridan, E. P., Brown, R. T., & Reed, G. W. (2001). Self-assessment in clinical health psychology: A model for ethical expansion of practice. *Professional Psychology: Research and Practice, 32,* 135–141.

Belar, C. D., & Deardorff, W. W. (1995). *Clinical psychology in medical settings: A practitioner's guidebook.* Washington, DC: American Psychological Association.

Berkman, L. F., & Syme, S. L. 1979). Social networks, host resistance, and mortality: A nine year follow-up study of Alameda County residents. *American Journal of Epidemiology, 109,* 186–204.

Blechman, E. A., & Brownell, K. D. (Eds.). (1998). *Behavioral medicine and women: A comprehensive handbook.* New York: Guilford Press.

Brown, R. T., Freeman, W. S., Belar, C. D., Hornyak, L. M., Rozensky, R. H., Brown, R. A., et al. (2002). The role of psychologists in health care delivery. *Professional Psychology: Research and Practice, 33,* 536–545.

Burish, T. G., Carey, M. P., Krozely, M. G., & Greco, F. A. (1987). Conditioned side effects lumbar puncture procedure on salivary cortisol, plasma vasopressin and osmolality induced by cancer chemotherapy: Prevention through behavioral treatment. *Journal of Consulting and Clinical Psychology, 55,* 42–48.

Camic, P. M., & Knight, S. J. (Eds.). (2004). *Clinical handbook of health psychology: A practical guide to effective interventions* (2nd ed.). Seattle, WA: Hogrefe and Huber.

Chapman, S. L. (1991). Chronic pain: Psychological assessment and treatment. In J. J. Sweet, R. H. Rozensky, & S. M. Tovian (Eds.), *Handbook of clinical psychology in medical settings* (pp. 603–614). New York: Plenum. p 401–420.

Chiles, J. A., Lambert, M. J., & Hatch, A. L. (1999). The impact of psychological interventions on medical cost offset: A meta-analytic review. *Clinical Psychology: Science and Practice, 6,* 204–220.

Compas, B. E., Haaga, D. A., Keefe, F. J., Leitenberg, H., & Williams, D. A. (1998). Sampling of empirical supported psychological treatment from health psychology: Smoking, chronic pain, cancer, and bulimia nervosa. *Journal of Clinical and Consulting Psychology, 66,* 89–112.

Davison, G. C. (2006). An invitation to Ausenandersetzen about the evidence-based practice in Psychology Task Force report. *The Clinical Psychologist, 59,* 1–4.

Dobson, K. S. (1989). A meta-analysis of the efficacy of cognitive therapy of depression. *Journal of Consulting and Clinical Psychology, 57,* 414–419.

Doleys, D. M. (2000). Chronic pain. In R. G. Frank & T. R. Elliott (Eds.), *Handbook of rehabilitation psychology* (pp. 185–203). Washington, DC: American Psychological Association.

Dworkin, S. F., Von Korff, M. R., & LeResche, L. (1992). Epidemiological studies of chronic pain: A dynamic-ecological perspective. *Annals of Behavioral Medicine, 14,* 3–11.

Engel, G. L. (1977). The need for a new medical model: A challenge for biomedicine. *Science, 196,* 129–136.

Frank, R. G., Baum, A., & Wallander, J. L. (2004). *Handbook of clinical and health psychology: Models and perspectives in health psychology.* Washington, DC: American Psychological Association.

Frank, R. G., & Elliot, T. R. (2000). *Handbook of rehabilitation psychology.* Washington, DC: American Psychological Association.

Friedman, H. S., & Adler, N. E. (2007). The history and background of health psychology. In H. S. Friedman & R. C. Silver (Eds.), *Foundations of health psychology* (pp. 3–18). Oxford, England: Oxford University Press.

Friedman, H. S., & Silver, R. C. (Eds.). (2007). *Foundations of health psychology.* Oxford, England: Oxford University Press.

Gatchel, R. J., & Blanchard, E. B. (Eds.). (1993). *Psychophysiological disorders: Research and clinical applications.* Washington, DC: American Psychological Association.

Gatchel, R. J., & Oordt, M. S. (2003). *Clinical health psychology and primary care: Practical advice and clinical guidance for successful collaboration.* Washington, DC: American Psychological Association.

Gunn, W. B., Seaburn, D., Lorenz, A., Gawinski, B., and Mauksch, L. B. (2000). Collaboration in action: Key strategies for mental health providers. In N. A. Cummings, J. L. Cummings, J. N. Johnson (Eds.) *Behavioral health in primary care: A guide for clinical integration* (pp. 103–120). Madison, CT: Psychological Press.

Helgeson, V. S., & Cohen, S. (1996). Social support and adjustment to cancer: Reconciling descriptive, correlational, and intervention research. *Health Psychology, 15,* 135–148.

Henderson, B. N., & Baum, A. (2002). Neoplasms. In S. B. Johnson, N. W. Perry, & R. H. Rozensky (Eds.), *Handbook of clinical health psychology: Vol. 1. Medical disorders and behavioral applications* (pp. 37–64). Washington, DC: American Psychological Association.

Institute of Medicine. (2001). *Crossing the quality chasm: A new health system for the 21st century.* Washington, DC: National Academy Press.

Jensen, M. P., Turner, J. A., & Romano, J. M. (2001). Changes in beliefs, catastrophizing, and coping are associated with improvement in multidisciplinary pain treatment. *Journal of Consulting Psychology, 69,* 655–662.

Johnson, S. B., Perry, N. W., & Rozensky, R. H. (Eds.). (2002). *Handbook of clinical health psychology: Vol. 1. Medical disorders and behavioral applications.* Washington, DC: American Psychological Association.

Joint Commission on the Accreditation of Healthcare Organizations (JCAHO; 2000). *Hospital accreditation standards.* Oakbrook Terrace, IL.

Kazak, A. E. (1989). Families of chronically ill children: A systems and social-ecological model of adaptation and challenge. *Journal of Consulting and Clinical Psychology, 57,* 25–30.

Lemanek, K. L., Kamps, J., & Chung, N. B. (2001). Empirically supported treatments in pediatric psychology: Regimen adherence. *Journal of Pediatric Psychology, 26*(5), 253–275.

Levant, R., Reed, G., Ragusa, S., Stout, C., DiCowden, M., Murphy, M., et al. (2001). Envisioning and accessing new roles for professional psychology. *Professional Psychology: Research and Practice, 32,* 79–87.

Linton, S. J., & Bradley, L. A. (1996). Strategies for the prevention of chronic pain. In R. J. Gatchel & D. C. Turk (Eds.), *Psychological approaches to pain management: A practitioner's handbook* (pp. 438–457). New York: Guilford Press.

Maunsell, E., Brisson, J., & Deschenes, L. (1995). Social support and survival among women with breast cancer. *Cancer, 76,* 631–637.

McDaniel, S. (1995). Collaboration between psychologists and family physicians: Implementing the biopsychosocial model. *Professional psychology: Research and practice, 26,* 117–122.

McDaniel, S. H., Johnson, S. B., & Sears, S. E. (2004). Psychologists promote biopsychosocial health for families. In R. H. Rozensky, N. G. Johnson, C. D. Goodheart, & W. R. Hammond (Eds.), *Psychology builds a healthy world: Opportunities for research and practice* (pp. 49–75). Washington, DC: American Psychological Association.

Melnyk, B. M., Feinstein, N. F., Moldenhouer, Z., & Small, L. (2001). Coping in parents of children who are chronically ill: Strategies for assessment and intervention. *Pediatric Nursing, 27,* 548–558.

Merskey, H., & Bogduk, M. (1994). *Classification of chronic pain: Description of chronic pain syndromes and definition of pain terms* (2nd ed.). Seattle, WA: International Association for the Study of Pain Press.

Mumford, E., Schlesinger, H. J., Glass, G. V., Patrick, C., & Cuerdon, T. (1984). A new look at evidence about reduced cost of medical utilization following mental health treatment. *American Journal of Psychiatry, 141,* 1145–1158.

Newman, R., & Rozensky, R. H. (1995). Psychology and primary care: Evolving traditions. *Journal of Clinical Psychology in Medical Settings, 2,* 3–6.

Nezu, A., Maguth, N. C., & Geller, P. (Eds.). (2003). *Handbook of psychology: Vol. 9. Health psychology.* Hoboken, NJ: Wiley.

Nicassio, P. M., & Smith, T. W. (Eds.). (1995). *Managing chronic illness: A biopsychosocial perspective.* Washington, DC: American Psychological Association.

Pace, T. M., Chaney, J. M., Mullins, L. L., & Olson, R. A. (1995). Psychological consultation with primary care physicians: Obstacles and opportunities in the medical setting. *Professional psychology: Research and practice, 26,* 123–131.

Papas, R. K., Belar, C. D., & Rozensky, R. H. (2004). The practice of clinical health psychology: Professional issues. In T. J. Boll, R. G. Frank, A. Baum, & J. Wallander (Eds.). *Handbook of clinical health psychology: Vol. 3. Models and perspectives in health psychology* (pp. 293–319). Washington, DC: American Psychological Association.

Prigatano, G., & Pliskin, N. (Eds.). (2003). *Clinical neuropsychology and cost outcome research.* New York: Psychology Press.

Resnick, R. J., & Rozensky, R. H. (Eds.). (1996). *Health psychology through the life span: Practice and research opportunities.* Washington, DC: American Psychological Association.

Rey, O. (2004). How the mind hurts and heals the body. *American Psychologist, 59,* 29–40.

Roberts, M., & Wright, L. (1982). Role of the pediatric psychologist as a consultant to pediatricians. In J. Tuma (Ed.), *Handbook for the practice of pediatric psychology* (pp. 251–289). New York: Wiley.

Robinson, J. D., & Baker, J. (2006). Psychological consultation and services in a general medical hospital. *Professional Psychology: Research and Practice, 37,* 264–267.

Robinson, J. D., & James, L. (2005). Assessing the patient's need for medical evaluation: A psychologist's guide. In L. James & R. Folen (Eds.), *The primary care consultant: The next frontier for psychologists in hospitals and clinics* (pp. 29–36). Washington, DC: American Psychological Association.

Rozensky, R. H. (1997). Medical staff membership and participation. In J. Morris & J. Banon (Eds.) *Rural psychologist: Hospital primer.* Washington, DC: American Psychological Association,

Rozensky, R. H. (1994). Clinical psychology in medical settings: Psychology's role in health care. *Journal of Clinical Psychology in Medical Settings, 1,* 1–5.

Rozensky, R. H. (2004). Freestanding psychology: The only way in academic health centers. *Journal of Clinical Psychology in Medical Settings, 11,* 127–133.

Rozensky, R. H. (2006a). An introduction to psychologists treating medically ill patients: Competent practice and seeking credentials in organized health care settings for routine or incidental practice. *Professional Psychology: Research and Practice, 37,* 260–263.

Rozensky, R. H. (2006b). Clinical psychology in medical settings: Celebrating our past, enjoying the present, building our future. *Journal of Clinical Psychology in Medical settings, 13,* 343–352.

Rozensky, R. H., Johnson, N. G., Goodheart, C. D., & Hammond, W. R. (2004). *Psychology builds a healthy world: Opportunities for research and practice.* Washington, DC: American Psychological Association.

Rozensky, R. H., Sweet, J. J., & Tovian, S. M. (1997). *Psychological assessment in medical settings.* New York: Plenum.

Sackett, D. L, Strauss, S. E., Richardson, W. S., Rosenberg, W., & Haynes, R. B. (2000). *Evidence based medicine: How to practice and teach EBM* (2nd ed.). London: Churchill Livingstone.

Sears, S. F., Kovacs, A. H., Azzarello, L., Larsen, K., & Conti, J. B. (2004). Innovations in health psychology: The psychosocial care of adults with implantable cardioverter defibrillators. *Professional Psychology: Research and Practice, 35,* 520–526.

Sears, S. F., Rodrigue, J. R., Greene, A. F., & Mills, R. M. (1995). Predicting quality of life with a pre-transplantation assessment battery: A prospective study of cardiac transplantation recipients. *Journal of Clinical Psychology in Medical Settings, 2,* 335–355.

Sobel, D. S. (1995). Rethinking medicine: Improving health outcomes with cost-effective psychosocial interventions. *Psychosomatic Medicine, 57,* 234–244.

Stanton, A. L. (1998). Cancer: Behavioral and psychosocial aspects. In E. A. Blechman & K. D. Brownell (Eds.), *Behavioral medicine and women, comprehensive handbook* (pp. 588–594). New York: Guilford Press.

Suchday, S., Tucker, D. L., & Krantz, D. S. (2002). Diseases of the circulatory system. In S. B. Johnson, N. W. Perry, & R. H. Rozensky (Eds.), *Handbook of clinical health psychology: Vol. 1. Medical disorders and behavioral applications* (pp. 203–238). Washington, DC: American Psychological Association.

Sweet, J. J., Rozensky, R. H., & Tovian, S. M. (1991). *The handbook of clinical psychology in medical settings.* New York: Plenum.

Sweet, J. J., Tovian, S. M., & Suchy, Y. (2003). Psychological assessment in medical settings. In J. Graham and J. Naglieri (Eds.), *Handbook of psychology: Vol. 10. Assessment psychology.* Hoboken, NJ: Wiley.

Tarter, R. E., Butters, M., & Beers, S. R. (2001). *Medical neuropsychology* (2nd ed.). New York: Klewer Academic/Plenum.

Taylor, D. N. (1995). Effects of a behavioral stress-management program on anxiety, mood, self-esteem, and t-cell count in HIV-positive men. *Psychological Reports, 76,* 451–457.

Taylor, S. E. (2006). Social support. In H. S. Friedmand & R. C. Silver (Eds.), *Foundations of health psychology* (pp. 145–171). Oxford, England: Oxford University Press.

Tovian, S. M. (2006). Interdisciplinary collaboration in outpatient practice. *Professional Psychology: Research and Practice, 37,* 268–272.

Tovian, S. M., Rozensky, R. H., & Sweet, J. J. (2003). A decade of clinical psychology in medical settings: The short longer view. *Journal of Clinical Psychology in Medical Settings, 10,* 1–8.

Turner, J., & Romano, J. (1990). Cognitive-behavioral therapy. In J. J. Bonica, C. R. Chapman, W. E. Fordyce, & J. D. Loeser (Eds.), *The management of pain in clinical practice* (2nd ed., pp. 1711–1721). Philadelphia: Lea & Febiger.

Wallander, J. L., & Thompson, R. J. Jr. (1995). Psychosocial adjustment of children with chronic physical conditions. In M. C. Roberts (Ed.), *Handbook of pediatric psychology* (2nd ed., pp. 124–141). New York: Guilford Press.

World Health Organization. (2005). Definition of palliative care. Retrieved September 15, 2006, from http://www.who.int/en.

Wright, L. (1982). Incorporating health care psychology into independent practice. *Independent Practitioner, 2,* 1–4.

Ziegelstein, R. C., Fauerbach, J. A., Stevens, S. S., Romanelli, J., Richter, D. P., & Bush, D. E. (2000). Patients with depression are less likely to follow recommendations to reduce cardiac risk during recovery from a myocardial infarction. *Archives of Internal Medicine, 160*(12), 1818–1823.

Chapter Two

HEALTHCARE IN THE NEW MILLENNIUM: THE CONVERGENCE OF THE MEDICAL, SPA, AND HOSPITALITY INDUSTRIES

Janice Gronvold, MS

> The ideal hospital would combine the best of spas with the best of hotels and the best of hospitals to become a truly healing environment.
> —Angelica Thieriot, Founder of Planetree Health Resource Center, 1978 (Alliance Community Hospital, n.d.)

Nearly three decades have passed since the founder of Planetree, an internationally recognized pioneer in patient-centered and community-based healthcare, envisioned a new type of hospital. Thieriot's prophetic vision is reflected in a growing convergence of industries today that bring together the best of diagnostic technologies, complementary and integrative medicine (CIM), complementary and alternative medicine (CAM), spa and traditional healing arts therapies, and service and programming concepts from the hospitality and travel industries. Examples of these developments are demonstrated with new categories of specialized hospitals, wellness centers, hospital spas, destination health resorts with medical services, hotels with wellness programs, medical spas, and spa life-style residential communities with medical and healthy living programs.

Across the United States, growing numbers of hospitals, universities, medical research centers, and community and real estate developers are partnering with spas, resorts, hotels, and residential communities to create a new—and some say a kindler, gentler—healthcare approach within new environments that are a clear departure from stark hospital rooms and impersonal doctor's offices many people associate with healthcare services. And like many trends, this emerging healthcare approach is consumer driven and largely sparked by economics, freedom of choice, and a transition from sickness management to wellness management healthcare models.

At the heart of the melding of spas, wellness, and healthcare is a shift away from the conventional medical system that focuses on treating sickness toward a system that promotes wellness. Unhappy with soaring healthcare costs, inadequate coverage for basic care, expensive tests and procedures, hurried office visits, and a shrinking pool of qualified hospital staff, consumers are demanding strategies that prevent disease and promote optimum wellness that will help them live longer and better, hopefully without the need of lengthy hospital stays.

According to Harvard Business School professor, Michael Porter, the "zero-sum" healthcare industry competition business model of the 1990s and 2000s "perpetuated inefficiency, substandard quality, drove up administrative costs, inhibited innovation, and resulted in alarming cost increases for patients, employers, and the government" (Porter & Teisberg, 2006, p. 197). According to Porter and Teisberg, the United States and other nations are on a collision course with an unsustainable healthcare business model burdened with many challenges. Their analysis of a system based on dysfunctional competition that restricts services and does not reward creation of true value for consumers is deeply flawed and vulnerable to outside forces and market trends. One of these forces is a new healthcare consumer who emerged in recent decades with the electronic age and globalization. With millions of people having access to medical information that would have been difficult to access prior to the existence of the Internet, hundreds of medical, wellness, and life-style sites such as WebMD, NetWellness, InteliHealth, Andrew Weil, and Spa Finder have been established, providing diverse sources of information for consumers seeking health and wellness resources outside of traditional healthcare settings. With some sites hosting millions of visitors a day, a new kind of information-empowered consumer demanding a different kind of healthcare experience based on information, choice, and partnership in the healthcare process is becoming a formidable economic force.

An example of the economic impact of the new healthcare consumer was first recognized by the government and medical community with the 1997 landmark study by David Eisenberg, director of the Center for Alternative Medicine and Research and Education at Beth Israel Deaconess and assistant professor of medicine at Harvard Medical School (Eisenberg et al., 1993).

The study identified 425 million consumers spending $12.2 billion out of pocket for unconventional therapies such as chiropractors, therapeutic massage, and acupuncture. This figure exceeded 386 million visits to conventional physicians who provided primary care in the same year. As a result of this survey, consumer trends supporting alternative and integrative medicine influenced allocation of funding and research by Congress and the creation, beginning in 1998, of organizations such as National Center for Complementary and Alternative Medicine to establish research programs, offer grants, and advance education in diverse medical and healthcare systems and practices not recognized in conventional medicine (National Center for Complementary and Alternative Medicine, 2006).

In the last decade, complementary and alternative medicine has become more mainstream, and now more than one in four hospitals in the United States (of 1,400 surveyed in 2005) offer alternative and complementary therapies such as acupuncture, homeopathy, and massage therapy. The *Health Forum 2005 Complementary and Alternative Medicine Survey of Hospitals,* released July 19, 2006, conducted and published by the American Hospital Association every two years, shows that the percentage of hospitals offering one or more CAM services increased from 8 percent in 1998 to 27 percent in 2005 ("Alternative Goes Mainstream," 2006). Survey results indicated the top six complementary and alternative medicine services offered on an outpatient basis among hospitals offering CAM were massage therapy (71%); tai chi, yoga, or chi gong (47%); relaxation training (43%); acupuncture (39%); guided imagery (32%); and therapeutic touch (30%). Top inpatient services were massage therapy (37%), music/art therapy (26%), therapeutic touch (25%), guided imagery (22%), relaxation training (20%), and acupuncture (11%) ("Alternative Goes Mainstream," 2006).

As more Americans pursue diverse complementary and alternative medicine therapies to reduce stress, improve overall wellness, treat minor ailments, and manage chronic disease, they are also seeking diverse environments for these services. Increasingly, these CAM-seeking consumers are receiving holistic programs and services (defined as those that focus on healing the whole body rather than the conventional allopathic approach that treats symptoms or diseases) in many nontraditional medical environments such as wellness centers, day and destination spas with medical services, hotels with medical alliances, and hospitals with spa facilities. Angelica Thieriot's vision of a new type of hospital has turned out to be startlingly prophetic. Indeed, as the millennium unfolds, many forces are converging to make hospitals and hotels more like spas and, conversely, spas more like hospitals and hotels.

THE HISTORY OF SPAS: HEALING WITH WATER

The trend for spas to be centers for health and healing is not a new notion. The foundation of spas as places that not only foster health and healing but also nurture the body, mind, and spirit has ancient roots around the globe. The word *spa* comes from the Latin phrase *salus per aquam,* which means "healing through water," and balneotherapy (water treatments designed to strengthen the immune system and stimulate blood and lymph circulation) has been associated with medicine, healing, religion, myth, and magic since the beginning of recorded history (Cribin-Bailey, Harcup, & Harrington, 2005). Records from ancient civilizations—Egyptian, Chinese, Greek, Persian, Babylonian, and Roman—all reference the miraculous powers of healing waters, and many historical architectural influences utilizing water in various forms and temperatures continue to influence contemporary spa design throughout the world to this day. Specific contemporary spa treatments for diverse health conditions can be traced to historical influences such as Indian Ayurvedic hydrotherapies dating back to 5000 B.C., the benefits of water and herbal remedies in Egypt in 3100–300 B.C., and steam and mud baths of ancient Persia during 600–300 B.C. (Cribin-Bailey et al., 2005) Homer and other Greek writers detailed a variety of bath and spalike treatments as early as 500 B.C., and in 217 A.D., records indicate the Baths of Caracalla, which accommodated up to 1,500 people a day, also included elaborate gyms, libraries, gardens, meeting rooms, and health facilities (Baths at Caracalla, n.d.).

Traditionally, spas were situated near natural springs, lakes, and the sea because water was believed to have profound healing properties. Hippocrates recognized the benefits of seawater by observing its effects on the injured hands of fishermen, and he encouraged thalassa cure therapies (*thalassa* is Greek for "sea") for various skin and health conditions (Grüner, 2002). Centuries later, facilities were established promoting the therapeutic use of seawater and marine by-products such as algae and seaweed. On the east coast of England, the first marine hospital (the Royal Sea-Bathing Infirmary) was established in 1791 by John Latham in Magate. At the same time, Richard Russell, also in Great Britain, authored a book on seawater therapy and coined the term thalassotherapy (Cribin-Bailey et al., 2005). In 1899, the first thalassotherapy center in France was established by Louis Bagot, with the industry growing to over 40 active centers, or thalassos, and a national association called the Fédération Mer et Santé, established in 1986 (Register, 2002).

The legend of Bath, England, first documented by the Romans, is founded on the properties of muddy thermal waters that healed a prince banished from the royal court who had contracted leprosy. Upon being healed, the prince was able to return to his court duties and later turned the thermal spring into a famous spa (Wechsbeerg, 1982, pp. 10–11). In 973 A.D., King Edgar assigned his physician, John de Villula, Bishop of Bath, the responsibilities of replacing a small abbey with a great cathedral and developing bath facilities so that people with poor health from all over England could bathe in the healing waters. Many monastic hospitals used the thermal waters to treat patients, and one of them, St. John's, founded in 1180, exists to this day (Wechsbeerg, 1982, pp. 11–12).

Most early spas centered on some form of hydrotherapy, the therapeutic use of water, to treat everything from paralysis and pneumonia to typhoid fever and tumors. Many modern-day hydrotherapies can be attributed to the research of Vicent Priessnitz (1799–1851), who established the first modern hydrotherapy spa concept with health package treatments (exercise, diet, and water treatments) in what is now Jesenik in the Czech Republic (Cribin-Bailey et al., 2005). By 1842, his work had influenced the establishment of over 40 hydropathic centers in Germany, Hungary, Poland, and Russia (Cribin-Bailey et al., 2005, p. 15). Priessnitz's work also had a profound impact on Sebastian Kneipp, a nineteenth-century German priest from Bavaria, afflicted with tuberculosis who had first learned about the benefits of hot and cold water-based therapies prescribed by Sigmund Hahn, author of *Cold Water Treatments*. Experimenting with water-based treatments combined with herbs, diet, and exercise prescribed by Hahn and Priessnitz, Kneipp treated his condition, completely recovered, and began to treat others with similar success (Vierille, 2006). Based on his research, documented with patient case studies, he became known as a hydrotherapist who authored several books, including *My Water Cure* in 1886 and *Thus Thou Shalt Live* in 1889 ("Sebastian Kneipp," 2006). On February 2, 1894, Kneipp's work was honored with the establishment of the International Association of Kneipp Physicians in Bad Wörishofen, outside of Munich (Bergel, n.d.). The organization later became the International Kneipp Association with private clinics and spas staffed with physicians trained in the Kneipp cure (often referred to as Kur spas) through-out Germany, Austria, Switzerland, Luxembourg, France, and South Africa (Bergel, n.d.). Kneipp water cures, baths, inhalation, packs, compresses, show-ers, ablutions, and wraps are practiced at many spas worldwide, with training and certification offered at the Sebastian Kneipp School of Physiotherapy in Bad Wörishofen (Vierille, 2006). In Germany alone, there are over 200 spas that offer the Kneipp System, which is valued as a preventative measure and is covered by medical insurance for some conditions (Vierille, 2006).

Kneipp's work was based on five pillars of health—hydrotherapy, kine-siotherapy, phytotherapy, nutrition, and regulative therapies—that were rec-ognized as the foundation for naturopathy, a system of treatments designed to strengthen an individual to overcome illness rather than by curing spe-cific diseases (Vierille, 2006). Each pillar had specific attributes and was believed to contribute to a balanced life and sense of well-being. The first pillar, hydrotherapy, is administered with varying temperatures of water baths, poultices, vapors, compresses, packs, and water jets. Kinesiotherapy applied to exercise, movement, and therapeutic massage. Phytotherapy, also called plant therapy, calls for herbs and plant-based extracts to be added to baths, applied to the skin, or taken orally. The fourth pillar emphasized a well-balanced low-protein, high-fiber diet that included modifications for individuals with weight and metabolic disorders. The last pillar integrates the other four, com-bined with exposure to sunlight, frequent water intake, and other practices addressing mental, emotional, seasonal, and cultural conditions that promote what Kneipp believed was "harmony" in life (Vierille, 2006).

Many early Kneipp sanitariums in the United States and Europe were associated with and staffed by religious organizations (Vierille, 2006). In 1894, a German physician, William Giermann, purchased 180 acres near Rome City, Indiana, and began to offer Kneipp treatments to patients from various Midwestern cities such as Chicago, Fort Wayne, Indiana, and Columbus, Ohio. Between 1901 and 1951, the facility—later purchased by the Sisters of the Precious Blood and affiliated with the Catholic Hospital Association, Indiana Hospital Association, and the American Hospital Association—administered Kneipp therapies to over 2,000 patients a year (Vierille, 2006).

In 1902, Benedict Lust, a German immigrant who had been healed of tuberculosis by Kneipp, purchased the rights to the term *naturopathy*, combining nature and homeopathy, from John H. Scheel, who had coined it in 1895. Encouraged by Kneipp to share his work, Lust opened the Kneipp Water-Cure Institute in New York City, which included a naturopathic sanatorium, college, retail store selling Kneipp products, and publication of a magazine on the subject of nature cures ("Healing Occurs Naturally," n.d.). This was the first of school of naturopathy—a healing discipline that focuses on water treatments along with diet, nutrition, light therapy, spinal manipulation, and herbal medicine—in the United States. Many of Kneipp's therapies are the foundation for spa therapies throughout the world, and it is not uncommon for naturopaths to be part of a clinic, health resort, or spa medical team.

HISTORICAL PERSPECTIVES OF U.S. SPAS AND HEALTH INSTITUTIONS

While spa traditions have been documented around the world—offering diverse treatments depending on location and local resources such as thermal waters, clay, and herbs said to have therapeutic properties—most early U.S. spas, established near hot springs, were mainly an outgrowth of European hydrotherapy-based spas by immigrants seeking to recreate spa traditions from their native countries. As of 1890, 694 mineral water spas were registered around the country, and in state of Missouri alone, there were over 80 mineral spring health resorts between the late 1800s and early 1900s (Bullard, 2004, pp. 23, 217–225). Some were simply enjoyed in their natural state; other locations were more sophisticated with accommodations and various water-based treatments combined with nutrition, exercise, and therapeutic programs that would be labeled holistic today.

Beginning in the 1830s, various health movements appeared, such as Thomsonianism, an early approach to modern Western herbalism founded by Samuel Thompson (1769–1843) ("History of Natural Health," 2006). Eclectic medicine, another alternative to conventional medicine, also emphasized the importance of herbal remedies and had over 20,000 practitioners during its peak ("Eclectic Medicine," n.d.). In 1851, the American Hydropathic Institute was established in New York and was reputed to be the first medical school founded on water cure principles (Cribin-Bailey et al., 2005). During this time, the Battle Creek Sanitarium in Michigan, originally called the Western Health Reform Institute, was one of the leading health institutions in the country—a reputation it held from the 1880s until 1929 when operations began to decline due to the stock market crash followed by the Great Depression and later World War II in 1939 ("Battle Creek Sanitarium," 2003). Its programs emphasized vitamin and protein-rich nutrition and focused on whole grains to foster good digestion and elimination, which was believed by staff physician John Kellogg, to be the cornerstone of optimum health. Advocating a low-calorie diet, Kellogg developed peanut butter, granola, and toasted flakes and cofounded a business producing whole grain cereals. This company was the foundation for the Kellogg Company, the leading producer of cereal and convenience foods established by his brother many years later ("Battle Creek Sanitarium," 2003).

Until World War II, people traveled to famous U.S. spas—such as in Hot Springs, Arkansas, and the elaborate Poland Springs House in Maine—seeking water cures claimed to treat various stomach, kidney, liver, and circulatory conditions (Holmes, n.d.). Saratoga Springs, established in New York in 1803, was referred to as the "queen of the spas," recognized as much for its European-inspired buildings as its mineral water therapies and its medical, and spa services (Saratoga Spa State Park, n.d.). Gurney's Inn Resort on Montauk in Long Island, New York, another European-inspired spa, was the first U.S. establishment to offer a thalassotherapy center with seawater, algae, and thermal baths (Gurney's Inn, n.d.). The famous healing waters of Greenbrier, in White Sulphur Springs, West Virginia, founded over 200 years ago, continues to offer health and rejuvenation spa packages in addition to preventative healthcare diagnostic evaluations at the Greenbrier Clinic, which was established in 1948 ("Welcome to the Greenbrier Clinic," 2003).

With the advent of World War II and a decline in customers, spas struggled to stay in business; many spas closed, properties were sold, fell into disrepair, or, in the case of Poland Springs, were destroyed by fire (Holmes, n.d.). After the war, until the 1960s, when health enthusiasts rediscovered the value of mineral springs, consumers gravitated toward modernization, pharmacology, and science-based medicine and turned their backs on old-world spas that had fallen into disrepair or closed altogether (Croutier, 1992, p. 155).

A DAY OF HEALTH INSPIRES A NEW GENERATION

The resurgence of interest in spas can be credited to several spa operations, and an exception to war-strained spa establishments was Rancho La Puerta, founded in the spring of 1940 in Tecate, Mexico (Szekely, 1990). What began more than six decades ago, and originally named the Essene School of Life, is now recognized as one of the top destination health spa resorts in the world. Honored by spa industry professionals and associations as a significant leader for North American spas in the twentieth century, it continues to pioneer new horizons (Spa Finder, 2006). Developed by Edmond Szekely and his wife Deborah near San Diego, California, Rancho La Puerta, as it was to later become, was selected for having a near-perfect year-round climate conducive for the gardens and orchards they envisioned for their school of life program. Szekely, originally from Hungary, was a prolific writer and scholar of ancient and modern languages and philosophies who had developed a following with his publications and various health retreat programs in Europe and the South Pacific before relocating to North America in the 1930s. He authored over 80 books, including the *Essene Science of Life,* offering guidelines for healthy living through nutrition, exercise, and various treatments influenced by his research of ancient cultures and exposure to spa therapies growing up in Eastern Europe ("Edmund Bordeaux Szekely," 2006).

Influenced by studies of ancient agriculturists and healing arts traditions, Rancho La Puerta became a learning center for synthesizing ancient and modern philosophies; physical disciplines such as yoga; and diverse programs such as special diets, fasting, massage, herbal wraps, and water therapies. In the early days, the remote destination was frequented by Americans as well as many European visitors seeking Kneipp-inspired therapies and nutrition and exercise programs they had heard about or experienced in European spas. These programs were continually refined and became the genesis of Rancho La Puerta's Health Day, a comprehensive program nurturing the body, mind, and spirit—a whole new concept for the emerging U.S. spa industry (Rancho La Puerta, 1996–2006).

Rancho La Puerta can be credited with offering programs that not only addressed outer health, but inner health as well. The Szekelys were pioneers in their recognition that true healing involves more than addressing a collection of symptoms or treating disease and should involve the mind and spirit in a truly holistic way. It was at Rancho La Puerta in 1960 where the Human Potential movement was celebrated during a five-day symposium led by Aldous Huxley (1894–1963), a prolific writer and leader of modern thought who gave lectures on "human potentialities" at universities and medical schools during the late 1950s and early 1960s (Szekely, 1990). The symposium featured notable thinkers and leaders in psychology, philosophy, music, movement, and the healing arts exploring revolutionary ideas, transformative practices, innovative art forms, and creativity. This pivotal event was part of a new movement emerging in the work of Alan Watts, Abraham Maslow, Fritz

Perls, Paul Tillich, Carl Rogers, Joseph Campbell and in the development of Esalen, a multidisciplinary center for humanistic education and research founded by Michael Murphy and Dick Price in 1962. In the years to follow, from this rich and varied milieu, thousands of people were exposed to humanistic psychology, a nonpathological view of a person and various mind-body methods, including biofeedback, tai chi, meditation, guided imagery, music, color therapy, and Feldenkrais. During the 1970s, the Feldenkrais body-mind awareness method was introduced at Esalen and universities throughout the United States by Moshé Feldenkrais, a physicist who developed a system for reducing physical pain and movement challenges. These diverse modalities—promoting physical and mental health, creativity, self-awareness and personal development—influenced a new spa generation that embraced the body, mind, and spirit, integrating traditional spa services with more esoteric programs designed to expand awareness, creativity, and human potential.

AN INDUSTRY IS BORN

In the 1980s and 1990s, globalization, the Internet, and worldwide travel contributed to increased consumer awareness and fueled demand for integrated wellness, spa, alternative medical services, and traditional healing arts from around the world. As visitors to health resorts such as Canyon Ranch in the United States or Chiva-Som in Thailand or to hotels with spa and medical services in spa cities such as Baden-Baden, Germany, sampled therapeutic benefits of such time-honored healing therapies ranging from traditional Chinese and Ayurvedic medicine, Kneipp therapies, acupuncture, nutrition, therapeutic massage, and exercise not typically offered at their conventional doctor's offices and hospitals, they began to seek out facilities offering diverse services in spa therapies, medical programs, and traditional healing arts in growing numbers.

Since the 1980s, influenced by pioneering destination spa resorts such as Rancho La Puerta, the Golden Door, Canyon Ranch, and Cal-a-Vie, thousands of day spas were established across the country, and, by the 1990s, the spa boom was in full swing, giving birth to industry associations, conferences, and trade publications. Growth has been fueled by consumer demand, and, as of 2006, U.S. spas were a $15 billion per year industry (Spa Finder, n.d.). As the fourth-largest leisure industry in the United States, it generates more revenue than ski resorts, amusement/theme parks, and box office receipts (Spa Finder, n.d.). That figure is expected to grow with continued industry expansion and diversification influencing secondary markets such as residential and commercial design and architecture, spa-inspired furnishings, personal care products, life-style accessories, travel and leisure industries, and real estate developments.

SPAS AS THE NEW HOSPITALS

As the industry continues to evolve, spas that bridge centuries of healing arts traditions with twenty-first-century healthcare have emerging as respected centers for integrative medicine—that is, places where wellness and spa treatments are offered side by side with medical diagnostics and prevention-based healthcare services. According to the International Spa Association, between 2002 and 2004, the medical spa segment expanded faster than any other segment, growing by 109 percent compared to 26 percent for the U.S. spa industry as a whole ("International Spa Association," n.d.). According to the International Spa Association, a medical spa is a facility that operates under the full-time, on-site supervision of a licensed healthcare professional whose primary purpose is to provide comprehensive medical and wellness care in an environment that integrates spa services as well as traditional, complementary, and alternative therapies and treatments. A medical spa facility operates within the scope of practice of its staff, which can include both aesthetic/cosmetic and prevention/wellness procedures and services (International Spa Association, 2004).

Healing-oriented spas have become a source of information about and inspiration for new ways to live and live well—where ideas, information, and resources about healing, fitness, nutrition, beauty, and spirituality converge. Spa categories continue to evolve, addressing broad and niche markets from day spas, wellness spas, aesthetic medicine spas, age management spas, dental spas, and hospitals spas to residential spa life-style communities. As the demand for optimizing health and managing stress grows and the healthcare industry transitions toward wellness and prevention, the spa industry is uniquely positioned to contribute centuries of spa culture to current and emerging wellness and healthcare models.

WHAT IS FUELING THE SURGE IN SPAS?

In an age when modern medicine usually means rushed office visits, a maze of fragmented services, and costly, invasive procedures, many consumers are finding that practitioners and health centers that offer a menu of nonmedical therapies along with medical treatments or diagnostic services that put them in charge of their own health are very appealing. In a growing number of cases, spas fill the bill because many are staffed by a host of practitioners—MDs, naturopaths, acupuncturists, chiropractors, nutritionists, and meditation teachers—who view patients as partners and are skilled in offering an array of therapy options customized to the needs of the individual, coordinated by a physician, nurse practitioner, or medical concierge professional. Again, the overall aim is not so much to treat disease but to provide an opportunity and environment with ongoing support for the body to heal itself. This approach is common in many non-Western medical modalities around the world, and, in 1978, the World Health Organization recognized holistic medical systems as "viewing humans in totality within a wide ecological spectrum, and emphasizing the view that ill health or disease is brought about by imbalance or disequilibrium of humans in the total ecological system and not only the causative agent and pathogenic mechanism" (Marcozzi, 2006, p. 11).

At a time when the long-term sustainability of the current high-cost U.S. healthcare system is in doubt, it is important to note that primary healthcare for 80 percent of the world's population utilizes modalities that are called "alternative medicine" in the United States—such as therapeutic approaches associated with health traditions of India, China, and Europe and medical systems such as chiropractic, homeopathy, herbal medicine, naturopathy, and osteopathy. These approaches stem from a philosophy that addresses the whole person in diagnosis, treatment of illness, disease and injury, and prevention of illness.

For managing minor pain conditions such as back pain, the leading cause of job-related disability in the United States, massage, a mainstay of spa menus, can be an attractive alternative to painkillers and a comforting treatment before and after medical procedures. Massage is the most requested treatment at spas, and, according to the Associated Bodywork and Massage Professionals (a national membership association for massage therapy and esthetic professionals), as of 2005, over 240,000 massage and bodywork professionals are licensed in the United States, providing 120 to 135 million massage sessions representing a $7 billion to $10 billion industry (Associated Bodywork & Massage Professionals, 2006). The Touch Therapy Institute at the University of Miami School of Medicine, the first center in the world devoted to the study of touch and its application in science and medicine, has identified various attributes and benefits of massage. These include reduced pain from migraines and arthritis; decreased glucose levels in patients with diabetes; greater attentiveness in children who have autism; less pain, nausea, and depression for oncology patients; improved immunity, stress reduction, and better work performance for employees receiving on-site massage treatments (Touch Research Institute, University of Miami School of Medicine, 1997). In the 2003 annual list of the 100 Best Companies for Working Mothers, published by *Working Mother* magazine, 77 of the top 100 companies offered work-site massage (Associated Bodywork & Massage Professionals, 2006).

More medical organizations are learning what spas have know for years: massage therapy is a highly effective means by which to manage all types of body pain, promote relaxation, manage stress, and promote the healing process. At the University of California, Los Angeles East-West Center in Santa Monica, 95 percent of patients who received massage indicated it was a "very important" part of their recovery. According to the director, Ka-Kit Hui, "Massage is a very important therapeutic approach which is underutilized and underappreciated. A lot of people think massage is good for aches and pains. But what we have found is that massage activates the body's own healing system" ("Immune Support," 2004).

EVOLUTION OF SPAS AS MODERN-DAY HEALING CENTERS

As spas continue to evolve and partner with hospitals, hotels, resorts, and research centers, more consumers can expect to find everything from high-tech MRI diagnostic scans and cholesterol-lowering strategies on the spa menu, alongside massage, stress management techniques such as meditation, yoga, and a host of other nondrug therapies and techniques. Whether Americans are seeking methods to cope with cancer, shed unwanted pounds, keep their hearts healthy, or stave off the effects of everyday stress, spas are emerging as a viable resource for services, guidelines, and support for healthy living practices.

Responding to increasing numbers of people affected by cancer, many spas specialize in programs that address this condition by teaching skills for managing pain and addressing challenging symptoms and side effects associated with radiation and chemotherapy. At the California-based Greet the Day program—partnered with Spa Gregories in Newport Beach, Pacific Water Spa at the Hyatt Regency in Huntington Beach, and nine participating hospitals—cancer patients receive a complimentary day of rejuvenation, relaxation, and empowerment; network with cancer survivors; and learn take-home tools for managing their health. According to Johnnette du Rand, Greet the Day cofounder, the program's goal is "to create a timeout from regular hospital visits and provide a place in which guests can reconnect with themselves as a whole" (Du Rand, 2006). A typical Greet the Day program begins with yoga or meditation, followed with spa treatments such as massage and facials and relaxation techniques. Social networking activities designed to minimize the feelings of isolation and disempowerment that often accompany radiation, surgery, and chemotherapy help establish a sense of community. Numerous studies confirm the importance of friends in the healing process, demonstrating that patients heal faster when they feel supported (Du Rand, 2006).

In addition to providing an extensive selection of therapies, with many customized to specific health problems, spas are also uniquely positioned to address life-style solutions for what experts have dubbed America's leading life-style diseases: obesity, heart disease, diabetes, and depression. To treat, prevent, and, in some cases, reverse these conditions, spas that help consumers make healthy life-style choices—dietary, fitness, and stress management among them—can be a powerful prescription.

Centers that offer a wide range of life-style strategies and customized programs especially for preventing and treating problems such as coronary heart disease (the leading cause of death in the United States) are in demand. Since opening its doors in 1970, Cooper Clinic at the Cooper Aerobics Center in Dallas, Texas, has helped over 70,000 people reduce their risk of heart disease and stress-related illness through nutrition, exercise, education, and motivation to live a healthy and active life-style (Cooper Wellness Program, n.d.).

Prevention appears to be especially important to the burgeoning aging population who want to live a full life not debilitated by chronic disease. According to the National Institute of Aging, nearly 8,000 people turn 60 each day (National Institute of Aging, n.d.). In addition, life expectancy continues to lengthen. As baby boomers look forward to living longer, they are eager for healthy life-style strategies and services to help them continue to function without being disabled by obesity, diabetes, heart disease, mental decline, and other chronic conditions. People want to feel and look fit, stay active, and remain independent well into their advanced senior years.

Looking as good as one feels is another priority for the aging population, and aesthetic services combined with wellness programs are predicted to be the largest growth segment for years to come. Many organizations offer hope and make impressive claims, but the results-oriented leaders of the future will be delivering science-based evaluations to assess biomarkers of aging, genomics testing (risk of developing age-related conditions such as heart disease, diabetes, and osteoporosis), and personalized programs for life-style enhancing services such as cosmetic procedures. The Miami Institute for Age Management and Intervention at the Four Seasons Hotel is an example of medical facilities within a hotel, offering personalized medical evaluations, hormone replacement therapy, weight management strategies, nutrition, exercise, and wellness programs in addition to noninvasive and surgical cosmetic procedures (Miami Institute for Age Management and Intervention, n.d.). Pritikin Longevity Center and Spa in Aventura, Florida, offers medically proven life-style programs. Examples have been demonstrated in lowering cholesterol that resulted in an average 23 percent drop in total cholesterol and a 23 percent drop in LDL (or so-called bad cholesterol) after analyzing 4,587 guests who participated in a three-week program (Pritikin Longevity Center and Spa, 2006a). A five-year follow-up of 64 guests who wanted to avoid bypass surgery found that 80 percent did not require surgery and 62 percent remained free of chest pain drugs (Pritikin Longevity Center and Spa, 2006a). The most comprehensive study of long-term weight loss ever conducted and published by the *Journal of American Dietetic Association* found nearly 4,500 participants lost an average of 66 pounds and kept it off for the duration of the six-year study (Pritikin Center and Spa, 2006c). More than 100 studies conducted by Harvard University, Stanford University, and other research centers and published in leading medical journals such as the *Journal of the American Medical Association,* the *New England Journal of Medicine* have demonstrated Pritikin's extraordinary success in helping thousands of people improve their health and quality of life (Pritikin Center and Spa, 2006b).

HEALTHCARE CONSUMERISM, OPTIMAL HEALING ENVIRONMENTS, AND EVIDENCE-BASED DESIGN

Harvard Business School professor Regina Herzlinger is a significant voice in healthcare reform and the author of two books on the subject: the best-selling *Market-Driven Healthcare* (1999) and *Consumer-Driven Healthcare* (2004). Emphasizing the needs for more personalized medicine, alternative approaches to conventional healthcare, innovative services to traditional medical insurance coverage, and an outline for restructuring the healthcare system for policymakers, she provides a vision for a creating a healthcare system that individuals, the business community, and government could afford and would be willing to pay for (Herzlinger, 2004).

While the merits of various types of consumer-driven programs are being debated across the country in board rooms, at medical conferences, within the insurance industry and organizations such as the American Medical Association, consumers are demanding effective health strategies, affordability, and access to information, choice, and alternatives. They are also seeking a different kind of healthcare experience and environment, and, for organizations seeking viability in the healthcare markets of the future, understanding these additional considerations will be critical.

Returning to the Planetree model, 10 components are recognized to promote a nurturing and healing environment for the physical, psychological, emotional, and spiritual dimensions of the healing process: (1) the importance of personalized human interaction; (2) empowering patients through information and choices; (3) family and social support; (4) the nutritional and nurturing aspects of food; (5) spirituality and the inner life; (6) the therapeutic benefits of human touch; (7) the value of art and music in the healing process; (8) balancing conventional medicine with mind-body medicine interventions such as meditation and healing guided imagery, therapeutic massage, acupuncture, and tai chi; (9) healing environments, architecture, and design conducive to health; and (10) bringing health and wellness information and resources to the larger community by working with schools, senior centers, and various community organizations (Alliance Community Hospital, n.d.).

Expanding upon Planetree's component for creating healing environments, the California-based Center for Healthcare Design is a leading research and advocacy organization of healthcare and design professionals with emphasis on research and resources supporting evidence-based healthcare design. A concept parallel to evidence-based medicine defines the philosophy and process for designing healthcare environments that are therapeutic, supportive of patient and family involvement, efficient for staff performance, restorative for employees under stress, and sensitive to diverse cultural nuances in health and healing. Measured through economic performance, clinical outcomes, staff productivity, and customer satisfaction, there are hundreds of design studies demonstrating the value of color, light, choice of materials, ergonomics, nature, nature, art, sound, and organizational design to optimize healing environments (Hamilton, 2003).

Another organization, the Samueli Institute, a nonprofit organization that conducts and supports healthcare research in CAM and patient-centered care approaches to healthcare, also addresses optimizing healing environments. In 2004, it sponsored a Toward Optimal Healing Environments in Health Care symposium, which addressed design guidelines in architecture, color, nature, sound, music, art, and light conducive for healing spaces combined with the benefits of applying collaborative patient-centered care services (Chez, Pelletier, & Jonas, 2004, p. 4).

In 1993, a *New York Times* article, "Hospitals Discovering Their Inner Spa," profiled various organizations such as the Integrative Health Center at the Rockefeller Pavilion in New York, the Hackensack University Medical Center in New Jersey, and Northwestern Hospital in Chicago that are pioneering innovative approaches to healthcare environments and services inspired from the spa, resort, and hospitality industries. Early adaptors in optimal healing environments for hospitals, as outlined in the article, often begin in maternity and women's healthcare departments (Ferla, 2000). Banner Good Samaritan Medical Center, the largest hospital in Arizona, recently expanded with three new Centers of Excellence: women's health, imaging, and a comprehensive cardiovascular center. Garden views are designed in waiting and public areas, complementing the architecture based on desert materials and imagery. The Oasis Spa, linked with the inpatient integrative therapy department, describes the philosophy of the spa on their Web site as "a hospital-based center providing a team of highly skilled, licensed practitioners who will access and individualize any therapy experience." Promoting holistic therapies, the therapeutic body treatments include oncology massage to minimize stress for patients undergoing chemotherapy; pre- and postnatal massage to reduce back pain, relieve swelling, and promote circulation; and reflexology to balance the body's energy systems (Banner Good Samaritan Medical Center, 2006).

In 2003, Memorial Hermann's Garden Spa in Houston, Texas, opened with a 5,200-square-foot facility adjacent to Memorial Hermann Southwest Hospital. The 15-room spa complements medical services and health screenings offered at the adjacent 80,000-square-foot wellness center. Offering tranquil surroundings and therapeutic services, they are the only Kneipp-affiliated facility in Texas offering Kneipp-based hydrotherapies, body wraps, nutrition education, and movement programs. The spa—which is open to the public and carries a variety of nutraceuticals, aromatherapy, books, music, fitness apparel, and other items to complement health and well-being—is an example of the increase of wellness themes appearing in hospital settings (Freshley, n.d.).

In 2004, Condell Medical Center in Libertyville, Illinois, opened a 190,000-square-foot addition housing a women's center, a New Life Maternity Center, a surgical services department, and one of the nation's first hospital spas called Inner Spa. Integrating Eastern and Western philosophies, the center offer's acupuncture, hydrotherapy, reflexology, Reiki, light therapy, and craniosacral treatments (a method for improving the functioning of the central nervous system developed by osteopathic physician, John Upledger). For cancer patients, special massage services are available, along with breast prostheses, wig fittings, and camouflage make-up lessons. Executive Health, a comprehensive medical exam provided by many hospitals and medical groups, is carefully coordinated by the center and is based on hotel customer service standards. Upon arrival to the Executive Health suite, a patient coordinator assists in arranging customized appointments and activities and accompanies the patient throughout the day. Between various tests, consultations, and a written report reviewed by a doctor with the patient at the end of the day, breakfast, lunch, and opportunities to relax are provided. In addition to services at the Inner Spa, patients can walk in an outdoor labyrinth, a healing tool with ancient roots that is effective for relaxation and meditative practices (Condell Medical Center Expansion, n.d.).

Receiving healthcare in high-touch nurturing environments is an attractive alternative for consumers who are dissatisfied with the typical stark, hurried, and impersonal atmosphere that has become standard in the age of managed care. Studies from the National Center for Health Statistics document most visits with a medical doctor average 16 minutes or less. Soothing fountains, dimmed lights, soft color palettes, and floor-to-ceiling windows with a view to nature that promote a sense of calm and well-being, common in spas and hotels, are appearing in more hospital developments. However, unless hospitals are reengineered on all levels of service delivery, with a focus on patient-centered care and a partnership model delivered in a multidisciplinary context, paradoxically they may fail to achieve better outcomes and patient satisfaction.

Spa culture has permeated the U.S. medical system in simple and profound ways, influencing even the most conservative healthcare institutions to explore new models of service and treatments. Considering that the words *hospital* and *hospitality* come from the same root, it is not surprising that consumer trends support a convergence of the medical, spa, and hospitality industries, blurring boundaries that were clearly delineated for many years. Undeniably, today's spa influences are transforming the healthcare system to be more hospitable and patient centered, and organizations such as Planetree, the Center for Healthcare Design, and the Samueli Institute, provide models, resources, and a framework for organizations seeking to understand these trends.

A VISION FOR THE FUTURE

As the current primary care system experiences a long-overdue reorganization, more spa, health, and wellness-based organizations will appear on the horizon and will change the face of healthcare. However, the place of greatest potential change is not with the government, medical community, spas, insurers, universities, or service providers, but within each individual. Through open access to information and education, consumers have a tremendous opportunity to enjoy good health individually and collectively and to support organizations and policymakers committed to offering the best of science, medicine, and technology balanced with practical tools and resources for healthy living.

The principles of spas and health have a long and rich history. Coming full circle from its ancient roots, the new horizon promises an inspiring vision of opportunity and possibility. The following examples of a destination spa resort, a medical facility, and two hotels illustrate how a new generation of organizations is expanding the concept of hospital, spa, and wellness, embracing an expanded definition of health services certain to influence an emerging era of wellness-based healthcare.

Canyon Ranch

Since establishing its first location in Tucson, Arizona, in 1979, Canyon Ranch has helped thousands of guests acquire the foundation for healthier and fuller lives through tools that show them how to manage aging, prevent disease, and cope with stress.

Over the years, Canyon Ranch has expanded to multiple locations with affiliations to various medical centers and universities such as Harvard Medical School, the University of Arizona Program for Integrative Medicine, and the Cleveland Clinic. In addition to providing customized preventative medicine, nutrition, behavioral health, movement therapies, healing arts, and exercise programs, the resort also sponsors continuing wellness education programs for medical professionals.

Expanding upon the success of its destination health resorts, Canyon Ranch is developing communities in cities nationwide designed to provide year-round spa living, where wellness is designed into the community. These spalike residential communities will offer health-conscious restaurants and fitness centers on the premises along with wellness services, life-style coaches, educational services, and retail stores. No longer just a fitness resort company, Canyon Ranch has become a life-style enhancement company that develops resorts, spa clubs, residential communities, educational programs, medical alliances, and life-style concept stores, all based on the company's commitment to healthy living programs and services (Canyon Ranch and Cleveland Clinic, n.d.).

The Medical Spa at Nova

The Medical Spa at Nova, an affiliate of the Nova Medical and Urgent Care Center, with four locations in Virginia, features spa services integrated into a comprehensive medical and wellness care program that offers an innovative prototype that could apply to the general delivery of outpatient medical care, including the hospital environment in the future. Their flagship location in Ashburn offers conventional and complementary medicine, acute care facilities, and therapeutic spa services. Board-certified internal medicine, family practice, and dermatology physicians work side by side with naturopaths, acupuncturists, clinical nutritionists, exercise physiologists, and massage therapists in the medical spa. Ongoing educational programs are provided for patients and available to the general community, and they address issues of nutrition, obesity, cancer, fibromyalgia, hormone replacement therapies, and prostate and breast health. Grace Keenan, medical director of Nova Medical Group, Nova Urgent Care, and the Medical Spa at Nova, has designed an integrative approach to patient care, using both conventional and CAM approaches aimed at general wellness as well as diagnosing and treating diverse acute and chronic medical conditions. As she explains, "Nova remains committed to the standard western approach to evaluating and diagnosing a patient, while offering complementary medicine modalities in addition to western approaches in both assessing and treatment by highly trained certified providers. In addition to managing acute medical illnesses, we focus on the long term effect of therapies and include an extensive battery of screening and preventative tests to optimize wellness. This approach limits drug side effects and interactions, by offering natural therapies as an option to prescription medications, a concept often neglected in today's health care delivery system" (Nova Medical Group, 2006).

Responsive to patient's requests for more choices in healthcare decisions, Keenan has been effective in developing a multidisciplinary team approach to evaluating patient conditions and cultivating a partnership model between mainstream Western-trained physicians and complementary providers, in both reviewing recommendations and selecting a treatment strategy. In treating high cholesterol, for example, patients are offered alternatives to cholesterol lowering drugs, including herbs and dietary interventions, while focusing on educating the patient and putting self care central to the healthcare process. With active input from the patient, "we decide together in a teamlike manner, on the best approach." According to Keenan, "cholesterol lowering drugs are not the only options available to a patient for effective treatment. Acupuncture, naturopathic services, dietary counseling and herbal medicine are frequently successful for lowering cholesterol levels in patients while avoiding pharmaceutical drugs altogether" (Nova Medical Group, 2006).

The California WellBeing Institute at the Four Seasons Hotel

Located at the Four Seasons Hotel and Spa in Westlake, California, the California WellBeing Institute is a medical facility that employs diagnostic methodologies to diagnosis and mange health challenges due to life-style choices, stress, and environmental factors. Corporate packages include comprehensive health evaluations, executive leadership programs, professional conferences, and well-being programs coordinated through institute physicians and wellness advisors. In addition to state-of-the art diagnostic services, the institute's Life Quality Profile focuses on determining the "quality of your whole life," addressing physical, mental, emotional, spiritual, and social considerations in patient assessments.

Consumer programs include comprehensive health evaluations, with specialty services and programs in areas of genetic screenings, cancer support, sleep disorders, obesity, diabetes, pain management, arthritis, cardiovascular health, and optimal aging. Accommodations include full-amenity services provided by one the world's leading operators of luxury hotels and resorts.

An example of the convergence of spa-medical-hotel and commercial products is the partnership with Dole World Headquarters, adjacent to the institute. The headquarters houses the Dole Nutrition Institute and research labs that actively contribute to the institute via seminars, food tasting events, demonstration kitchens, cooking classes, a television production studio, and instructional DVDs. With consumer trends supporting health and longevity-related services and products, the institute's comprehensive wellness approach is likely to be emulated by spas and hospitality organizations.

Peninsula Hotels

In 2006, Peninsula Hotels launched "Peninsula Wellness"—a lifestyle program designed to address guests' well-being, both during their stay and beyond—at locations in Hong Kong, Bangkok, Beverly Hills, Chicago, New York, Beijing, Manila, and Tokyo in 2007. In collaboration with international spa consultancy ESPA, headed by renowned spa authority Susan Harmsworth, programs and services draw upon Eastern and Western wellness philosophies. Healthy dining options are developed with the hotels' award-winning chefs and guest clinical nutritionist, Gabrielle Tusher, who also offers individual guest consultations to develop personalized daily menus to meet a guest's individual taste and health requirements. The innovative Peninsula Academy—offering learning experiences and introductions to the local cultures of each Peninsula location—coordinates programs with wellness-themed spa packages and "Naturally Peninsula" cooking classes for hotel guests (Peninsula Hotels, 2007).

EDUCATING FUTURE HEALTHCARE PROVIDERS

Education and information will be critical components to the evolution of new healthcare and wellness models. Just as the medical, spa, and hospitality industries have converged, new alliances between education, research, and wellness-based healthcare organizations will continue to grow as CAM programs are introduced into the curriculum of more medical and healing arts institutions. A few examples are identified below.

The Center for Integrative Medicine at the Cleveland Clinic, in partnership with Canyon Ranch, offers continuing education to physicians, nurses, and professionals in nutrition, exercise physiology, stress management, and integrative wellness so they can effectively assess specific needs of guests. Each participant receives a customized "lifestyle prescription" (Canyon Ranch and Cleveland Clinic, n.d.).

The Tai Sophia Institute in Laurel, Maryland, a graduate school for acupuncture, herbal medicine, and applied healing arts, collaborates with the University of Pennsylvania School of Medicine to research clinical applications of CAM therapies. This alliance will include the creation of a master's degree in complementary and alternative medicine to be offered by the Tai Sophia Institute and developed in collaboration with Penn's School of Medicine faculty. "This degree program is one of the first of its kind in the nation," states Alfred P. Fishman, MD, Senior Associate Dean for Program Development at Penn's School of Medicine and codirector of the collaboration. "It will afford a solid background for Penn's medical and nursing students in their understanding of alternative healing arts." In addition to the master's degree, a program that will integrate the best practices in cardiac care and complementary and alternative medicine for patient care, to be known as Optimal Healing Environments, will be formed by the Division of Cardiology at Penn's Presbyterian Medical Center and Tai Sophia Institute (Tai Sophia Institute, 2006).

Tai Sophia's curriculum includes community programs in healing arts and offers a nondegree program called Redefining Health, which provides a framework for addressing the importance of language and communication in the healing process. Provided to medical and nonmedical professionals, the program is offered on campus or on site at various medical facilities such as Kennedy Krieger Institute in Maryland.

The University of Minnesota has added a complementary therapies and healing practices program to the required curricula for its Medical School, College of Pharmacy, and School of Nursing. Courses include overviews of CAM, spirituality in healthcare, healing touch, traditional Chinese medicine, botanical medicine, clinical aromatherapy, clinical hypnosis, mediation, yoga, and osteopathy. Students have access to various online resources, including a tool designed to complement the PBS documentary "The New Medicine" at www.thenewmedicine.org (Tai Sophia Institute, 2006).

In 2001, Georgetown University received a five-year $1.7 million grant from the National Institutes of Health to develop and implement a comprehensive program in the School of Medicine curriculum designed to improve the level of awareness and advances about CAM (Tai Sophia Institute, 2006).

The Mount Sinai School of Medicine offers a program called Integrative Approaches to Health in Clinical Practice. The program combines Western medicine with complementary/alternative modalities such as acupuncture, nutrition, homeopathy, vibrational medicine, and mind-body techniques (Tai Sophia Institute, 2006).

In addition to conventional medical schools, naturopathic schools are also uniquely positioned to prepare students for future opportunities in the wellness industry. The principles of naturopathic medicine are utilized by spas throughout the world, and opportunities for naturopathic schools to collaborate with academic, research, medical, spa, and hospitality organizations are increasing. Arizona's Southwest College of Naturopathic Medicine with centers in environmental medicine, women's medicine, pediatric and geriatric medicine, has numerous collaborations with conventional medical institutions to conduct research projects. Their on-site medical center offers multidisciplinary primary medical care for common, serious, and chronic health conditions with a staff of naturopathic and allopathic physicians, chiropractors, and nutritionists.

Bastyr University, located north of Seattle, is another leading center for natural health science education, with doctorate programs in naturopathic, acupuncture, and Oriental medicine, master of science in nutrition and clinical health psychology, in addition to various undergraduate health science degrees. In 1994, the NIH selected Bastyr University as the national center for research on alternative treatments for HIV/AIDS with a million dollar grant. With continued funding for various research projects and formal recognition by the federal government of the legitimacy and significance of naturopathic medicine, schools such as Bastyr and the Southwest College of Naturopathic Medicine are contributing to national research studies and renewed interest in the development of a patient-centered system of healthcare delivery focused on restoring individual and community health while preventing illness.

Organizations such as Canyon Ranch and the Nova Medical Group are examples of organizations utilizing naturopathic medicine in their service programming. As demand for naturopathic and patient-centered models becomes more widespread, schools such as the Southwest College of Naturopathic Medicine, Bastyr University, and Tai Sophia are positioned to participate with conventional medical schools to prepare healthcare professionals for growing employment opportunities in the wellness industry.

CONCLUSION

Trends in consumer-driven healthcare, spa, wellness, and healthy life-style industries presented in this chapter are just a few examples of the many forces that are demonstrating new paradigms emerging on the U.S. health-care landscape. Returning to Angelica Thieriot's quote, "the ideal hospital would combine the best of spas with the best of hotels and the best of hospitals to become a truly healing environment," has now become a reality with many organizations across the country. But there is much work to be done in engineering a transition from a sickness and episodic model of healthcare that is expensive, fragmented, and dysfunctional with millions of individuals uninsured to a preventative wellness model that is affordable, functional, and available to all.

In 2007, Dick Davidson, the second longest serving president of the American Hospital Association will retire. Under his leadership, the association went through one of the most tumultuous periods of legislative change in hospitals and attempts at healthcare reform in the United States. When asked about his perspective of healthcare in the next millennium, he replied,

> Patient-centered care must be human-centered care, delivered in a supportive hospital environment that continues to provide the best and most appropriate care that medical science has to offer, without neglecting the emotional and spiritual aspects of illness. As traditional monuments to human empathy and benevolence, hospitals must remain houses of healing. (Cassel, 1991, p. 69)

To aspire to Davidson's goal, hospitals and the healthcare industry will face significant challenges for decades to come. Harvard Business School professors, Michael Porter and Regina Herzlinger provide countless examples in their books, referenced earlier in this chapter, indicating that U.S. healthcare is on a collision course with public needs and economic reality. Ironically, the solution to the crisis they address lies in refocusing the healthcare system on health. Simply stated, better health is less expensive than poor health. Strategic organizational changes will be required by all stakeholders, at every level—such as schools, food manufacturers, medical and nursing schools, research institutions, hospitals and policymakers—to be compelled and rewarded to focus on creating value for consumers and a new culture of health.

The Cooper Clinic in Texas, which has treated thousands of patients, was founded by Kenneth Cooper, who has dedicated his career to providing patients with the tools, education, and motivation to live healthy and active life-styles. His quote, "It is easier to maintain good health through proper exercise, diet, and emotional balance than to regain it once it is lost," provides insight for organizations seeking to be relevant in the present healthcare system and emerging wellness industry of the future (Cooper Wellness Program, n.d.).

TOOL KIT FOR CHANGE

Role and Perspective of the Healthcare Professional

1. Healthy life-style programs and multidisciplinary approaches to patient-centered care incorporate conventional and nontraditional approaches. How do you integrate conventional and nontraditional modalities? Do you include staff training and ongoing education to support this integration?
2. Assess the effectiveness of your approach to providing healthcare services to consumers seeking wellness and prevention-based services in a patient-centered model.
3. Identify areas where you can enhance the patient's experience in terms of quality of time they have with you and other providers, depth of discussion concerning choices and recommended services and therapies available, and your process for developing a treatment and follow-up plan.

Role and Perspective of the Participant

1. Market trends and demographic changes confirm that consumers are having a profound impact on the changing landscape of healthcare as they seek a wider range of choices, services, and environments combined with more participation in treatment strategies. Please identify examples of market trends and demographic changes that are impacting your healthcare choices.
2. Prepare a list of resources that you would use to locate organizations offering a partnership model in healthcare.
3. Determine and identify what elements and expectations are most important to you when you see a medical or healing arts professional.
4. Define what the terms conventional medicine, CAM, and CIM mean to you personally.
5. Discern what considerations influence the provider or medical facility you choose to visit. Price, convenience, location, services offered, reputation of providers, environment, insurance coverage, degree of customer service?

Interconnection: The Global Perspective

1. Diverse healthcare business models will continue to emerge within conventional healthcare organizations and nontraditional environments, such as spas, health resorts, wellness centers, and hotels. Can you identify five projects, not mentioned in this chapter, that illustrate examples of convergence of the medical, spa, and hospitality industries?
2. Referencing the 10 components of the Planetree model outlined in this chapter, and described in more detail on its Web site, http://www.planetree.org/about/components.htm, utilize this framework to design a patient-centered care medical center concept that would incorporate each component.

REFERENCES

Alliance Community Hospital. (n.d). *Planetree at Alliance Community Hospital.* Retrieved October 15, 2006, from http://www.achosp.org/Planetree.aspx.

Associated Bodywork & Massage Professionals. (2006). Massage therapy fast facts. Retrieved September 12, 2006, from http://www.massagetherapy.com/_content/images/Media/Factsheet1.pdf.

Banner Good Samaritan Medical Center. (2006). Retrieved October 3, 2006, from http://www.bannerhealth.com/Locations/Arizona/Banner+Desert+Medical+Center/The+Oasis+Spa/The+Oasis+Spa.htm

Baths at Caracalla. (n.d.). *ItalyGuides.it.* Retrieved September 12, 2006, from http://www.italyguides.it/us/roma/baths_of_caracalla.htm.

Battle creek sanitarium years, faith, breakfast and the Kellogg legacy. (2003). Defense Logistics Information Service. Retrieved October 18, 2006, from www.dlis.dla.mil/Federal-Center/Sanyears.asp

Bergel, R. (n.d.). *The healing power of water.* Retrieved October 18, 2006, from http://www.dayspaassociation.com/mainpages/water.htm.

Bullard, L. (2004). *Healing waters, Missouri's historic mineral springs and spas.* Columbia: University of Missouri Press.

Canyon Ranch and Cleveland Clinic. (n.d.). *Cleveland Clinic/Canyon Ranch Executive Health Program.* Retrieved October 18, 2006, from http://www.executivehealthpro gram.com/about-our-partnership.asp.

Cassel, E. (1991). *The nature of suffering and the goals of medicine.* New York: Oxford University Press.

Chez, R., Pelletier, K., & Jonas, W. (2004). *Toward optimal healing environments in health care.* [New Rochelle, NY: Mary Ann Liebert.

Condell Medical Center Expansion: Spa. (n.d.). Pratt Design Studio. Retrieved October 18, 2006, from http://www.prattdesign.com/site/epage/13356_417.htm.

Cooper Wellness Program. (n.d.). *Cooper Wellness Program, fitness, weight loss, stress management.* Retrieved October 18, 2006, from http://www.cooperaerobics.com/wellness.

Cribin-Bailey J., Harcup, J., & Harrington, J. (2005). *The spa book: The official guide to spa therapy.* Clifton, NY: Thompson Delmar Learning.

Croutier, L., (1992). *Taking the waters: Spirit, art, sensibility.* [New York: Abbeville Press.

du Rand, J. (2006) Interview, Newport Beach, California, November 2006

Eclectic medicine. (n.d.). Answers.com. Retrieved October 18, 2006, from http://www.answers.com/topic/eclectic-medicine.

Edmund Bordeaux Szekely: Life. (2006). Retrieved October 3, 2006, from http://en.wikipedia.org/wiki/Edmund_Bordeaux_Szekely.

Eisenberg, D., Kessler, R., Foster, C., Norlock, F., Calkins, D., & Delbanco, T. (1993). Unconventional medicine in the United States: Prevalence, costs, patterns of use. *New England Journal of Medicine, 328,* 246–252.

Freshley, C. (n.d.). *Day spas: A new trend in healthcare.* Retrieved October 12, 2006, from http://www.kaiser.net/articledetail.cfm?article_id=57

Grüner, M. (2002). Paresis, historical therapy in the perspective of Caelius Aurelianus, with special reference to the use of hydrotherapy in antiquity. *J Hist Neurosci, 11*(2), 105–109.

Gurney's Inn. (n.d.). What you always wanted to know about thalasso. Retrieved September 12, 2006, from http://www.gurneys-inn.com/Spa/Thalasso.htm?menu=seawaterspa.

Hamilton, D. K. (2003). Four levels of evidence-based design practice. Retrieved August 26, 2006, from http://www.healthdesign.org/aboutus/mission/EBD_definition.php.

Healing occurs naturally: Naturopathy in America. (n.d.). Coalition for Natural Health. Retrieved October 18, 2006, from http://www.naturalhealth.org/tradnaturo/history2.html.

Herzlinger, R. (1999). *Market-driven healthcare: Who wins, who loses in the transformation of America's largest service industry.* Reading, MA: Addison-Wesley.

Herzlinger, R. (2004). *Consumer driven health care: Implications for providers, payers, and policy* makers. San Francisco: Jossey Bass.

History of natural health, the popular health movement. (2006, October 18) Retrieved October 19, 2006, from http://en.wikipedia.org/wiki/Natural_therapy.

Holmes, D. (n.d.). Maine's Poland spring: This source of famed bottled water was a legendary resort in years gone by. The Old House Web. Retrieved September 12, 2006, from http://www.oldhouseweb.com/stories/Detailed/12127.shtml.

Immune support: hospitals getting a grip: massage therapy finds place in patient care for fm and more (2004, December 28). Retrieved October 20, 2006 from http://www.immunesupport.com/library/showarticle.cfm/ID/6151/e/1/T/CFIDS_FM/

International Spa Association. (2004, November 15). How fast is the spa industry growing? *ISPA 2004 spa industry study.* Retrieved September 12, 2006, from http://www.experienceispa.com/ISPA/Media+Room/Press+Releases/2004+Industry+Study+Summary.htm

International Spa Association. (n.d.). Retrieved from http://en.wikipedia.org/wiki/Spa

La Ferla, R. (2000, August 13). Hospitals are discovering their inner spa. *New York Times.* Retrieved September 12, 2006, from http://www.nytimes.com/library/style/weekend/081300medical-spa.html.

MacGregor, H. (2004, December 28). Hospitals getting a grip: Massage therapy finds place in patient care for FM and more. ImmuneSupport.com. Retrieved October 18, 2006, from http://www.immunesupport.com/library/showarticle.cfm/ID/6151/e/1/T/CFIDS_FM.

Marcozzi, M. (2004). Culture and complementary medicine. *Seminars in Integrative Medicine, 2*(3), 11.

Miami Institute for Age Management and Intervention. (n.d.). Services. Retrieved October 15, 2006, from http://www.miami-institute.com

National Center for Complementary and Alternative Medicine. (2006). Mission and history. Retrieved October 29, 2006, from http://nccam.nih.gov/about.

National Center for Health Statistics. (n.d.). *Maximize face-to-face doctor time: Analyze your logbook.* Retrieved October 15, 2006, from http://www.medscape.com/viewarticle/537265.

National Institute of Aging. (n.d.). *Health and aging.* Retrieved October 15, 2006, from http://www.nia.nih.gov.

Nova Medical Group. (2006). *Interview with Grace Keenan, MD July 11, 2006.* Retrieved August 12, 2006, from http://www.novamedgroup.com/about.php?PHPSESSID=35bd462893d8023aa3ed126c62e601da.

Peninsula Hotels. (2006, April 28). *Introducing "Peninsula Wellness."* Retrieved August 12, 2006, from www.asiatraveltips.com/news06/284-PeninsulaHotels.shtml

Porter M., & Teisberg E. (2006). *Redefining health care: Creating value-based competition on results.* Cambridge, MA: Harvard Business School Press.

Pritikin Longevity Center & Spa. (2006a). Reduce high cholesterol: Diet for high LDL cholesterol. Retrieved October 14, 2006, from http://www.pritikin.com/benefits/benefits_Cholesterol.shtml.

Pritikin Longevity Center & Spa. (2006b). Medical studies/Proven research. Retrieved October 14, 2006, from http://www.pritikin.com/research/research_StudiesResearch.shtml.

Pritikin Center and Spa. (2006c). Weight loss: Safe, healthy & natural. Retrieved October 14, 2006, from http://www.pritikin.com/benefits/benefits_WeightLoss.shtml.

Rancho La Puerta. (1996–2006). About us. Retrieved August 3, 2006, from http://www.rancholapuerta.com/About/index.html.

Register, J. (2002). Thalasso center at Paraiso de la Bonita in Puerto Morelos, Mexico: Thallassotherapy history. Retrieved September 12, 2006, from http://spas.about.com/library/weekly/aa110802.htm.

Saratoga Spa State Park (n.d.). Springs: History of the mineral waters. Retrieved September 12, 2006, from http://www.saratogaspastatepark.org/springs.html.

Schneider, L. (n.d.). Battle creek sanitarium, early health spa. Retrieved October 18, 2006, from http://www.faqs.org/nutrition/Ar-Bu/Battle-Creek-Sanitarium-Early-Health-Spa.html.

Sebastian Kneipp. (2006). Retrieved September 23, 2006, from http://en.wikipedia.org/wiki/Sebastian_Kneipp.

Spa Finder. (n.d.). *Rancho La Puerta highlights and awards.* Retrieved September 12, 2006, from http://www.spafinder.com/Spas/overview.jsp?spaID=37&pageType=highlights.

Spa Finder. (2006). *Spa history.* Retrieved September 12, 2006, from http://www.spafinder.com/spalifestyle/spa101/history.jsp.

Szekely, D. (1990). *Vegetarian spa cuisine from Rancho La Puerta.* Rancho La Puerta, Author.

Tai Sophia Institute. (2006, Summer/Fall). The report A3. *4*(2)

Touch Research Institute, University of Miami School of Medicine. (1997). *General information about TRI research.* Retrieved September 12, 2006, from http://www6.miami.edu/touch-research.

Vierille, J. (2006). Hydrotherapy: Washes, wraps, packs and herbs. Kneipp USA. Retrieved August 12, 2006, from http://www.kneippus.com/Hydrotherapy-%11-The-Water-Cure/The-Water-Cure/Der-Wasser-Kur-%28The-Water-Course%29.html.

Warner, Jennifer. Reviewed by Louise Chang, M.D. © 2006, WebMD Inc. Alternative medicine goes mainstream: 1 in 4 hospitals offer services such as acupuncture, yoga and homeopathy. (2006, July 20). CBS News. Retrieved October 15, 2006, from http://www.cbsnews.com/stories/2006/07/20/health/webmd/main1823747.shtml.

Wechsbeerg J. (1982). *The lost world of the great spas.* New York: Harper & Row.

Welcome to the Greenbrier Clinic. (2003). Retrieved October 3, 2006, from http://www.greenbrierclinic.com.

Chapter Three

EMOTION AND DISEASE: INTERFACING PSYCHOLOGY AND HEALTH USING A BIOPSYCHOSOCIAL MODEL

Antonio E. Puente, PhD and A. Griffin Pollock, BA

Psychology's history has seen two faces of the discipline, one academic/ research and the other applied or clinical. Due to its origin within the psychiatry departments of the Veterans Administration system after World War II, the application of psychology quickly become focused—indeed synonymous— with mental health. With the advent of licensing laws and third-party reimbursement, the focus of clinical psychology has been largely, if not exclusively, on mental health. After all, the origins of clinical psychology were largely centered on psychiatric services.

In recent years, the expansion of clinical psychology outside the boundaries of mental health has yielded a number of theoretical and practical opportunities that have expanded the horizons of clinical psychology and, subsequently, of psychology itself. Of the expansions, one of the more robust has been the application of psychological principles to health and medicine. For the purposes of this chapter, health will be considered as all that is disease free but is biological and pertaining to humans, whereas medicine will be focused on the disease process. In many ways, this resembles the difference between health psychology, which often focuses on healthy behaviors, and behavioral medicine, which almost exclusively focuses on the amelioration or control of a disease process.

This chapter focuses on the interface between the application of psychology and the disease process. Of particular interest is the relationship between emotion and disease. Whereas the traditional area of psychosomatic medicine has a long history of attending to this interface, its focus has historically been "medical" and psychiatric. The current focus is on how emotion affects the disease process and, in turn, how the disease process affects emotion. Further, as a means of providing a model for how this reciprocal deterministic model of disease and psychology interact, the primary focus will be on neurological diseases. These diseases are by far the most challenging for medicine as a whole, especially when the rehabilitation and control, including pharmaceutical, are involved. In addition, this focus is in greater synchrony with psychology because the role of mental processes is more directly involved (versus, for example, digestive diseases).

The chapter first defines emotion—including traditional versions—explaining the similarities and differences between positive and negative emotion and couching the concept of emotion within a neuropsychological perspective. Next, the chapter reviews the interface between emotion and disease process using a health psychology/neuropsychological perspective. The third section focuses on immunological diseases, especially multiple sclerosis and HIV/AIDS. This section will set the foundation for determining how their understanding has, in turn, helped develop viable theories of emotion and disease. The fifth section addresses alternative methods of understanding and altering immunity. A summary section reviews the major points developed in the chapter and provides methodological, clinical, and theoretical perspectives for the future.

DEFINING EMOTION

Emotion can be defined in numerous ways: traditional interpretations, based on concepts of valance, and neuropsychological. Whereas the concept of emotion has been defined repeatedly in the history of psychology and popularized by researchers such as Cannon and Selye, more modern and empirical interpretations such as those provided by Carver, Scheier, and colleagues as well as Taylor may be more applicable to the purposes of this chapter. Carver, Scheier and Weintraub (1989) have suggested that emotion is a response to stressors that are often environmental and overt and just as powerful as internal ones. In many respects, this concept follows Selye's ideas of a load being placed on a system and that system's ability to handle the load. The assumption would be that the lighter the perceived load is (since the perception may be more critical than the reality in terms of a response), the lower the emotionality associated with the load would be. A more cognitive perspective has been developed by Taylor and colleagues (1983) and continues to evolve. This perspective suggests that the individual's adjustment to a threatening event results in a cognitive adaptation, whether it be a habituation (as in the case of Wolpe's systematic desensitization) or a more resilient understanding and redirecting of goal-directed activity (as in the case of Meichenbaum's cognitive restructuring).

Regardless, there are now widespread understanding and acceptance that stressful life events, such as those measured by the Holmes and Rahe scale (e.g., death, divorce, etc.) ultimately, directly or indirectly, affect physical functioning and thus the development and/or exacerbation of disease. Indeed, health psychology and behavioral medicine have no more than a quarter of a century of history. However, the acceptance of the interface between emotion and disease has seeped down to the level of insurance reimbursement (e.g., see the new health and behavior assessment and intervention codes from the American Medical Association's Current Procedural Terminology manual, 2007). The assumption held by most is relatively straightforward: strong emotion, especially over the long term, will eventually produce serious, sometimes irreversible, and, in some cases, lethal results.

What is not so clear, however, is that emotion can be perceived by the recipient of change or threat as either positive or negative. Indeed, something as positive as a holiday or celebratory event (e.g., wedding) can produce significant changes that, in the long run, appear to produce similar undesirable effects to both the body and the mind. In other words, too much of a good thing, especially for a long period, can be in the end rather negative. Further, the existence of positive emotion can be prophylactic as well as restorative. In summary, cognitions about one's health and the perception of the disease process and the development of its symptoms can be affected by emotion.

Negative emotions have historically been reported to be associated with morbidity and mortality (Friedman & Booth-Kelley 1987). In groundbreaking work with cardiovascular disease, Friedman and colleagues reported that psychological stress, especially negative and long term, could be associated with the development of cardiovascular disease. Further, Friedman and colleagues postulated that a pattern of personality and of coping with stress, such as the Type A personality, could inevitably result in altered physiological functioning, including cortisol levels, and subsequently with the development of significant cardiovascular disease—including, but not limited to, hypertension, congestive heart failure, and myocardial infarctions. Since the development of the original concepts of Type A personality, a shift to determining what types of individuals and what types of specific emotional experiences, primarily negative, would be associated with the development of a "cardiovascular" personality disorder.

More recent efforts, partially spurred by the positive psychology movement of Seligman (2005), have focused on positive rather than negative emotion and the impact of such on the understanding and control of disease. Richman and colleagues (2005) have explored the relationship between two positive emotions—hope and curiosity—and three diseases—hypertension, diabetes mellitus, and respiratory tract infections. Hope and curiosity can be considered to be emotions related to "interest." Hope motivates actions and has a subsequent effect on both thought and behavior. It is a forward-looking emotion that is accompanied by positive expectations about the future. Curiosity is a desire to explore, to understand as well as to integrate new experiences and new knowledge. Presumably, such information would, in turn, affect the evolution of goal-directed behavior. Their findings, as well as the findings of others, suggest a strong correlation between positive affect and enhanced immunological functioning. They reported evidence that positive emotions may have a protective effect on the disease process, which included cardiovascular, metabolic, and respiratory systems.

According to Chesney and colleagues (2005), the effects of positive emotion seem to do more than counteract or cancel the effects of negative emotion. Positive emotion has its own protective value, independent of negative emotion. Further, these authors postulate that the experience of positive emotion may actually boost the body's immune system. Positive emotion may ensure the individual to engage in healthy behavior and to seek help when help is needed. Also, positive emotion may assist in helping one adapt in a healthy way to new or stressful situations. Nevertheless, the interface between emotion and disease should be considered, at least relative to the interface between negative emotion and disease, to be in its early stages of development.

The relationship between emotion and neuropsychology is even less developed than that of positive emotion and disease. Examination of the neuropsychological literature indicates a preponderance, to a fault, of cognition as the primary, if not the sole, factor in neuropsychological processes. For example, over the first decade of publication of the highly regarded journal *Neuropsychology Review*, only two articles focused on the role of emotion in neuropsychological processes. Historically, emotion, almost exclusively negative, was a result of diminished capacity due to the acquisition of a brain dysfunction. For example, individuals became depressed as cognitive capacity (e.g., memory) was reduced secondary to a dementing process such as Alzheimer's disease. However, the pioneering research of Sperry (1982) with split-brain patients provided an initial glimpse into the right hemisphere. It turns out that this hemisphere, though relatively "silent" due to the language centers being primarily in the left (or dominant) hemisphere, is directly associated with emotion. The first author has seen unpublished or undistributed films of the emotion emitted but denied (at least verbally) by male split-brain patients who had been shown sexually explicit films to the right hemisphere. There is increasing clinical and more recent empirical evidence that alteration of right hemisphere integrity (e.g., head trauma) results in perceived positive emotional changes such as disinhibition and, in other cases, negative emotional changes such as emotional flatness or inability to express or understand emotional stimuli.

THE EMPIRICAL INTERFACE OF HEALTH AND NEUROPSYCHOLOGY WITH EMOTION

This section focuses on the idea that emotion can be positive or negative and that such emotion can be either directly or indirectly associated with the disease process. As mentioned previously, the primary focus is on how this relationship expresses itself in diseases that are associated with or are a function of nervous system dysfunction.

Research on HIV/AIDS has produced a wealth of information that illustrates the close relationship between emotion and diseases that affect the nervous system (Kemeny et al., 1994). Recent studies have described the close link between immunological processes and emotion, especially in diseases of or affecting the nervous system. Marques-Deak, Cizza, and Sternberg (2005), described multiple neuroendocrine pathways, including the hormones of the hypothalamic-pituitary-adrenal (HPA), hypothalamic-pituitary-gonadal (HPG), hypothalamic-pituitary-thyroid (HPT), and the hypothalamic-growth hormone axes and how they interface with the immune system. The HPA axis is modulated by glucocorticoids. These substances suppress, enhance, and modulate the immune system. Thus, indirectly, emotion plays a pivotal role in immunity to disease and inflammation. Extreme or prolonged stress of the HPA axis results in extended activation of glucocorticoids, which, in turn, inhibit the immune system. Such an inhibition increases the likelihood of susceptibility to infection. Examples of diseases that are more likely to be developed or exacerbated include inflammatory arthritis, systemic lupus erythematosus, allergic asthma, and atopic dermatitis. Further, it was thought originally that glucocorticoids were only immunosuppressive. However, there is mounting evidence that they are important in immunomodulation and immunoenhancement as well, in a way similar to the dichotomy between negative and positive emotion.

The HPT axis hormones have been shown to directly stimulate immune cells. The hormones included thyroid-releasing hormone (tSH), triiodothyronine (T3), and thyroxine (T4). The effects of these thyroid hormones on immunity can result from either the HPT axis itself or from an interaction between the HPT and HPA axes. The HPG axis modulates the immune system in two ways. It directly affects the sex hormone effect on the immune cells. Indirectly, it does so through interactions between the HPG and HPA axes. The probability of this occurring is increased during periods of stress and may contribute to changes in one's susceptibility to autoimmune and inflammatory diseases as well as the expression of those diseases.

Major depressive disorder appears to cause a disruption of communication between the neuroendocrine and immune systems. Cohen, Doyle, Turner, Alper, and Skoner (2003) have reported that emotional style affects susceptibility to the common cold. The opposite also appears to be true. That is, a positive style of coping decreases the likelihood of disease or the expression of disease. This has especially been found in work with cardiovascular disease. Gallo, Ghaed, and Bracken (2004) reported on both risks and resiliency as well as social contexts in the interface between emotion, cognition, and coronary heart disease. Ray (2004) provided a provocative and comprehensive review on the topic. The title of the article is as descriptive of the contents as any paraphrasing of the material could be: "How the mind hurts and heals the body."

Two diseases that exhibit a close interface between emotion, immunological processes, and brain function are multiple sclerosis and HIV/AIDS. In multiple sclerosis, ample evidence suggests the existence of depression secondary to the development of the disease. However, a review of some of the findings indicates that much of the literature appears to confuse symptoms of depression with symptoms of physical, emotional, and cognitive fatigue. In general, more commonly seen is a deregulation of emotion, including, but not limited to, emotional flatness or even agnosia, where there is little understanding or interest in emotional information. In other cases, there is an emotional deregulation where there is little connection between the emotion and the social context. For example, an individual may cry over a particularly provocative commercial but may cognitively consider the act of crying to be foolish.

The HIV/AIDS literature is replete with information on the interface between emotion and the disease process. Sikkema, Hansen, Meade, and Lee (2005) reported that psychological health is related to disease progression, HIV-related symptoms, and even death. The researchers examined HIV-infected individuals who had suffered from the loss of a partner or other type of close friend or relative due to an AIDS-related death. The authors examined the possibility that coping group intervention could improve the lives of these individuals. Using the Functional Assessment of HIV Infection scale, they examined physical health status and symptomatology. Those in the intervention group showed a significant improvement in general health-related quality of life and in health issues/symptoms specifically associated with HIV/AIDS.

In a related study, Stein and Rotheram-Borus (2004) examined different coping styles: positive, passive, depressive withdrawal, and escapist. They examined the relationships among environmental stress, self-esteem, social support, coping style, AIDS symptoms, and CD4 count. Results indicated that CD4 counts were not related to coping styles. However, AIDS-related symptoms were predicted only by the passive coping style but not by the others.

The authors conclude that greater self-esteem may lead to improved coping skills, which, in turn, may lead to better health outcomes. Leslie, Stein, and Rotheram-Borus (2002) found that emotional distress directly influenced distress related to HIV/AIDS symptoms. Emotional distress was able to predict greater HIV/AIDS symptoms and may make physical symptoms worse.

Reed, Kemeny, Taylor, Wang, and Visscher (1994) reported that gay men with AIDS who scored high on realistic acceptance died nine months earlier than those who scored low. The research suggests that positive expectation, even unrealistic expectations, may increase longevity. In a similar vein, Reed, Kemeny, Taylor, and Visscher 1999) reported that high scores on HIV-specific expectancies were associated with a greater likelihood of symptom development. Negative HIV-specific expectancies were significant predictors of the onset of prognostically relevant symptoms of AIDS among previously asymptomatic HIV seropositive gay men. In this study, negative expectations are associated not only with a more rapid progression toward death among those diagnosed with AIDS, but also with a more rapid onset of symptoms in those who had previously been asymptomatic.

These findings have been reported by other laboratories and thus appear to reflect an intricate and bidirectional relationship between emotion and disease (e.g., Friedland, Renwick, & McColl, 1996; Taylor, Kemeny, Reed, Bower, & Gruenewald, 2000; Weitz, 1989).

DEVELOPMENT OF THEORIES OF THE INTERFACE BETWEEN EMOTION AND DISEASE

The interface between emotion and disease processes has yielded a robust and evolving research literature. In the wake of the emerging body of information have come several viable theories of how emotion and disease interface. Futterman, Kemeny, Shapiro, and Fahey (1994) were some of the first researchers to postulate viable theories linking positive and negative emotions with disease. They postulate that physiological changes affecting immunological capacity, and vice versa, were induced with positive and negative mood. Taylor and colleagues (2000) suggested that optimistic beliefs concerning the future, even unrealistic ones, may help protect one's health and are associated with a slowing of the illness process. Positive illusions seem to have a protective psychological effect that can be crucial in one's reaction to extremely threatening or negative events. Intervention in the form of encouraging positive emotion may be useful in slowing down the progression of disease. Taylor and colleagues (2000) posited that there are several probable routes by which emotional states affect disease. The practice of habits that improve health (such as exercise) or make health worse (such as smoking or excessive alcohol consumption) can have direct and critical impact. In addition, appropriate use of healthcare services as well as the inclusion of social support and encouragement may have a positive effect. The authors indicate that, at present, there is no empirical support for these probable routes. They conclude, however, that, while the exact biopsychosocial pathways through which the protective effects of positive emotion take place are not yet known, there is evidence that they do, in fact, exist. In another attempt at developing a comprehensive theory of (especially positive) emotion, Taylor (1983 postulated that cognitive adaptation, including a positive attitude, may directly modulate the disease process.

Research linking positive emotion to long-term outcome is becoming increasingly common in the literature. Stone, Cox, Valdimarsdottir, Jandorf, and Neale (1987) reported that secretory IgA antibody is directly tied to daily mood. Further, there is evidence that positive emotional states result in long-term positive physiological changes.

Research by Cohen and Herbert (1996) indicates that negative emotional states are directly linked to physiological changes prognostic for illness and to the development of several chronic diseases. Specifically, in an earlier work, Herbert and Cohen (1993) reported that depression and anxiety are indisputably linked to the immune system.

Barefoot and colleagues (2000) reported that depressive symptoms were directly correlated with the development of coronary disease. Specifically, depression was closely tied to the existence of increased risks of coronary artery disease. Although the study was correlational, the findings focus specifically on negative emotion in the development of serious heart disease. However, no clear evidence has been reported, at least until recently, of the long-term effects of negative emotion and cardiovascular disease. Recent research by Morrill, Richardson, Keith, and Puente (in press) reported that the best predictor of morbidity 10 years after coronary artery bypass surgery is presurgical anxiety. Thus, the original theory of Friedman and colleagues with the development of theories associated with Type A behavior have slowly evolved to address a more specific relationship between emotion and disease. The theory proposed by contemporary workers in the field, such as Shelley, provide room for both negative (as in the case of the original research on cardiovascular disorders) and positive (as in the more recent research on HIV/AIDS) emotion and the interplay of both in the development and progression of disease.

Alternative methods for changing immunity may also affect emotional status and, subsequently, disease expression. Molassiotis and Maneesakorn (2004) reported that quality of life and psychological status in individuals living with AIDS could be altered by the regular practice of meditation. The authors examined the interrelationship between anxiety, depression, coping, and quality of life. Emotion-focused meditation was found to be related to higher quality of life, though not a decrease of AIDS symptoms.

CONCLUSION

Despite increasing interest in the relationship of emotion and disease over the last 100 years, the focus on research and clinical practice has evolved essentially only over the last 25 years. That focus has been almost exclusively on the concept that emotion is often secondary to a disease process and that negative emotion hastens the development or evolution of the disease process. As a result, a plethora of research focused on emotion as a negative mediator of disease. However, there is increasing evidence that emotion has a primary effect on the development of disease. More recent research has explored the idea that positive emotion can have a protective impact on disease. Further, there is additional evidence that emotion does not exist in a void from cognition. Indeed, the opposite appears to occur. Specifically, cognitive (or least perceptual) processes interact with emotional ones to produce mediating effects on disease.

Methodological issues remain to be resolved. Emotion is difficult to record, especially if it is self-reported. Further, emotion is broadly and often idiosyncratically defined, both by the researchers as well as the subjects involved in studies. The interface between paper-and-pencil measures, such as questionnaires of emotion, and more direct physiological measures, such as corticosteroid levels and/or psychophysiological recordings, may increase the likelihood of a closer connection between emotion and disease and the reliability of measurement of both.

Increasing evidence shows that emotion and disease are intractably related. In fact, the possibility exists that a Cartesian dualism may not be the most robust approach to understanding how emotion and disease are related. An alternative approach would be to consider that disease and emotion are merely different faces of the same coin. In doing so, the dualistic interpretation of mind and body may be replaced with a continuum with emotion at one end and disease at the other. That alternative interpretation would, however, not resolve the problem of timing or evolution of the two—that is, which one comes first. It could very well be that, when all is said and done, such questions are irrelevant because the two may, as previously suggested, be two sides of the same coin.

TOOL KIT FOR CHANGE

Perspective of the Healthcare Professional

1. The interplay between emotion and disease is subtle but will have a powerful impact on the development and expression of disease.

2. Negative emotion will increase the likelihood of a disease being expressed or make the symptoms more intense.
3. Positive emotion will have a protective impact and may assist in the amelioration of symptoms.
4. Positive emotions can be either explicit or implicit and may take some time to have an eventual impact on the disease process.
5. The perception of the patient may be more powerful than the reality of the situation.

Perspective of the Patient

1. Embrace the idea that the mind and the body are unified, especially when it comes to the disease process.
2. Accept the possibility that emotions, whether negative and/or positive, can impact disease.
3. Understand that negative emotions can both cause a decrease in overall health and increase the possibility of the disease process appearing or worsening.
4. Appreciate that positive emotions may have a critical impact on disease.
5. Positive emotions are what make you happy and content, not what others believe should make you happy and content.

The Larger Perspective

1. Public healthcare policy has to understand the continuum between mind and body, especially with regard to disease.
2. Emotional issues need to be given parity with physical issues, especially in light of the continuum indicated in point 1.
3. Health and healthcare will improve substantially, especially for those in difficult circumstances (e.g., poverty) when this continuum is acknowledged and bridged.

REFERENCES

American Medical Association. (2007). *Current procedural terminology.* Chicago: Author.
Barefoot, J. C., Brummett, B. H., Helms, M. J., Mark, D. B., Siegler, I. C., & Williams, R. B. (2000). Depressive symptoms and survival of patients with coronary artery disease. *Psychosomatic Medicine, 62*(6), 790–795.
Carver, C. S., Scheier, M. F., & Weintraub, J. K. (1989). Assessing coping strategies: A theoretically based approach. *Journal of Personality and Social Psychology, 56*(2), 267–283.
Chesney, M. A., Darbes, L. A., Hoerster, K., Taylor, J. M., Chambers, D. B., & Anderson, D. E. (2005). Positive emotions: Exploring the other hemisphere in behavioral medicine. *International Journal of Behavioral Medicine, 12*(2), 50–58.
Cohen, S., Doyle, W. J., Turner, R. B., Alper, C. M., & Skoner, D. P. (2003). Emotional style and susceptibility to the common cold. *Psychosomatic Medicine, 65*(4), 652–657.
Cohen, S., & Herbert, T. B. (1996). Health psychology: Psychological factors and physical disease from the perspective of human psychoneuroimmunology. *Annual Review of Psychology, 47,* 113–142.
Friedland, J., Renwick, R., & McColl, M. (1996). Coping and social support as determinants of quality of life in HIV/AIDS. *AIDS Care, 8*(1), 15–31.
Friedman, H. S., & Booth-Kewley, S. (1987). The "disease prone personality": A meta-analytic view of the construct. *American Psychologist, 42*(6), 539–555.

Futterman, A. D., Kemeny, M. E., Shapiro, D., & Fahey, J. L. (1994). Immunological and physiological changes associated with induced positive and negative mood. *Psychosomatic Medicine, 56*(6), 499–511.

Gallo, L. C., Ghaed, S. G., & Bracken, W. S. (2004). Emotions and cognitions in coronary heart disease: Risk, resilience, and social context. *Cognitive Therapy and Research, 28*(5), 669–694.

Herbert, T. B., & Cohen, S. (1993). Depression and immunity: A meta-analytic review. *Psychological Bulletin, 113*(3), 472–486.

Kemeny, M. E., Weiner, H., Taylor, S. E., Schneider, S., Visscher, B., & Fahey, J. L. (1994). Repeated bereavement, depressed mood, and immune parameters in HIV seropositive and seronegative gay men. *Health Psychology, 13*(1), 14–24.

Leslie, M. B., Stein, J. A., & Rotheram-Borus, M. J. (2002). The impact of coping strategies, personal relationships, and emotional distress on health-related outcomes of parents living with HIV or AIDS. *Journal of Social and Personal Relationships, 19*(1), 45–66.

Marques-Deak, A., Cizza, G., & Sternberg, E. (2005). Brain-immune interactions and disease susceptibility. *Molecular Psychiatry, 10*, 239–250.

Molassiotis, A., & Maneesakorn, S. (2004). Quality of life, coping and psychological status of Thai people living with AIDS. *Psychology, Health and Medicine 9*(3), 350–361.

Morrill, E., Richardson, E., Keith, J., & Puente, A. E. (in press). Anxiety as a determinant of morbidity 10 years post coronary artery bypass surgery. *Journal of Clinical Psychology in Medical Settings.*

Ray, O. (2004). How the mind hurts and heals the body. *American Psychologist, 59*(1), 29–40.

Reed, G. M., Kemeny, M. E., Taylor, S E., & Visscher, B. R. (1999). Negative HIV-specific expectancies and AIDS-related bereavement as predictors of symptom onset in asymptomatic HIV-positive gay men. *Health Psychology, 18*(4), 354–363.

Reed, G. M., Kemeny, M. E., Taylor, S. E., Wang, H. Y. J., & Visscher, B. R. (1994). Realistic acceptance as a predictor of decreased survival time in gay men with AIDS. *Health Psychology, 13*(4), 299–307.

Richman, L. S., Kubzansky, L., Maselko, J., Kawachi, I., Choo, P., & Bauer, M. (2005). Positive emotion and health: Going beyond the negative. *Health Psychology, 24*(4), 422–429.

Seligman, M.E.P., Steen, T. A., Park, N., & Peterson, C. (2005). Positive psychology progress: Empirical validation of interventions. *American Psychologist, 60*(5), 410–421.

Sikkema, K. J., Hansen, N. B., Meade, C. S., & Lee, R. S. (2005). Improvements in health related quality of life following a group intervention for coping with AIDS-bereavement among HIV-infected men and women. *Quality of Life Research, 14*(4), 991–1005.

Sperry, R. W. (1982). Some effects of disconnecting the cerebral hemispheres. *Bioscience Reports, 2*(5), 265–276.

Stein, J. A., & Rotheram-Borus, M. J. (2004). Cross-sectional and longitudinal associations in coping strategies and physical health outcomes among HIV-positive youth. *Psychology and Health, 19*(3), 321–336.

Stone, A. A., Cox, D. S., Valdimarsdottir, H., Jandorf, L., & Neale, J. M. (1987). Evidence that secretory IgA antibody is associated with daily mood. *Journal of Personality and Social Psychology, 52*(5), 988–993.

Taylor, S. E. (1983). Adjustment to threatening events: A theory of cognitive adaptation. *American Psychologist, 38*(11), 1161–1173.

Taylor, S. E., Kemeny, M. E., Reed, G. M., Bower, J. E., & Gruenewald, T. L. (2000). Psychological resources, positive illusions, and health. *American Psychologist, 55*(1), 99–109.

Weitz, R. (1989). Uncertainty and the lives of persons with AIDS. *Journal of Health and Social Behavior, 30,* 270–281.

Chapter Four

MULTIMODAL IMAGERY AND HEALTHCARE

Kirwan Rockefeller, PhD, Ilene A. Serlin, PhD, ADTR, and John Fox, CPT

A PICTURE IS WORTH A THOUSAND WORDS

Imagery is a term used to describe a simultaneous information processing mode that underlies the holistic, synthetic, pattern thinking of the unconscious mind. As a mental thought process, imagery has sensory elements; imagery is something we see, hear, taste, smell, touch, or feel. Imagery has been shown to affect almost all physiologic control systems of the body, including respiration, heart rate, blood pressure, metabolic rates in cells, gastrointestinal mobility and secretion, sexual function, cortisol levels, blood lipids, and even immunity responsiveness (Rockefeller, 2007; Rossman, 2004).

This chapter addresses imagery as a technique that can aid healthcare professionals and patients in accessing the power of imagery for healing. Because not all people use visual imagery and because humans tend to use a variety of imagery modes, we address guided imagery, kinaesthetic imagery, and verbal imagery.

GUIDED IMAGERY

Imagery has an ancient lineage for healing that applies across a wide diversity of cultures. The benefits of healing imagery are evident in Ayurvedic, Chinese, Japanese, European, Native American, and various indigenous healing cultures (Achterberg, Dossey, & Kolkmeier, 1994; Rossman, 2000, 2003). Indeed, according to Micozzi (2004), "what some in the United States call 'alternative medicine' [including imagery] constitutes primary health care for 80% of humans worldwide" (p. 90).

The dramatic increase among consumers in the use of complementary and alternative, or integrated, treatments attests to a paradigm shift incorporating a holistic approach to healthcare, prevention, and wellness (Hyman, 2004). Imagery often ranks high on lists of the most popular and accessible integrative modalities that resonate across different sociocultural ethnicities.

Any activity that requires looking ahead to the future or planning ahead begins with a picture in one's mind, or an *image*. Beliefs, feelings, attitudes, and ideas are represented and deeply rooted in *imagery*. Imagery can be thought of initially as pictures in one's mind; yet imagery is so much more. It is a full sensory experience made up of thoughts that one can see, feel, hear, taste, and smell. Imagery can be about events that have happened in the past or have yet to happen. Rich in symbols, imagery tells us how we see ourselves, how we see others, and how we plan for the future. Imagery is a window into one's inner world—the world of dreams, daydreams, fantasies, and the creative imagination. Imagery is also a reflection of one's outer world, the world of self-image. Imagery is important in whole person healthcare because it is low cost, noninvasive, easy to learn, and can empower a patient to be a part of a treatment protocol (Rockefeller, 2007).

Martin Rossman, a physician and board-certified acupuncturist who has practiced holistic medicine since 1972, states in *Guided Imagery for Self-Healing* (2000, p. 7), "literally thousands of scientific studies have demonstrated the attitudinal, emotional, and behavioral effects" using the natural healing abilities of imagination. Research in eye movement desensitization and reprocessing, biofeedback, hypnosis, prayer, yoga, meditation, and creative visualization has documented a remarkable capacity for humans to use visualization and guided imagery in a relaxed state of mind. Yet, as Rossman states, there is still resistance in the medical community and among the general population to the idea that the body and the mind are connected.

Barnes, Powell-Griner, and Nahin (2004), in conducting the Centers for Disease Control's most comprehensive assessment to date of complementary and alternative medicine (CAM) in the United States, found that 62 percent of all American adults used some form of CAM therapy, when prayer was included in the definition, including imagery. They estimate that the U.S. public spent between $36 billion and $47 billion on CAM therapies in 1997. Of this amount, between $12.2 billion and $19.6 billion was paid out of pocket for the services of CAM healthcare providers. These fees are more than the U.S. public paid out of pocket for all hospitalizations in 1997 and about half that paid for all out-of-pocket physician services. The authors state that CAM use was more likely used among older adults than younger adults; Asian adults were more likely (43.1%) to use CAM than white adults (35.9%) or black adults (26.2%); and adults who live in urban areas are more likely than adults in rural areas to use CAM.

A growing body of research supports the effectiveness of guided imagery for a variety of complaints, increasing feelings of well-being and self-efficacy. Guided imagery has been shown to be effective in reducing depression and anxiety (Baider, Peretz, Hadani, & Koch, 2000; Bisson, 1995; McDonald & Hilgendorf, 1986), reducing pain and the need for pain medication (Syrjala et al., 1997), changing life-style habits associated with hypertension (Agras, 1981; Barabasz & Spiegel, 1989; Cochrane & Friesen, 1992; Wynd, 1992), finding meaning in the experience of cancer (Brown-Saltzman, 1997; Dahlquist, 1985; Krystal & Zweben, 1989; Richardson, Post-White, & Grimm, 1997; Rossman, 2003), increasing comfort in women with fibromyalgia (Fors, Sexton, & Gunnar, 2002), early stage breast cancer undergoing radiation therapy (Kolcaba & Fox, 1999), alleviating symptoms associated with congestive heart failure (Klaus, Beniaminovitz, Choi, Greenfied, Whitworth, Oz & Mancini, 2000), cognitive-behavioral interventions on life quality in persons with HIV (Antoni et al., 1991; Auerback, Oleson, & Solomon, 1992; Eller, 1999); and in lowering anxiety in phase II cardiac rehabilitation programs (Collins and Rice, 1997).

There is a wide body of literature supporting the use of guided imagery for pain control and relief, including pain from cancer treatment (Carr, 1995), pain following anterior cruciate ligament reconstruction (Cupal & Brewer, 2000); chronic pain in outpatient groups (Newshan & Balamuth, 1990–1991); pain, anxiety, and cardiac surgery (Tusek, Cwynar, & Cosgrove, 1999); pain in colorectal surgery (Tusek, Church, Strong, Grass, & Fazio, 1997); acute preoperative pain (Manyande et al., 1995; Tusek, Church, & Fazio, 1997), chronic headaches (Mannix, Chandurkar, Rybicki, Tusek, & Solomon, 1999); cancer pain (Arathuzik, 1994; Graffam & Johnson, 1987; Sloman, 1995); pain from fibromyalgia (Creamer, Singh, Hochberg, & Berman, 2000); pediatric pain (Krueger, 1987), and pain from rheumatoid arthritis (Kerns, Turk, Holzman, & Rudy, 1986). In the field of pain management, two distinct goals of guided imagery treatment strategies are identified: to reduce or block the pain sensation and to enhance tolerance to pain (Bresler, personal communication, March 31, 2005).

Baird & Sands (2004) studied 28 women 65 years to 93 years of age with a diagnosis of osteoarthritis who were randomly assigned to either a treatment or control group. The treatment consisted of listening twice a day to a 10- to 15-minute audiotape that guided the women in guided imagery and progressive muscular relaxation. The authors report that, after one week, the treatment group reported a significant reduction in pain and mobility difficulties when compared to the control group.

A well-designed guided imagery protocol for pain management can be found in the work of Fors, Sexton, and Gotestam (2002). The authors explored the use of *pleasant guided imagery* (that distracts participants away from a pain experience) and *attention imagery* (that focuses attention on the active workings of the body's internal pain control systems) on daily fibromyalgia pain. Fifty-five women participated in the study: n = 17 in the pleasant imagery group; n = 21 in the attention imagery group; and n = 17 in the control group. Additionally, all women were randomly assigned to a group that received 50 mg of amitriptyline per day or a placebo group. The slopes of diary pain ratings over a four-week period were used as the outcome measures. The level of pain reported by the pleasant imagery group declined significantly when compared with the control group, but the level of pain reported by the attention imagery group did not. There was neither a difference between the amitriptyline and placebo slopes, leading the researchers to conclude that pleasant guided imagery was an effective intervention in reducing fibromyalgic pain during the 28-day study period.

Baider, Uziely, and De-Nour (1994) used progressive muscular relaxation and guided imagery to study immediate and long-term effects on psychological distress and pain of self-referred cancer patients. Of the 123 cancer patients who began the study, 70 percent (n = 86) completed the full intervention and showed marked improvement on the Brief Symptom Inventory and the Impact of Events Scale. Improvements were maintained over the next six months for 58 patients who continued assessment through the follow-up period.

Lawlis, Achterberg, Kenner, and Kopetz (1984) studied 60 African American, Mexican American, and white patients with chronic spinal pain, among whom 10 men and 10 women had persistent spinal pain for over one year. Results showed ethnic differences on the ischemic test (a psychological scaling technique used to approximate clinical pain and pain tolerance), with Mexican Americans describing the highest levels. Women of all ethnic groups tended to be perceived as emphasizing their pain more than men, based on judgment of their pain behaviors and on their own numerical estimates of pain. It was determined that, while ethnic and sex differences were found, stereotypic responses were not uniform.

Moore and Spiegel (1999) explored cross-cultural narrative experiences of metastatic breast cancer and cancer pain in a population of African American and white women who had survived metastatic breast cancer. The authors report that women were drawn to guided imagery not only to cope and manage cancer-related anxiety and pain, but as a vehicle for reconnecting to the self and as a means of finding meaning within their experiences of breast cancer.

GUIDED IMAGERY AND PAIN MANAGEMENT

Pain is a universal of human condition. A multifaceted and subjective experience, pain operates on a sensory continuum and can be neurological, musculoskeletal, psychological, and/or emotional. As pain intensifies for an individual, it expands into psychological territory containing existential elements of uncertainty, fear, and suffering. Throughout history, humans have attempted to guard against pain, prepare for pain, medicate pain, endure pain, place blame for pain, attach personal narrative to the meaning of pain, and transcend pain.

In addition to the physiological and psychological realms, pain has inherently social, political, and moral implications within specific historical and cultural backgrounds. The perception, experience, responses to, and treatment of pain come together as a unified embodiment affecting not only the patient, but family, friends, and co-workers who all shape the experiential world of the suffering patient. These contextual interactions transform the very meaning of life, including painful relationships, pained feelings, and decreased function in a painful world (Kleinman, Brodwin, Good, & DelVecchio-Good, 1992; Moore & Spiegel, 1999).

The experience of pain can also cause a split between one's sense of reality and the reality of other people and, in many cases, between the person and one's own body (Moore, 1999; Scarry, 1985; Spiegel, 1995). As Achterberg, Dossey, and Kolkmeier (1994) eloquently state, "When asked what they fear most about injury or illness, most people name pain" (p. 96).

In the United States, pain is the most frequent reason for physician consultation (Abbott & Fraser, 1998). It is estimated that up to 105 million Americans have a chronic pain condition (Harstall, 2003). Turk and Burwinkle (2004) state that pain is not only prevalent, but costly. It has been suggested that the healthcare costs of patients with chronic pain exceeds those for patients with coronary artery disease, cancer, and AIDS; lost income and productivity are estimated to be between $50 billion and $100 billion annually (Carpenter, 2002; Cousins, 1995).

If untreated, pain can cause increases in psychological and physiological symptoms such as depression, mood disturbance, and anxiety. Chronic pain can cause fatigue, depress the immune system, and has been linked to decreased survival rates. Full of symbolic meaning, unrelieved pain can shatter lives and destroy worlds (Lang & Pratt, 1994; Scarry, 1985; Spiegel & Moore, 1997).

Voluminous research exists on pain. A Medline and Psychinfo Internet search yielded over 100,000 citations. It is beyond the scope of this discussion to adequately review pain as it applies to the human condition. However, given guided imagery's low cost, the fact that it carries no side effects, and is an easy-to-learn strategy, it is a highly appropriate intervention for adults seeking whole person healthcare.

KINAESTHETIC IMAGERY

Kinaesthetic imagery has common roots with other forms of imagery and yet is distinctive. We will first compare it with visual imagery, and then will describe its unique nature.

Imagery has been defined as "a mental picture of something not actually present, a mental conception symbolic of a basic attitude, orientation or attribute. Feelings, beliefs, and ideas are represented and vested in images, symbols and mental pictures which become part of our personal narrative" (Rockefeller, 2005).

The groundbreaking work of Candace Pert in psychoneuroimmunology provides a physiological and biochemical base for imagery in the neuropeptide receptors (Pert, 1997). Indeed, a whole range of psychological methods are already based on images such as creative visualization, active imagination, Gestalt therapy, and creative arts therapies. Finally, the use of imagery for psychological and physical health has been shown to be a significant and cost-effective healing practice (Baider et al., 2000; Bisson, 1995; Fors et al., 2002; Hyman, 2004; Moore & Spiegel, 1999).

Kinaesthesia comes from the Greek word meaning the sensation and impressions arising from body movement. A kinaesthetic image is difficult to describe in words, because it is more of a sensation than a visual image. It doesn't have the clear boundaries of a visual image, and in fact has been called a "fuzzy image" (Sheets-Johnstone, 1978) or a "form" (Merleau-Ponty, 1963). It is dynamic rather than static and so is difficult to pin down or document. When they are embodied, kinaesthetic images tend to flow in a continuous stream of "expressive gestures" (Merleau-Ponty, 1963) that form a language or text (Serlin, 1996).

In nonverbal communication, it is useful to distinguish among types of kinaesthetic images. When using kinaesthetic imagery in therapy, the question of what certain images mean or communicate is important. As with other forms of imagery, a therapist using kinaesthetic imagery must stay sensitive to the individual meaning of the client, and not impose his or her meaning system on the image. As a language, kinaesthetic imagery can be metaphoric, symbolic, archetypal, or spiritual.

Metaphoric images, like metaphoric phrases, are characterized by the word *like*. A gesture is like another situation; the action of the gesture mirrors reality. For example, a student explored her dance with another student as a metaphor for her relationship with her boyfriend:

> Did mirror with a partner. I felt that we began to move as one, not as leader-follower. But I didn't really feel a genuine felt-sense. It was there on a shallow level, but deep

down I guess I wanted more. It's like my relationship with Ron…I'm not exactly sure of what I want from him, but I have a feeling of what he wants from me. (Serlin, 1996, p. 29)

In a support group for women with breast cancer, movement was used to explore themes of courage, fear, and facing mortality (Serlin, Classen, Frances, & Angell, 2000).

Symbolic images have a more dreamlike quality, and they are not about everyday actions or events. Susanne Langer (1953) described them as pulsating forms of expressiveness or "patterns of sentience" (p. 187). Another student explored the symbol of goddess in her movement:

> All my joints softened. Without taking a step I could feel the weight of my body making a hundred little adjustments, a tiny current of energy flowing through every pathway, down to the earth, up to the crown, back and forth…I was aware of the fleshiness of the bottoms of my feet, how far I could "step into them"…The dance took a serpentine shape, turning back and forth on a line with the feet barely leaving the ground, but the knees fluid. (Serlin, 1996, p. 30)

In the support group, women explored their Warrior, Bad Girl, Queen, and Healer selves. Taking the image into their whole bodies allowed them to experience a new state of being or amplify a part of themselves associated with self-assertion and resilience.

Finally, spiritual images may have specific religious content, but also may be transcendent and numinous. French philosopher Paul Ricoeur (1976) described these images in terms of time and space: "The preverbal character of such an experience is attested to by the very modulations of space and time as sacred space or sacred time, which result and which are inscribed beneath language at the aesthetic level of experience" (p. 61). Another student said about her movements:

> When I move in circular motion, all parts of me move, I feel a great sense of centeredness, of wholeness, a soothing gentleness. I felt moved and inspired by feeling myself extended out into the universe. As the primitive saw himself as a conglomeration of parts into a whole, as his tribal space was the universe and his body the earth and sky all else, I can feel the wonder of existence surge through me. (Serlin, 1996, p. 30).

In the breast cancer support group, sometimes just holding hands in a circle gave group members a palpable sense of support and safety. The circle is an ancient form for connection and wholeness.

THE PROBLEM OF INTERPRETATION: WHAT DOES A KINAESTHETIC IMAGE MEAN?

Kinaesthetic images resist interpretation: for example, what is the meaning of a movement of strength or vulnerability? While the movement may look one way to an observer, it may have quite a different feel or association to the mover. Instead of prematurely rushing to understand a movement, continuing to develop and amplify the essence of the movement will reveal its meaning. Movement itself is a process of meaning-making; a student reported, "I don't know what happened during the session, but something shifted and felt right. I feel different now than when I came in; I know that a perceptual shift has happened and that I worked something through" (Serlin, 1996, p. 31).

Kinaesthetic Knowing

Like visual images, kinaesthetic images are encoded in a nonlinear and nonlogical way. Kinaesthetic knowing comes from a kinaesthetic intelligence (Gardner, 1983) and a felt-sense that moves into felt-images and felt-understanding. (Serlin & Stern, 1998) and enters into dialogical relationship with others (Serlin, 1989). It is a way of knowing with the whole body that is difficult to put into words. The most reliable descriptions, appearing in a student paper from a course taught by this author in Israel during 2006 war in Lebanon are those of a student learning this process. The following description evokes the experience of kinaesthetic knowing.

The Moment I Knew

During this split moment "knowing" was different from anything I have ever known before .... A sweet pain filled my body and soul.

It was the first day of the course. The war outside is making me more sensitive to myself, more sensitive to noises from outside .... I have no idea why, but I got up and joined B ... moving with him, entering his mood, his rhythm .... At that moment, I was feeling a void in me, feeling that I had no idea what should I do .... Suddenly I knew, out of the movement, that freedom is not enough for me. I said, "I want to create something out of this freedom."

This sentence did not come from my head, from my mind. It came from somewhere else inside me. "So create ..." the leader said, inviting me with her eyes, again, to keep on going. How do I create something just with my body, a thought crossed my mind. Do not think, act, I said to myself, finding this new place of not thinking a calm place to be.

I was working with my hands, as if I was trying to shape something with them. The leader and B joined me in a small circle, inside the large circle of the group, moving their hands with me, in my rhythm. I could feel the energy between my hands, amplified by the leader's presence. It was real. I was not thinking. I was just moving my hands according to some inner knowledge or inner sense. I was giving up all control of my body and mind; I gave up thinking in this unfamiliar situation, just letting things happen.

Suddenly it was there, striking like a lightning, like a boost of extra energy. The book was in front of me, between my hands, real as much as non-existing object can be. Out of so many planned projects that I have now, this book, I clearly knew at that moment is the thing that I so badly want to create out of my freedom.

The void in my body and mind filled up with unknown energy, with a feeling of power and gratitude, all mixed in an unfamiliar way.

KINAESTHETIC IMAGERY EXERCISES

The shape and experience of the body can reveal much about a person and is often an invaluable diagnostic tool. For example, a patient who faces a life-threatening illness may express his or her sense of helplessness in slumped shoulders, constricted breathing, or other physical images. Further, the experience of having slumped shoulders and constricted breathing can bring about an experience of hopelessness; this cycle of hopelessness can be changed anywhere in the cycle. Thus cognitive therapy works to change the cognition of hopelessness, while kinaesthetic imagery works to change the experience of hopelessness.

Once someone is aware of his or her experience of hopelessness, and can give voice to that experience in the form of an image, then that person can begin to take control of his or her experience and even try new experiences. In this way, the patient becomes an active participant in his or her healing process, discovering his or her unique images of healing.

The following is a brief exercise for you to experience your own kinaesthetic imagery:

1. Close your eyes, focusing on the sensation of weight as you sink into your chair. Notice where you are pressing into that chair and, on each exhalation, release more of your weight into those places. Focus only on the exhalations, letting the inbreath come in by itself. As you sink further into the chair, let more of your body relax. Notice which parts of your body usually hold tension, and find the points that let that tension go. Don't forget your hands, your legs, your face, your eyes, your jaw...keep finding new places to relax. (2 minutes).
2. Now, can you imagine yourself or someone you know as hopeless about a medical condition? How does hopeless feel? Where do you experience it in your body? Now exaggerate it, amplify the image. (2 minutes).
3. Now begin to reverse that image. Begin to mobilize your breathing, your weight, your contact with the chair. Begin to feel your strength and flexibility. Breathe deeply and experience a sense of hope. (2 minutes).
4. Now go back and forth between these two postures, experiencing both and what it takes to make the changes. Feel how it is to bring awareness and more control into your coping. (2 minutes).
5. Take a moment and reflect on how this gave you insight into your own patterns of hopelessness and hope, and how it could be applied to one of your clinical cases. (2 minutes).

Kinaesthetic imagery is not as well understood as visual imagery, but it has strong potential for working with nonverbal and bodily traumas. Through training programs that teach kinaesthetic awareness and good clinical skills, the practitioner can contribute to healthy communities.

VERBAL IMAGERY: GIVING NEW LIFE TO WORDS

Underneath

What language can't reach
is so much.
The hook dangles
from the fishline,
while the fish
swim by.
The sea urchins
are un-interested,
the kelp waves,
a whole world
expands.
The hook finds
a few slender
words,
pulls them
to light.
Maybe I
can cook them.

(Barbara McEnerney, in Myers, 1999, p. 143)

"Underneath" is one of the first poems Barbara McEnerney ever wrote. With the image of a fishing line and hook that drops below the surface of the water, she enters poetry's world of verbal imagery to describe what it is like to face the blank page. We know or can likely imagine what it is like to not get even a nibble.

Right then, in that moment, the vivid power of verbal imagery begins to reveal itself. The poet recognizes that much of her experience of life occurs beyond, or perhaps more accurate to say *below*, language. The picture she paints of fish swimming by and uninterested sea urchins provide a rich sense for what she is feeling. Where are the words that can truly describe her experience? Is there anything to say because the words are elusive?

Suddenly, after acknowledging this difficulty, something shifts, something begins to happen in the creative process. A new thought/image arrives on the page when the poet imagines "the kelp waves,/a whole world/expands." She drops down deeper into the embryonic moments of the creative process. It's not only about catching fish—that is, finding words. Images themselves begin to speak: "The kelp waves,/a whole world/expands."

Here is a moment of pure, expansive being. Image takes us to that place with the poet. This poem is really about entering into the creative experience. It is about seeing all of what's there. It is not only about finding words to describe experience. Rather, the poet becomes, through the use of the image, the experience itself. She gets a sense of the depths, her depths. Through the image of the waving kelp, *being* comes to the foreground. There are energetic connections made at this moment. There is a sense of greeting and welcome: the kelp *waves*.

From here the energetic connection afforded to the poet by the image of waving kelp, there is a larger field of consciousness into which she now has access that leads her toward the next lines of the poem:

> The hook finds
> a few slender
> words,
> pulls them
> to light.
> Maybe I
> can cook them.

Gaston Bachelard (1994) in the introduction to his classic, *The Poetics of Space*, writes, "It is as though the poem through its exuberance, awakened new depths in us" (p. xix). I have shared this poem in all regions of the United States and in other countries. I can see on the faces of those who hear it a particular kind of satisfaction and insight with the verb "cook" applied to words. There is something powerful about this instant conveyance, the intuitive sense of cooking words. We can savor what might happen, a freshwater trout sizzling in a pan. For Bachelard (1994), "the image in its simplicity has no need of scholarship" (p. xv).

Through reading and imaging the images in Barbara's poem—fishing line, dangling hook, uninterested fish and sea urchin, waving kelp, expanding world, slender words that can be cooked—we join with the poet in the feeling experience directly. We let go of trying to explain and understand and enter a space that is whole, full of creative insight and feeling.

My words here *about* her poem are at some remove from the vitality and vividness of these few words Barbara chooses to express. To really enter it, the image asks us to not analyze but rather to do what the poet Donald Hall (Moon and Schoenholtz, 1994) suggests,

> I would tell him, for instance, that he should not ask for a poem to do any particular thing. I would ask him to relax and listen and float. I would ask him to allow himself to associate .... To read the poem, you must stop paraphrasing, stop "thinking" in the conventional way, and do some receiving instead. (pp. 187–188)

As Bachelard (1994) continues:

> The image offered us by reading the poem now become really our own. It takes root in us. It has been given to us by another, but we begin to have the impression that we could have created it, that we should have created it. It becomes a new being in our language, expressing us by making us what it expresses; in other words, it is at once a becoming of expression and a becoming of our being. Here expression creates being. (p. xix).

In writing this chapter, I spoke with Barbara McEnerney to request her permission to use her poem. She reminded me that when she wrote this poem in our poetry circle, I had asked her if she could name one or two lines in the poem that most attracted her, that she gravitated toward. She said, without any conscious thought, the lines about the kelp.

Verbal images, when used in a healing and therapeutic way, can help the writer to develop a new relationship with his or her writing. It can help therapist and client to address and apply the salve of nonjudgment and encouragement to old wounds. We may recall critical comments by teachers or parents about how our writing "should" be done or how a poem must rhyme, contain a particular meter, etc. Too often, whatever we did wasn't right or very good.

The blank page can be scary and leave one facing a blankness inside. Judgments from others—whether teachers, parents, or friends—about writing echo in a writer's heart and mind. Who cares anyway? For Barbara, this feeling finds expression when she writes: "the fish swim by. The sea urchins are un-interested."

It is not only the writer who will benefit from the letting go of judgment, of allowing for a sense of being rather than doing. But the poetry therapist, too, needs to do this fully and deeply. It is the only way that the deeper levels, the unconscious and unknown levels, of the poem will be revealed.

In addition to a lack of judgment, a spirit of curiosity and admiration are helpful. There is a generative act that can welcome insight. Once again, Bachelard (1994) in *The Poetics of Space* writes,

> We can admire more or less, but a sincere impulse, a little impulse towards admiration, is always necessary if we are to receive the phenomenological benefit of the poetic image. The slightest critical consideration arrests this impulse by putting the mind in second position, destroying the primitivity of the imagination. (p. xxii)

What *can* be said about grief, joy, love, beauty, fear—experiences that are felt kinesthetically or somewhere in the body or in the deep silence of the soul or in the keening, inarticulate, and powerful cry of one's heart.

Gary Snyder, a practitioner of Zen and a nature poet, created this image about what it is like to approach the creative voice within himself:

How Poetry Comes To Me

It comes blundering over the
Boulders at night, it stays
Frightened outside the
Range of my campfire
I go to meet it at the
Edge of the light.

(Snyder, 1999, p. 557)

It is a kind of deep humility and wisdom to recognize that words can be limited in the realm of feeling and sensation and mystery. If we want to be in touch with that, to listen to the body and the heart, we need to be willing to take our time to approach those feelings at the edges of life and with some awareness, to feel those feelings rather than icing them over with words.

Verbal imagery can help people to stay in contact with the feelings, sensations, and the mystery at the edge. A poem that communicates this edge, the staying close to feeling to people, in both a visceral and intuitive way, is one by Martin Jude Farawell.

If I Sing

If I sing, I weep.
If I sing joy, even sing joy, I weep.
If I weep, if I weep, if cries splatter from me,
if I sputter snot and spit
down my chin, my shirt, your shirt,
if I shake and shake until you fear I'll shake apart,
don't be afraid for me, don't be ashamed;
I will not break from this, will not die,
but from lack of it, from the closing,
and I will not close anymore, will not deny anymore
the child I was who could not
cry out has kept crying in
me. And now that I can cry I will sing,
even if my song comes shoved out
on the wave of snot and spit I swallowed not
to cry, I will sing.

(Farawell, in Bosveld, 1998, p.160)

I urge you to read this poem aloud. I would further suggest that you stand up to read it. Read it more than once. Pay attention to the repetitions in the poem, the way the poem recapitulates in a few words and stays close to the profound and essential desire to express oneself. How tactile and tangible words are: snot, spit, tears, splatter, child, shirt, weep, cry, and sing. This is a poem that arises in the body and is felt there.

Walt Whitman was fierce about this—that the poem is not just in the letters that make up the words, but is felt. The words are a somatic, bodily awareness and experience. For a man who was so expansive (and some might say excessive) in the use of words, Whitman realizes there is an origin to words that is organic and alive, elemental and breathing, rooted and that flourishes into something more:

A song of the rolling earth, and of words according
Were you thinking that those were the words, those upright lines?

those curves, angles and dots?
No, those are not the words, the substantial words are in the ground and sea,
They are in the air, they are in you.
Were you thinking those were the words, those delicious sounds
    out of your friend's mouths?
No, the real words are more delicious than they.
Human bodies are words, myriad of words...

(Whitman, 1891–1892, p. 179)

The depth of these images and the real experience of a word is much more meaningful and more sacred and healing than the mental agribusiness of a media-saturated culture generally acknowledges. It is more than what our educational system often acknowledges. But it is necessary to explore this possibility to discover whether what I am saying is true.

One afternoon I spent many hours in a restaurant, actually going deep into the evening, with a deep longing to find words that felt wholly true. Words so often are like wet matches and because of that, useless. I was exploring how words, the universe and my own aliveness and longing for connection in my body might find a way to express together. The images that came to me distilled into this: body, word, fire, star. It's important to say that I took my time with this poem. I gave my time to it. I let the poem/writing speak to me about what it wanted to be. I learned that it wanted to be compact and brief. I don't often write in rhyme but it wanted to come in rhyme:

There Is an Origin

For each true poem born there is an origin:
Blessed ignorance of words that turn
To splendid fire, as stars in space will yearn
To find on earth their up stretched twin.

(Fox, 1989, on an audiotape)

I found in this poem a deep and living memory of my true nature. In yoga, that memory is linked to the sacred and called *smriti*, a Sanskrit word for "divine memory." Another way of putting it is that writing this poem and the poem itself helped me return to the magic of words. A magic that we lose as children and in doing deep therapeutic work through the creative arts we have the chance to reclaim.

Marilyn Krysl, in her dynamic poem *Saying Things*, reminds us that a word itself has a body. It is permeable. We enter it. It is made of our breath. Our voice gives life to that word. There is, in fact, magic and pleasure that is discoverable in words, pleasure and magic that all too often we begin to forget about as soon as we take our first spelling test. Krysl's poem encourages the reader to experience the magic and pleasure of the image created by the word:

> Say bellows, say sledge,
> say threshold, cottonmouth, Russian leather,
> say ash, picot, fallow deer, saxophone, say kitchen sink.
> This is a birthday party for the mouth—it's better than ice cream,
> say waterlilly, refrigerator, hartebeest, Prussian blue
> and the word will take you, if you let it,
> the word will take you along across the air of your head
> so that you're there as it settles into the thing it was made for,
> adding to it a shimmer and the bird song of its sound,
> sound that comes from you, the hand letting go
> its dove, yours the mouth speaking the thing into existence,
> this is what I'm talking about, this is called saying things.*

—Marilyn Krysl (Krysl, 1980, p. 19)

When I use the word *sacred*, I am not suggesting that we can only write about God, things that keep us comfortable, or appear to us as good. Rainer Rilke said, "We must give birth to our images, they are the future waiting to be born" (p. Rilke, from Moon and Schoenholtz, 2004, p. xvii)). The idea of birth must suggest to us that this process can be, and usually is, messy and painful. I am not leaving out the possibility of postpartum depression either. But generally speaking, there could be deep joy as well, a joy born of speaking what's true, even if it is difficult to say it, in this giving birth to images.

What I mean by images that are born of speaking what's true, I mean the images that flow to you, through you, that celebrate, rage, cry out, touch what's true, and speak that truth—these images can grow out of life's real grit and a place of mystery and grace.

These Days

Whatever you have to say, leave
the roots on, let them
dangle

And the dirt

Just to make clear
where they come from[†]

—Charles Olson (Olson, 1987, p.106)

---

* Reprinted with permission from the Cleveland State University Poetry Center.

† From *The Collected Poems of Charles Olson*, by Charles Olson, (edited by George Butterick), © 1987 The Estate of Charles Olson. Published by the University of California Press. Reprinted with permission.

TOOL KIT FOR CHANGE

Role and Perspective of the Healthcare Professional

1. Discover the nonverbal forms in a physical or psychological symptom.
2. Let the nonverbal movement "speak" so that the visual, kinaesthetic, or verbal imagery is amplified and made conscious.
3. Let the meaning or association come from the client.
4. Help the client discover more constructive kinaesthetic images that aid in healing.

Role and Perspective of the Participant

1. Imagery will naturally arise from within your world of sensations and emotions. Pay attention to the slightest thought that allows an image to form.
2. Imagery—visual, kinaesthetic, or verbal—has a depth of meaning that is apparent to you, the images arise from within you and are carriers of great depth.

Interconnection: The Global Perspective

1. Imagery is as old as humans. All humans have repositories of personal imagery that can help guide them through difficult transitions.
2. Imagery, being both personal and collective, is ideally suited for use in global healthcare.

REFERENCES

Abbott, F. V., & Fraser, M. I. (1998). Use and abuse of over-the-counter analgesic agents. *Journal of Psychiatry Neuroscience, 23*(1), 13–34.

Achterberg, J., Dossey, B., & Kolkmeier, L. (1994). *Rituals of healing: Using imagery for health and wellness.* New York: Bantam Books.

Agras, W. S. (1981). Behavioral approaches to the treatment of essential hypertension. *International Journal of Obesity, 5*, 173–181.

Antoni, M. H., Baggett, L., Ironson, G., LaPerriere, A., August, S., Klimas, N., Schneiderman, N., & Fletcher, M. (1991). Cognitive-behavioral stress management buffers distress responses and immunologic changes following notification of HIV-1 seropositivity. *Journal of Consulting and Clinical Psychology, 59,* 906–915.

Arathuzik, D. (1994). Effects of cognitive-behavioral strategies on pain in cancer patients. *Cancer Nursing, 17,* 207–214.

Auerback, J. E., Oleson, T., & Solomon, G. (1992). A behavioral medicine intervention as an adjunctive treatment for HIV-related illness. *Psychology and Health, 6,* 325–334.

Bachelard, G. (1994). *The poetics of space.* Boston: Beacon Press.

Baider, L., Peretz, T., Hadani, P. E., & Koch, U. (2000). Psychological intervention in cancer patients: A randomized study. *General Hospital Psychiatry, 23,* 272–277.

Baider, L., Uziely, B., & De-Nour, A. K. (1994). Progressive muscular relaxation and guided imagery in cancer patients. *General Hospital Psychiatry, 16,* 340–347.

Baird, C. L., & Sands, L. (2004). A pilot study of the effectiveness of guided imagery with progressive muscle relaxation to reduce chronic pain and mobility difficulties of osteoarthritis. *Pain Management Nursing, 5* (3), 97–104.

Barabasz, M. A., & Spiegel, D. (1989). Hypnotizability and weight loss in obese subjects. *International Journal of Eating Disorders, 8,* 335–341.

Barnes, P. M., Powell-Griner, E., & Nahin, R. L. (2004, May 27). Complementary and alternative medicine use among adults: United States, 2002. *Advance data from vital and health statistics*, No. 343. Atlanta, GA: Centers for Disease Control and Prevention.

Bisson, J. I. (1995). Taped imaginal exposure as a treatment for post-traumatic stress reduction. *Journal of the Royal Army Medical Corps, 141*, 20–25.

Bosveld, J. (1998). Prayers to protest: Poems that center and bless us. Johnstown, OH: Pudding House.

Brown-Saltzman, K. (1997). Replenishing the spirit by meditative prayer and guided imagery. *Seminars in Oncology Nursing, 13*: 255–259.

Carpenter, S. (2002). Hope on the horizon: Behavioral researchers are uncovering promising new ways to treat chronic pain. *Monitor on Psychology, 33*(4). Washington, DC: American Psychological Association.

Carr, J. E. (1995). Relaxation and imagery and cognitive-behavioral training reduces pain during cancer treatments: A controlled clinical trial. *Pain, 63*(2), 189–198.

Cochrane, G., & Friesen, J. (1992). Hypnotherapy in weight loss treatment. *Journal of Consulting and Clinical Psychology, 54*, 489–492.

Collins, J. A., & Rice, V. H. (1997). Effects of relaxation intervention in phase II cardiac rehabilitation: Replication and extension. *Heart & Lung, 26*(1), 31–44.

Cousins, M. J. (1995). Back pain in the workplace: management of disability in nonspecific conditions. In W. E. Fordyce (Ed.) *Task Force Report* (p. ix). Seattle, WA: IASP Press.

Creamer, P., Singh, B. B., Hochberg, M. C., & Berman, B. M. (2000). Sustained improvement produced by non-pharmacologic intervention in fibromyalgia: Results of a pilot study. *Arthritis Care and Research, 13*, 198–204.

Cupal, D. D., & Brewer, B. W. (2001). Effects of relaxation and guided imagery on knee strength, reinjury anxiety and pain following anterior cruciate ligament reconstruction. *Rehabilitation Psychology, 46*(1), 28–43.

Dahlquist, L. M. (1985). Behavioral management of children in distress during chemotherapy. *Journal of Behavioral Therapy in Experimental Psychiatry, 16*, 325–329. Eller, L. S. (1999). Effects of cognitive-behavioral interventions on quality of life in persons with HIV. *International Journal of Nursing Studies, 36*, 223–233.

Fors, E. A., Sexton, H., & Gotestam, K. G. (2002). The effect of guided imagery and amitriptyline on daily fibromyalgia pain: A prospective, randomized, control trial. *Journal of Psychiatric Research, 36*(3), 179–187.

Fox, J. (1989). *When jewels sing*. Palo Alto, CA: Open Heart Press.

Fox, J. (1997). *Poetic medicine: The healing art of poem-making*. New York: Jeremy P. Tarcher.

Gardner, H. (1983). *Frames of mind: The theory of multiple intelligences*. New York: Basic Books.

Graffam, S., & Johnson, A. (1987). A comparison of two relaxation strategies for the relief of pain and its distress. *Journal of Pain & Symptom Management, 2*, 229–231.

Harstall, C. (2003). How prevalent is chronic pain? *Pain: Clinical Updates, 11*, 1–4.

Hyman, M. (2004). Paradigm shift: The end of "normal science" in medicine. *Alternative Therapies in Health and Medicine, 10*(5), 10–15, 90–94.

Kerns, R. D., Turk, D. C., Holzman, A. D., & Rudy, T. E. (1986). Comparison of cognitive-behavioral and behavioral approaches to the outpatient treatment of chronic pain. *Clinical Journal of Pain, 1*, 195–203.

Klaus, L., Beniaminovitz, A., Choi, L, Greenfield, F., Whitworth, G. C., , Oz, M. C., & Mancini, D. M. (2000). Pilot study of guided imagery use in patients with severe heart failure. *American Journal of Cardiology, 86*, 101–104.

Kleinman, A., Brodwin, P. E., Good, B. J., & DelVecchio-Good, M. J. (1992). Pain as human experience: An introduction. In *Pain as a human experience: An anthropological perspective* Del-Vecchio, M. J., Brodwin, P. E., Good, B. J., & Kleinman, A. (Eds). (p. 1028). Berkeley: University of California Press.

Kolcaba, K., & Fox, C. (1999). The effects of guided imagery on comfort of women with early stage breast cancer undergoing radiation therapy. *Oncology Nursing Forum, 26*(1), 67–72.

Krysl, M. (1980). *More palamino, please, more fuchsia.* Cleveland, OH: Cleveland State University Center.

Krystal, S., & Zweben, J. (1989). The use of visualization as a means of integrating the spiritual dimension into treatment: II. Working with emotions. *Journal of Substance Abuse Treatment, 6,* 223–228.

Krueger, L. C. (1987). Pediatric pain and imagery. *Journal of Child & Adolescent Psychotherapy, 4*(1), 32–41.

Langer, S. (1953). *Feeling and form.* New York: Scribner.

Lang, S., & Pratt, R. B. (1994). *You don't have to suffer: A complete guide to relieving cancer pain for patients and their families.* New York: Oxford University Press.

Lawlis, G. F., Achterberg, J., Kenner, L., & Kopetz, K. (1984). Ethnic and sex differences in response to clinical and induced pain in chronic spinal pain patients. *Spine, 9*(7), 751–754.

Mannix, L. K., Chandurkar, R. S., Rybicki, L. A., Tusek, D. L., & Solomon, G. D. (1999). Effect of guided imagery on quality of life for patients with chronic tension-type headache. *Headache, 39,* 326–334.

Manyande, A., Berg, S., Gettins, D., Stanford, S. C., Mazhero, S., Marks, D. F., et al. (1995). Preoperative rehearsal of active coping imagery influences subjective and hormonal responses to abdominal surgery. *Psychosomatic Medicine, 57*(2), 177–182.

McDonald, R. T., & Hilgendorf, W. A. (1986). Death imagery and death anxiety. *Journal of Clinical Psychology, 42,* 87–91.

Merleau-Ponty, M. (1963). *The structure of behavior.* Boston: Beacon Press.

Micozzi, M. S. (2004). Culture and complementary medicine. *Seminars in Integrative Medicine, 2*(3), 89–91.

Moon, B., & Schoenholtz, R. (1994). *Word pictures: The poetry and art of art therapists.* Springfield, IL: Charles C. Thomas.

Moore, R. J., & Spiegel, D. (1999). Uses of guided imagery for pain control by African American and white women with metastatic breast cancer. *Integrative Medicine, 2*(2/3), 115–126.

Moore, R. J. (1999). African-American women and breast cancer: Failures of Western biomedicine? In D.D. Weiner (Ed.) *Preventing and controlling cancer* (pp. 37–54). Westport, CT; Praeger.

Myers, T. O. (1999). *The soul of creativity.* Novato, CA: New World Library.

Newshan, G., & Balamuth, R. (1990–1991). Use of imagery in a chronic pain outpatient group. *Imagination, Cognition & Personality, 10*(1), 25–38.

Olson, C. 1987). *The collected poems of Charles Olson.* Berkeley: University of California Press.

Pert, C. (1997). *Molecules of emotion: Why you feel the way you feel.* New York: Scribner.

Richardson, M. A., Post-White, J. Grimm, E. A., Moye, L. A., Singletary, S. E., & Justice, B. (1997). Coping, life attitudes, and immune response to imagery and group support after breast cancer treatment. *Alternative Therapies in Health Medicine, 3,* 62–70.

Ricoeur, P. (1976). *Interpretation theory: Discourse and the surplus of meaning.* Fort Worth: Texas Christian University Press.

Rockefeller, K. (2005, February 3). *Imagery and relaxation: Doorways to health.* Lecture presented at the Susan Samueli Center for Integrative Medicine Colloquium Lecture Series, University of California, Irvine.

Rockefeller, K. (2007). *Visualize confidence: How to use guided imagery to overcome self-doubt.* Oakland, CA: New Harbinger Publications.

Rossman, M. L. (2000). *Guided imagery for self-healing: An essential resource for anyone seeking wellness.* Tiburon, CA: H. J. Kramer Books.

Rossman, M. L. (2003). *Fighting cancer from within: How to use the power of your mind for healing.* New York: Henry Holt.

Rossman, M. L. (2004). Guided imagery in cancer care. *Seminars in Integrative Medicine, 2*(3), 99–106.

Scarry, E. (1985). *The body in pain.* New York: Oxford University Press.

Serlin, I. A., (1989). Choreography of a verbal session. In A. Robbins (Ed.), *The psychoaesthetic experience: An approach to depth-oriented psychotherapy* (pp. 45–57). New York: Human Sciences Press.

Serlin, I. A. (1996). Kinaesthetic imagining. *Journal of Humanistic Psychology, 36*(2), 25–33.

Serlin, I., Classen, C., Frances, B., & Angell, K. (2000). Support groups for women with breast cancer: Traditional and alternative expressive approaches. *The Arts in Psychotherapy, 27*(2), 123–138.

Serlin, I. A., & Stern, E. M. (1998). The dialogue of movement: An interview/conversation. In K. Hays (Ed.), *Integrating exercise, sports, movement and mind* (pp. 47–52). New York: Haworth Press.

Sheets-Johnstone, M. (1978). *The passage rites of the body—A phenomenological account of change in dance.* Unpublished manuscript.

Sloman, R. (1995). Relaxation and the relief of cancer pain. *Nursing Clinics of North America, 30*, 697–709.

Snyder, G. (1999). *The Gary Snyder reader.* Berkeley, CA: Counterpoint Press.

Spiegel, D. (1995). *Living beyond limits: New hope and health for facing life threatening illness.* New York: Time Books.

Spiegel, D., & Moore, R. J. (1997). Imagery and hypnosis in the treatment of cancer pain. *Oncology, 11*(8), 1179–1190.

Syrjala, K. L., Donaldson, G. W., Davis, M. W., Kippes, M. E., Tusek, D. L., Church, J. M., et al. (1997). Guided imagery as a coping strategy for perioperative patients. *ANORN Journal, 66*, 644–649.

Turk, D., & Burwinkle, T. (2004). Treatment of chronic pain suffers—An antidote to mural dyslexia. *The Pain Practitioner, 14*(3), 20–25.

Tusek, D. L., Church, J. M., & Fazio, V. W. (1997). Guided imagery as a coping strategy for perioperative patients. *ANORN Journal, 66*, 644–649.

Tusek, D. L., Church, J. M., Strong, S. A., Grass, J. A., & Fazio, V. W. (1997). Guided imagery: A significant advance in the care of patients undergoing elective colorectal surgery. *Diseases of the Colon and Rectum, 40*(2), 172–178.

Tusek, D. L., Cwynar, R., & Cosgrove, D. M. (1999). Effect of guided imagery on length of stay, pain and anxiety in cardiac surgery. *Journal of Cardiovascular Management, 10*(2), 22–28.

Whitman, W. (1891-1892). *Leaves of grass.* New York: Modern Library.

Wynd, C. A. (1992). Relaxation imagery used for stress reduction in the prevention of smoking relapse. *Journal of Advanced Nursing, 17*, 29.

Chapter Five

MEANING AND ILLNESS

Tamara McClintock Greenberg, PsyD, MS

Health is not valued till Sickness comes.

—Thomas Fuller (1732)

Medical illness exists in an individual context that involves both physical and psychological realms. This context includes all aspects of patients' lives, because illness often affects work, relationships, finances, as well as psychological and emotional functioning. How one thinks about illness—that is, the meaning that is ascribed to it—is an important part of the illness process. The meaning of illness is often far more complicated than the psychological sequelae of illness. For example, common sequelae of medical illnesses are depression and anxiety, which are discrete diagnostic entities that define how one might react to illness. However, these diagnostic constructs do not fully capture the unique experiences of patients who experience acute or chronic illness. In other words, how patients think of their individual illness may not be reflected in the diagnoses ascribed to patients. For example, consider the following vignette:

Susan is a 35-year-old investment banker who was diagnosed with a serious and rare form of leukemia. She was diagnosed with depression while in the hospital and was started on an antidepressant. When I first met with her in the hospital, she talked about the shock of her illness. She was an accomplished athlete and often competed in her sport. She appeared depressed but was also very anxious and found herself constantly worried about whether she would return to the same kind of work once she was in remission. These thoughts kept her awake at night. She had trouble focusing on her present circumstances and longed to be able to exercise, which was the primary way (before her illness) that she managed the anxiety and stress associated with her job. After we met a few times, she told me that her worries in the middle of the night were related not only to her vocational future, but that she thought about what may have caused her leukemia. She said,

> I lay here at night when it's quiet and I think about what I did to cause this. I know it's crazy, but I think that painting my house last year was the cause, or maybe that I am on the cell phone all of the time. I try to calculate all of the risks in my environment, such as the electromagnetic fields from the technology I use, or the fact that when I was younger I used to have a cigarette or two at a party, or that I drink wine with dinner, and I try to think of how I may have prevented this from happening to me. I say to myself, "I must have done something wrong."

Although Susan's diagnosis of depression was accurate, her reasons for being depressed were related to her sense that she caused her illness, the loss of exercise as a way to manage stress, and the worry that her anxiety about how she developed her illness made her appear crazy. Susan's responses illustrate that, although depression is an understandable consequence to a severe and life-threatening illness, her unique understanding of the implications of and cause of her illness is far more complex than the diagnosis of depression would suggest. Susan worried that she caused her illness and hoped that by figuring out specifically what caused her blood cancer, she could attribute meaning to this unfair and random event.

This chapter addresses some of the issues that arise in persons diagnosed with a serious illness and how illness disrupts one's sense of identity, stability, and ultimately affects the sense of self. Illness requires an abrupt reconfiguration of meaning for some and challenges preexisting ideas of meaning for others. However, meaning is interpreted differently based on different individual circumstances, the severity and nature of illness, and individual conceptualizations of meaning prior to illness. I will first discuss the complexity and difficulty with the definition of meaning as it relates to medically ill patients. Following this discussion, I will briefly present some of the research that has attempted to capture the physical and psychological implications of meanings developed by patients with illness and then will present common psychological dynamics related to meaning in working with medically ill patients.

A FRAMEWORK FOR THE CONCEPT OF MEANING

Because of its subjective nature, meaning in the context of illness is difficult to describe. One way to describe it is to say that meaning involves an awareness of thoughts and feelings that result in individual interpretations and appraisals about disease. Although illness appraisal may impact and involve the employment of specific coping strategies (Lazarus & Folkman, 1984) and sense of meaning influences a number of aspects of illness adaptations, individual interpretations of illness may differ substantially. Kleinman (1980) proposed an explanatory model of illness that encompasses ideas and beliefs about illness that helps persons understand illness within an individual and cultural context. Individual experiences of illness may match what we might expect patients to think about (e.g., the meaning of life and suffering). However, what is meaningful for one person is not necessarily meaningful for another. For example, the way Susan thought about her illness was by focusing on what caused her disease and, specifically, how she might have prevented her disease. Other patients, however, may not think about how they caused their disease; they may describe their illness as bad luck. The conclusions that are arrived at in response to thinking about illness are one aspect of meaning, but meaning involves both cognitive (explanatory) elements and emotional elements. Susan's sense that she caused her illness was associated with distress, anxiety, and sense of responsibility. Blaming herself for her illness seemed to be a major factor in understanding Susan's anxiety and depression. Feeling the weight of responsibility for her illness caused her to have unrelenting thoughts about how she may have prevented it and caused her to feel that she had been careless and, ironically, increased her sense of control over her illness. (This latter issue of control will be discussed in a subsequent section.) The meaning ascribed to illness impacts how people adjust to and cope with illness but often involves unique interpretations that are related to how the world was viewed before illness.

A few authors have attempted to describe the nature of meaning as it might apply it to the psychological impact of illness. Although Frankl (1985) described meaning as a "primary motivational force" (p. 104), in human beings, coming up with a precise definition of meaning is difficult and complicated. The search for meaning has been described as the need to understand why a crisis has occurred and what its impact is (Taylor, 1983). An earlier attempt to describe the meaning of medical illness was developed by Lipowski (1970), who said that eight ideas encompassed the personal meanings of illness: challenges of illness, illness as an enemy, illness reflecting punishment, illness reflecting weakness, the relief of illness, illness as strategy, the value of illness, and illness as loss or damage. Lipowski also said that coping with illness is dependent on intrapersonal factors, disease-related factors, and environmental factors. Meaning has also been linked to identity (Marris, 1974) as well as to existential issues such as the meaning of life and death. Fife (1994) described two fundamental dimensions of meaning: self-meaning, which pertains to the perceived effect of an event of aspects of identity; and contextual meaning, which pertains to the perceived characteristics of an event as well as the social circumstances surrounding it. The trauma literature has long addressed the impact of meaning in the face of traumatic events, and, more recently, severe life-threatening illness has been addressed in relation to the development of post-traumatic stress disorder, which is common in a number of medically ill patients (e.g., Doerfler & Paraskos, 2005; Kangas, Henry, & Bryant, 2002, 2005). Trauma causes people to question meaning, which can include the randomness of events, identity, level of control, and the inevitability of death (Serlin & Cannon, 2004). These issues are all important considerations in persons who develop a serious illness. The meaning of illness can encompass all of these aspects: Illness is traumatic, illness affects identity, and illness involves and disrupts social relationships.

Meaning can be conceptualized in a variety of ways, and what is meaningful to one person may not be meaningful to another. In other words, meaning is in the eye of the beholder. Although many might argue that coming to terms with death is an important aspect of meaning for a patient diagnosed with a serious or life-threatening illness, not all patients are concerned about this issue. For example, I once worked with a woman dying from a gynecological cancer. She was resigned to the inevitability of death but was very concerned about the possibility that her husband might remarry after her death. This issue was so important to her that she found herself pleading with her husband to never marry again. Because this was a promise he could not honestly make, the couple argued about this extensively, which negatively impacted the couple's last weeks together. For this woman, meaning was addressed in this context (her worry about and the meaning of her husband remarrying) and was the focus of our work. One could argue that this woman was in denial or that the focus on her husband was an attempt to avoid thinking about her own mortality. Although this may be the case, it is important to recognize that meaning is what patients bring forth, what is on their mind, and what their present worries are.

Patients who have a serious illness often respond to illness in a way that is consistent with how they have responded to other stressors. For example, if a patient tended to blame herself for negative events in the past, her response to illness will likely be similar. Returning to Susan, I saw Susan as an outpatient a year after she completed her cancer treatment. She had been cleared medically to go back to work and was working part-time. She was doing well physically and had adopted a healthy life-style (even more so than she had before her illness) that involved eating organic foods, meditation, and frequent exercise, which included yoga. Yet she was consumed with thoughts about her illness recurring. She said, "I think about it all the time, what I eat and what I am putting in my body. I feel that if I make a mistake, a wrong move, I will re-invite the cancer back into my body."

Susan's comments illustrate her difficult and painful thoughts related to causing her illness. An important part of her therapy involved addressing these thoughts and helping her to realize that she was not responsible for her illness. Although there are often common themes in the impact and meaning of illness, what is important in working with medically ill patients is what is meaningful to them. We may not understand their meanings, but the psychological work with this population should focus on helping to elucidate the meaning of illness in an individual context.

RESEARCH ON MEANING ON HEALTH

In the literature on coping with illness, meaning is often addressed superficially (Fife, 1994). Additionally, clinical psychology and psychosocial oncology have become increasingly cognitive in emphasis (White, 2004). Although a cognitive emphasis in research illuminates the impact of thoughts on coping behaviors and other outcomes in medically ill patients, one risk of a cognitive emphasis in the research is that it does not fully capture the extent of emotional experiences patients with serious illnesses have. A related issue is that, despite a large body of literature addressing coping with illness, adjustment to illness, and the psychological impact (as well as psychological antecedents) of illness, few articles address the issue of meaning directly. This is likely due in part to the difficulties in developing a common definition of meaning, as described above, because many aspects of meaning that extend beyond cognitions and appraisals are difficult to describe.

Although it is difficult to fully and accurately define meaning, some research has attempted to capture this complex concept. Some of the constructs that are related to meaning are negativity and pessimism, optimism, the ability to find benefit through the process of being diagnosed and treated for an illness, and the use of religion as a way to enhance meaning. These constructs are important because one aspect of meaning as it relates to illness is illness expectation. Some patients are diagnosed with a serious illness and take it in stride. They are aware of the severity of the illness but are hopeful that they can fight it. Other patients, however, immediately upon being diagnosed with an illness, are negative; they believe that the illness will kill them and they have no chance of a cure. One patient exemplified this latter belief when he told me about being diagnosed with Type-II (adult onset) diabetes. He said, "I heard the word diabetes and I thought, 'That's it. I am going to have an amputation and I am going to die.'"

In some medically ill populations, negativity is associated with a more rapid disease progression. For example, for men with HIV, negative expectations regarding the course of the disease were associated with disease decline, including the onset of symptoms in previously asymptomatic patients (Reed, Kemeny, Taylor, & Visscher, 1999). Pessimism is another construct that is related to negativity. Pessimists not only tend to see the glass as half empty (and thus likely to have negative expectations regarding illness outcome), they also tend to be harsh on themselves and blame themselves for negative events. In elderly adults, a pessimistic attitude was associated with reductions in cell-mediated immunity, which theoretically could increase susceptibility to illness (Kamen-Siegel, Rodin, Seligman, & Dwyer, 1991). In patients with heart disease, persons with more pessimistic traits tended to have slower recovery following coronary artery bypass surgery and were more likely to be rehospitalized within the next six months (Scheier et al., 1999).

Another way of looking at negativity is to examine the impact of its opposite—what we might think of as positive coping styles, such as optimism. People with optimistic personalities have an easier time accessing social support, are more motivated to cope with illness in an active way, and are less prone to depression and hopelessness in the face of a stressful illness. Specifically, optimism is associated with faster recovery from coronary artery bypass surgery (King, Bowe, & Kimble, 1998; Scheier et al., 1989). Optimists are less likely to develop heart disease (Kubzansky, Sparrow, Vokonas, & Kawachi, 2001) and are less likely to die of cardiovascular disease (Giltay, Geleijnse, Zitman, Hoekstra, & Schouten, 2004). Additionally, optimistic attitudes were found to be protective against the progression of atherosclerosis in women (Matthews, Räikkönen, Sutton-Tyrrell, & Kuller, 2004). Kivimäki and colleagues (2005) found that optimists tended to be healthier and recover faster from illness in the months following a stressful life event.

An additional facet to optimism and perhaps even more closely linked with meaning is *benefit finding.* An example of this is a patient describing that, although his struggle with heart disease has been difficult and frightening, the experience has helped him recognize his sense of purpose and place greater value on the importance of primary relationships. Another example is some patients who report that their illness has made them realize that they have been working too much and have been overlooking aspects of their life that they consider equally or more important. Research suggests that finding benefit in one's illness has physical implications. A randomized trial by Stanton and colleagues (2002) found that four sessions of written expressive disclosure or benefit finding resulted in fewer reports of physical symptoms and medical appointments among breast cancer patients. A longitudinal study with HIV-positive gay men found that men who were able to find meaning through bereavement of a partner or a close friend had a slower rate of CD4 cell decline and had lower AIDS-related mortality at two- to three-year follow-up (Bower, Kemeny, Taylor, & Fahey, 1998).

There is also evidence that thinking about the meaning of illness can improve psychosocial variables. For example, Lee, Cohen, Edgar, Laizner, and Gagnon

(2006) found that four sessions of encouraging breast and colorectal cancer patients to think about the meaning and the context of their illness resulted in improved self-esteem, optimism, and self-efficacy. Additionally, Carver and Antoni (2004) found that breast cancer patients who were able to attribute some kind of benefit and meaning to their disease in the first year were in less distress five to eight years after diagnosis and reported fewer symptoms of depression.

Religion is another source of meaning for many people, and, although a complete discussion of religion and meaning is beyond the scope of this chapter (religion is addressed in other chapters in this volume), it is important to mention that religion has been studied in terms of its impact on coping with illness. Praying, the sense of a personal relationship with God, and the sense of knowing what will happen to them when they die are all comforting to medical patients who are religious. Research suggests that for some patients for whom religion is an important part of their lives, religious beliefs and perhaps the meanings provided by religious understandings increase coping ability and reduce distress. Conversely, religious beliefs can also be unhelpful. Indeed, this has been the case for some patients who report feeling abandoned by God, blaming God for their difficulties, or feeling that they are being punished for some wrongdoing in the past. Because of the different ways persons utilize religion, religious coping has been divided into two categories: positive religious coping and negative religious coping. In a review of 147 studies by Smith, McCullough, and Poll (2003) examining the correlations between religion and depression, it was determined that positive religious coping is associated with fewer depressive symptoms, especially in times of stress. This same review found that negative religious coping was associated with an increase of depressive symptoms. The use of religion has also been found to reduce distress and disability in end-stage pulmonary patients as well as to reduce anxiety in heart disease patients (Burker, Evon, Sedway, & Eagan, 2004; Hughes et al., 2004).

A confounding variable in evaluating the impact of religion is social support. Positive social support is linked with better psychological and physical outcomes, and, because religion often involves social contacts such as attending religious services and developing friendships with persons who have similar religious beliefs, it is difficult to fully gain a sense of what this research means. Nevertheless, religious-beliefs often provide a sense of meaning. Not only can positive religious coping be soothing in times of stress, many religions have an explanation of causal events, right and wrong, and the meaning of life and death. It is conceivable that these explanations offered by religion can serve as important explanations for patients who are faced with medical illness, which can seem cruel and random. Religion may help to organize the impact of illness and thus promote meaning.

INDIVIDUAL RESPONSES TO ILLNESS

Although the cited research attempts to capture some of the important dynamics related to meaning and illness, the personal nature of illness and the tragedy of severe, life-threatening, and/or incapacitating illness is difficult to quantify.

The sixth definition of tragedy in Webster's dictionary (1996) is "a lamentable, dreadful or fatal event or affair; calamity; disaster" (p. 2006). Illness is a tragic event. It can be a surprise for those who develop a serious illness, and they may have little time to prepare. Many patients who develop sudden illness speak of a sense of disorientation that their experience of life can shift so quickly. This is not unlike the reaction of people who have experienced other kinds of trauma, such as natural disasters, violent crime, or serious car accidents. Especially when illness strikes suddenly, life is normal one minute and not normal at all the next. This is an important aspect related to the trauma of illness. This sudden change requires patients to integrate new information regarding medical treatments, preparation for surgery, and thoughts about how they need to alter their life to accommodate the limitations imposed by illness. Illness alters the routines of daily life. Work, social contacts, and intimate relationships are all impacted by illness. These disruptions can be as pragmatic as having to miss work because of a hospitalization or frequent doctor appointments, or as subtle as being preoccupied and worried about one's health when spending time with friends and family.

Illness is also an intrusion. As stated above, illness requires people to change their routines and alter their life-styles, and it impinges on relationships; it also involves the concrete and literal intrusions associated with diagnostic procedures and medical treatments. Blood is drawn, scopes are placed into the body, and new medications are put into the body. Hospitalized patients have to deal with the loss of privacy as health professionals enter their rooms without warning. People who patients do not know well touch them to examine them. All of these facets of illness are routine for health professionals, but not for patients. These experiences are constant reminders to patients that their bodies are no longer the same. For medical patients, one's body becomes a kind of public property. Although necessary for the diagnosis and treatment of illness, patients are impacted by these contacts. In the hospital, patients often complain that they have no privacy. For patients who have had medical events that impact the way they can take care of themselves, this is especially meaningful. For example, a neurological rehabilitation patient who was paralyzed and needed help learning how to maneuver her body to use the bathroom told me, "It is so humiliating to have going to the bathroom, which used to be a private affair, suddenly become something that I have to have help with. It's as if everyone knows everything that I am doing." The process of being a medical patient requires patients to tolerate changes in the kind of physical contact in which they allow themselves and others to engage. Additionally, patients often have very little choice and control regarding these changes.

In addition to being an intrusion, illness is sometimes a surprise. Although most people are aware on some level of the limitations of their bodies, illness is often not something for which people are prepared. For example, a patient may be aware that breast cancer is prevalent in her family, yet be surprised to learn that she has the disease. This is not abnormal, as one could argue that people who go through life worried about getting a serious illness could significantly impact their quality of life and create a sense of uncertainty that prevents them from feeling productive and happy. Thus, it could be argued that not trying to predict when illness may strike is healthy and normal. Yet illness is inevitable for most people. Because most people cope with the inevitability of illness by not becoming overly worried about it, most patients who become ill face the task of trying to cope with the surprise of illness. Many patients who are newly diagnosed with a serious illness are in shock. Although their physicians might ask me to see them to determine whether these patients have an anxiety or depressive disorder, this is often difficult to determine in the early phase of illness because patients are still in the process of trying to integrate and understand the implications of their diagnosis. Additionally, many patients who are newly diagnosed with illness are quite physically ill and uncomfortable. The attention demanded by the body when it is ill can make it difficult for patients to be aware of and focus on emotional responses. Anyone who has not had a serious illness but who has been sick with the flu might be able to relate to this notion. Simply put, when people feel terrible physically, it is hard to pay attention to how they are feeling emotionally.

That patients may be relatively less emotionally distressed due to the physical demands of illness has led me to conclude that, for many patients, depression and anxiety tend to be less of a problem during the diagnostic phase of illness and for some during the process of active medical treatment when they are engaging in active medical treatment to combat their disease (Greenberg, 2007). When acutely and seriously ill, many patients are too preoccupied with their bodies to develop severe depression and anxiety disorders. However, the issues of adjusting to the surprise of illness—including the intrusiveness of diagnostic tests, medical treatments, and becoming aware of the implications of illness and prognosis—depend on personality factors. These personality factors include past coping mechanisms, ability to tolerate vulnerability, relationship with one's body, need for control, and comfort level with relying on internal and emotional resources. These issues are described in the next sections.

SENSE OF SELF AND ILLNESS

Illness profoundly affects the experience of the self, which includes identity. Illness changes the way people can count on the use of their bodies, and in some cases radically changes how people can function physically and vocationally. The emotional ramifications of these changes are profound and can contribute to an enormous sense of loss. Consider the following example:

Jeff is a 55-year-old married man who worked as a delivery person. He collapsed one morning while on his delivery route as the result of a stroke. He was paralyzed on the left side of his body and couldn't walk. When I initially met him in the hospital, he spoke mainly of how worried he was about money and his inability to provide for his family. He frequently asked his doctors when he could go back to work, and his physicians told him they were not sure that he would be able to resume his job ever again. Jeff was devastated. He frequently talked about how he "didn't know who he was anymore," that "everything seemed different," and that his stroke made him "less of a man." Although his wife frequently reassured him that his stoke didn't change her feelings for him and that she didn't think any less of him as a man, Jeff felt emasculated and embarrassed.

Jeff's experience demonstrates a number of important issues. Although he had underlying arthrosclerosis, he was unaware of being ill and felt fine. His stroke was without warning. Within one day, life as he knew it had changed. However, Jeff quite quickly developed a sense of meaning of his stroke, at least in terms of its consequences. He thought that his masculinity had been stolen from him, and, because that happened, he was unsure what to live for. Jeff became plagued with self-doubt, because he could not imagine a life with a body that didn't work as it used to. Jeff's use of his body was essential to his work, and he was terrified that because of his paralysis that he would never again be able to use his body to work. In subsequent interviews, it became clear that Jeff not only relied on his body to work and to earn money for his family, but that his physical strength was something on which he prided himself. His ability to lift and carry his deliveries made him feel strong and purposeful. He said "My work is valuable. This stuff I have to carry for people, they couldn't do it themselves. I help them and they need me. Now, I can't do anything; I need help getting up to sit in a chair."

These comments illustrate the importance of Jeff's use of his body in his work, but also how his use of his body was related to his self-esteem. This is a common response to illness. Whether we rely on our bodies for manual labor or for getting us to work, we expect that our bodies are there to serve us. When this ability is lost, feelings of emptiness can develop. This seems particularly true for people who rely on their bodies to a great extent. For example, some people cope with stress by becoming more physically active; they may exercise more, work longer hours, or organize their house more. For some people who use their bodies in this way, it is at the expense of having an active emotional life. Some people who rely more on their bodies than their minds are not accustomed to thinking about their feelings or even being aware of thoughts that have emotional consequences. For these individuals, an illness that limits their physical functioning is devastating not only because they are unable to use their body for coping, but also because a loss in bodily functioning often requires an increased reliance on the mind—something for which many people are unprepared. For such persons, it is only when a physical illness strikes that there is an increase in the need for an internal and emotional life to help make sense of the experience. Such patients often need to learn to develop an "emotional language" to describe their experiences.

Jeff's comments illustrate this difficulty: Jeff was wheelchair-bound a few months after his stroke, although he continued to make progress in physical therapy. He came to see me because he had developed intense anxiety that was present especially in the morning. When I asked him if there were thoughts that accompanied his anxious feelings, he said that there weren't. In fact, although he came to see me for help, he was unable to articulate the nature of his distress. He said, "I like to come and see you, it's just that I don't know what to say to you. I come here and I just don't have anything to say." I asked him if it was difficult to talk with me because he didn't know what his thoughts were. He said, "Yeah, it's like, I never talked about myself before this happened, what I am supposed to come up with now?"

Such comments are common in persons who, prior to illness, have not spent a lot of time thinking about their internal lives. Additionally, major bodily changes are disorienting, and, once illness and limitations become chronic, patients often articulate feeling "lost," which is an expression of how disjointed the sense of self can become following a serious illness. The need for an increased sense of emotional understanding becomes important for coping and adjustment.

There are many implications for therapeutic interventions for patients with issues such as Jeff's. First, it is important to be more active in sessions. While the space created by psychotherapy is soothing for some patients, for people like Jeff, the quiet moments in therapy can create a lot of fear. Therefore, I tend to take a more active stance: talking more, asking questions, and sometimes structuring the session by bringing up issues to discuss. For people who do not readily access their internal life, a therapist who can model thinking can create a sense of safety for patients and can show patients what emotional reflection looks like. Additionally, I often explain the goals of therapy very directly. For patients such as Jeff I may say something like, "I think you feel lost because you can't use your body like you used to. I want to help you figure out other ways to soothe yourself, and part of that involves being able to rely on your mind.

I think therapy can help you do that." It is also important to talk with patients about their bodies. Many people, including therapists, believe that therapy is a place to talk solely about one's mind and that the details of bodily functioning are off limits. Discussing concrete issues related to bodily functioning (such as what it is like to need help showering-and-not being able to walk) not only is soothing for patients, but also helps to introduce the connection between physical functioning and emotions.

ILLNESS AS AN UNFAIR AND RANDOM EVENT

Although we are able to predict some illness—for example, smoking is predictive of lung cancer and a high-cholesterol diet predicts atherosclerosis—illness is and is often experienced by patients as a random event, and this idea is not entirely unreasonable. In the example of smoking cigarettes, about one-third of patients who smoke will develop lung cancer. Patients who have smoked cigarettes and develop lung cancer-often remark that they knew of the risks but that they didn't think that lung cancer would happen to them. Although these patients may be in denial about the contribution of smoking, they may also have a point. How can we explain the two-thirds of smokers who don't develop lung cancer? Additionally, although relatively rare, people who have never smoked can develop lung cancer. The fact is, although we can explain some illnesses as being related to poor health behaviors, some patients who engage in these poor behaviors do not develop illness. Patients who engage in high-risk health behaviors are often aware (even if it is only a vague understanding) of the odds of developing disease related to their health behaviors. Yet when it happens to them, patients are still surprised that they are in the unfortunate group who develop illness. This raises a number of important issues related to illness. The fact is, although we can make some predictions about who will develop illness, it is still random. In many ways, the development of illness is subject to chance. Some people are more prone to illness than others, and, although health behaviors-such as smoking, excessive alcohol use, diet, and exercise-do play a role in the development of many illnesses, the development of illness is also dependent on genetic factors and heritability, which are factors that cannot be controlled.

Patients develop a number of different meanings regarding the random aspects of illness. Susan felt that she had caused her cancer. These thoughts tortured her but also increased her sense of control over her worries about relapse. Some sense of control regarding the prevention of illness or relapse makes sense, and awareness of factors that can be controlled is linked with better psychological adjustment to illness. There are ways that we can take care of ourselves to reduce the chances of illness; however, as stated above, illness tends to be random in many cases. How people come to terms with this and the meanings they develop is can predict how they will cope with and adjust to illness.

Susan's belief that she could control whether she relapsed was related to an increase in her self-care. This increase in self-care was not associated with a reduction in anxiety, however. She was also constantly worried about whether she would get cancer again. She developed ways to try to increase her sense of control, yet these ways were based on magical thinking. For example, she had routine CT scans to check her remission. As with all cancer patients, these follow-up exams were associated with a great deal of apprehension and fear. In one session, we were discussing an upcoming scan and check-up. Regarding the scan, she said, "I tell myself that the scan will show that I have relapsed as a way to assure that I won't have relapsed." I asked her what she meant and she said, "It's like a trick, I tell myself the outcome will be bad so that will mean that the outcome will be good. If I prepare myself for the worst, then it won't happen."

Susan's response to these anxiety-provoking examinations reflected her desire to control the outcome of something that in reality she had little control over. Susan had already taken control of the factors that she could control by watching her diet, managing stress, and coming to psychotherapy. Other aspects related to whether she would relapse were beyond her control. I learned from working with Susan that she had never been accustomed to feeling out of control. She worked in a high-power, prestigious position where she had a lot of control. But it was also clear that Susan tended to feel that she had control over many things that she actually did not or could not control. Her use of cognitive tricks as a way of coping with her routine follow-up examinations demonstrated how desperately she wanted to control the possibility of relapsing. A major part of the therapeutic work with Susan involved helping her to develop a more realistic sense of what she could control. It seemed helpful to point out to her that, while her cognitive tricks did have some short-term effect of managing her intense anxiety, she paid a price for this in the long term, because she knew on some level that she could not control some aspects of whether her disease would return. This also involved a realization of fear and helplessness that is often a part of coping with illness.

As was the case for Susan, many people who have trouble coming to terms with the randomness of illness are tormented with unrelenting worries that can lead to overwhelming anxiety. Yet acknowledging that illness sometimes involves being the victim of bad luck requires an acknowledgement of vulnerability. Acknowledgement of this vulnerability requires a relinquishment of control. For some people, this is very difficult and seems to be more so in persons from abusive or chaotic backgrounds in which they have had to be in control of neglectful or abusive parents. Additionally, this issue is tied closely to guilt feelings associated with having survived an illness—especially an illness that takes some lives but not others.

SURVIVOR GUILT

The concept of survivor guilt has long been associated with guilt that is manifested by survivors of war and other traumas in which some persons are spared (often arbitrarily) from death. The term survivor guilt was first used by Niederland (1968) to describe reactions of concentration camp survivors. Survivor guilt involves a sense of disorientation and confusion about why and how the trauma was survived. Additionally, feeling happy or relieved about having been spared death when others have perished can result in overwhelming guilt feelings and can prohibit survivors from feeling entitled to live happy lives.

The concept of survivor guilt has also been applied to chronic illness (e.g., Vamos, 1997). Major illness such as cancer, strokes, heart attacks, and renal disease seem to spare lives and take lives in a way that can seem—and often is—random. For example, if someone has a heart attack in a crowded place, the likelihood that someone will be present to perform CPR or call for help is high and the chance for survival is increased. On the other hand, a person who has a heart attack alone at home when no one is likely to drop by has a decreased chance of receiving help and the chance of survival is decreased. These random events are something that patients often think a lot about, and adjusting to illness often involves coming to terms with the meaning of how and why they were able to survive. Additionally, feeling relieved about living can feel crazy for patients who are struggling with sadness and resentment that they became ill at all. Further, allowing oneself to be happy when others have suffered can feel to patients that they are being aggressive. Sometimes people deal with this by becoming angry or consumed with aggressive feelings. Consider the example of Joe:

Joe was an undergraduate when he was diagnosed with a rare cancer. He underwent extensive treatment and surgery and did well. When I met him, he had been disease free for two years. Yet he continued to be consumed with anger regarding the fact that he had gotten cancer and felt that no one around him understood his anger. He said,

> I try to tell people that I am really pissed off, you know, that this shouldn't have happened to me. But what people say back is that I should feel lucky that I survived it—that I am okay now and should just move on. I feel like they don't want to hear it.

While Joe has a good point, his anger also reflected his difficulty about feeling entitled to move on and have a good life despite this tragic event. Although he had been seriously ill, he was now well and there was no reason that Joe couldn't try to focus on future goals. It turned out that Joe had other factors that exacerbated his difficulties, including having grown up in a poor and chaotic family in which his parents had little time for him. His guilt of having a better life than his parents was another factor at play, but his focus on his cancer and his anger made addressing these other issues difficult. Usually with patients such as Joe, it is important for the therapist to be able to listen and provide understanding regarding the anger the patient is expressing. Acknowledging anger eventually allows room for other emotions that patients feel they cannot express until their anger is understood. When friends, family, and therapists cannot tolerate a patient's anger, the patient feels more compelled to hold on to angry feelings.

Anger is one consequence of survivor guilt; depression is another. Blacher (2000) described in his work with cardiac surgery patients that many of these patients awoke from surgery surprised that they hadn't died, but that also many of these patients became depressed and felt unable to celebrate having lived through surgery. Often these individuals had family members who had died from heart disease, and they were conflicted about having survived a difficult surgery. Blacher found that, by acknowledging this understandable conflict, patients felt freer to allow themselves to be happy about having survived surgery and they felt less impacted by guilt.

Patients with survivor guilt often feel crazy. They are in the bind of trying to make sense of having survived an illness, and this survival feels random. Random events are hard to make sense of because it is difficult to develop a sense of meaning when one feels the victim of arbitrary events. Additionally, feeling happy when other others have died from a disease may create a sense of betrayal. Patients may express this by saying, "How can I feel good when other people have died?"

Developing a sense of meaning regarding why one was spared—even if it means acknowledging that factors out of the patient's control, such as genetics—often helps to diffuse some of the conflicted and chaotic feelings of people who have survived an illness. This can also give permission to patients to think about the possibilities for the future and to feel entitled to live happier lives.

CONCLUSION

Illness impacts every aspect of patients' lives. Medical illness involves a number of emotional upheavals. Diagnostic labels such as depression and anxiety, although common in medically ill populations, do not fully capture the emotional experience of adapting to illness. Illness disrupts sense of self and identity, forces many people to have an increased reliance on emotional functioning, and requires survivors of illness to endure guilt feelings about living when others have died. Although meaning is difficult to describe and is subjective, facing an illness requires patients to emotionally adapt to and accept the losses associated with decreases in physical functioning. Illness is tragic and unfair, and, even in cases in which illness can be predicted, it often involves elements that cannot be controlled. It is understandably difficult for patients to come to terms with these facts. However, developing a sense of meaning and an explanation regarding illness is crucial to adapting to the event of illness. Developing a sense of meaning is also likely tied to an increased sense of control. By realizing what aspects of illness over which patients do have control—such as health behaviors, coping responses, and accessing social support—patients can focus on factors that may decrease illness recurrence or exacerbation. Finally, having an understanding of what an illness means, and even seeing the potential benefits of an illness, can allow patients to cope better with the normative emotional struggles in illness.

TOOL KIT FOR CHANGE

Role and Perspective of the Healthcare Professional

1. Healthcare professionals should help patients explore the meaning of illness.
2. Medical illness impacts the identity of patients and may require clinical attention to address self-image and coping.
3. Although anxiety and depression are common responses to illness, helping patients cope involves understanding the individual context in which illness takes place.

Role and Perspective of the Participant

1. Developing a sense of meaning in response to illness appears to be important for psychological, and possibly physical, health.
2. To avoid self-blame, patients need to acknowledge that illness involves some aspects of randomness and bad luck.
3. Patients should develop a network of close persons with whom they can discuss the meaning and impact of illness.

Interconnection: The Global Perspective

1. Encouraging patients to develop a sense of meaning about illness helps reduce psychological symptoms.
2. The psychological responses and symptoms of medically ill patients are as important as other medical symptoms.
3. Psychological interventions with medically ill patients are an important part of healthcare, and mental health professionals should be an active part of the multidisciplinary team.

REFERENCES

Blacher, R. S. (2000). "It isn't fair": Post operative depression and other manifestations of survivor guilt. *General Hospital Psychiatry, 22,* 43–48.
Bower, J. E., Kemeny, M. E., Taylor, S. E., & Fahey, J. L. (1998). Cognitive processing discovery of meaning, CD4 decline and AIDS related mortality among bereaved

HIV seropositive men. *Journal of Consulting and Clinical Psychology, 66*(6), 979–986.

Burker, E. J., Evon, D. M., Sedway, J. A., & Eagan, T. (2004). Religious coping, psychological distress and disability among patients with end stage pulmonary disease. *Journal of Clinical Psychology in Medical Settings, 11*(3),179–193.

Carver, C. S., & Antoni, M. H. (2004). Finding benefit in breast cancer during the first year after diagnosis predicts better adjustment 5–8 years after diagnosis. *Health Psychology, 23*(6), 595–598.

Doerfler, L. A., & Paraskos J. A. (2005). Posttraumatic stress disorder in patients with coronary artery disease: Screening and management implications. *Canadian Journal of Cardiology, 21,* 689–697.

Fife, B. L. (1994). The conceptualization of meaning in illness. *Social Science and Medicine, 38*(2), 309–316.

Frankl, V. (1985). *Man's search for meaning.* New York: Pocket Books.

Fuller, T. (1732). Comp., *Gnomologia: Adages and Proverbs,* 2478.

Giltay, E. J., Geleijnse, J. M., Zitman, F. G., Hoekstra, T., & Schouten, E. G. (2004). Dispositional optimism and all-cause and cardiovascular mortality in a prospective cohort of elderly Dutch men and women. *Archives of General Psychiatry, 61,* 1126–1135.

Greenberg, T. M. (2007). *The psychological impact of acute and chronic illness.* New York: Springer.

Hughes, J. W., Tomlinson, A., Blumenthal, J. A., Davidson, J., Sketch, M. H., & Watkins, L. L. (2004). Social support and religiosity as coping strategies for anxiety in hospitalized cardiac patients. *Annals of Behavioral Medicine, 28*(3),179–185.

Kamen-Siegel, L., Rodin, J., Seligman, M. E., & Dwyer, J. (1991). Explanatory style and cell mediated immunity in elderly men and women. *Health Psychology, 10,* 229–235.

Kangas, M., Henry, J. L., & Bryant R. A. (2002). Posttraumatic stress disorder following cancer: A conceptual and empirical review. *Clinical Psychology Review, 22,* 499–524.

Kangas, M., Henry J. L., & Bryant, R. A. (2005). The relationship between acute stress disorder and posttraumatic stress disorder following cancer. *Journal of Consulting and Clinical Psychology, 73,* 360–364.

King, K. B., Bowe, M. A., & Kimble L. P.(1998). Optimism, coping and long-term recovery from coronary artery bypass in women. *Research in Nursing and Health, 21,* 15–26.

Kivimäki, M., Vahtera, J., Elovainio, M., Helenius, H., Singh-Manoux, A., & Pentti, J. (2005). Optimism and pessimism as predictors of change in health after death or onset of severe illness in family. *Health Psychology, 24*(4), 413–421.

Kleinman, A. (1980). *Patients and healers in the context of culture: An exploration of the borderland between anthropology, medicine, and psychiatry.* Berkeley: University of California Press.

Kubzansky, L. D., Sparrow, D., Vokonas, P., & Kawachi, I. (2001). Is the glass half empty or half full? A prospective study of optimism and coronary heart disease in the normative aging study. *Psychosomatic Medicine, 63,* 910–916.

Lazarus, R. S., & Folkman, S. (1984). *Stress, appraisal and coping.* New York: Springer.

Lee, V., Cohen, S. R., Edgar, L., Laizner, A. M., & Gagnon, A. J. (2006). Meaning-making intervention during breast or colorectal cancer treatment improves self-esteem, optimism, and self efficacy. *Social Science and Medicine, 62*(12), 3133–3145.

Lipowski, Z. J. (1970). Physical illness, the individual and the coping process. *Psychiatry Medicine, 1*, 91–102.

Marris, P. (1974). *Loss and change.* New York: Random House.

Matthews, K. A., Räikkönen, K., Sutton-Tyrrell, K., & Kuller, L. H. (2004). Optimistic attitudes protect against progression of carotid atherosclerosis in healthy middle-aged women. *Psychosomatic Medicine, 66*, 640–644.

Niederland, W. G. (1968) Clinical observations of the "survivor syndrome." *International Journal of Psychoanalysis, 49*(2), 313–315.

Reed, G. M., Kemeny, M. E., Taylor, S. E., & Visscher, B. R. (1999). Negative HIV specific expectancies and AIDS related bereavement as predictors of symptom onset in asymptomatic HIV positive gay men. *Health Psychology, 18*, 354–363.

Scheier, M. F., Matthews, K. A., Owens, J., Magovern, G. J., Lefebvre, R. C., Abbott, R. A., et al. (1989). Dispositional optimism and recovery from coronary artery bypass surgery: The beneficial effects on physical and psychological well-being. *Journal of Personality and Social Psychology, 57*, 1024–1040.

Scheier, M. F., Matthews, K. A., Owens, J. F., Schulz, M. W., Bridges, G. J., Magovern, C. S., et al. (1999). Optimism and rehospitalization after coronary artery bypass graft surgery. *Archives of Internal Medicine, 159*(8), 829–835.

Serlin, I., & Cannon, J. (2004). A humanistic approach to the psychology of trauma. In D. Knafo (Ed.), *Living with terror, working with trauma: A clinician's handbook* (pp. 313–330). New York: Jason Aronson.

Smith, T. B., McCullough, M. E., & Poll, J. (2003). Religiousness and depression: Evidence for a main effect and the moderating influence of life events. *Psychological Bulletin, 129*(4), 614–636.

Stanton, A. L., Danoff-Burg, S., Sworowski, L. A., Collins, C. A., Branstetter, A. D., Rodriquez-Hanley, A., et al. (2002). Randomized controlled trial of written emotional expression and benefit finding in breast cancer patients. *Journal of Clinical Oncology, 20*, 4160–4468.

Taylor, S. E. (1983). Adjustment to threatening events: A theory of cognitive adaptation. *American Psychologist, 38*, 1161–1173.

Vamos, M. (1997). Survivor guilt and chronic illness. *Australia and New Zealand Journal of Psychiatry, 31*(4), 592–596.

Webster's new universal unabridged dictionary. (1996). New York: Barnes and Noble.

White, C. A. (2004). Meaning and its measurement in psychosocial oncology. *Psycho-oncology, 13*, 468–481.

Chapter Six

SPIRITUALITY, HEALTH, AND MENTAL HEALTH: A HOLISTIC MODEL

Betty Ervin-Cox, PhD, Louis Hoffman, PhD, Christopher S. M. Grimes, PsyD, and Stephen Fehl, MA

DEFINITIONS

What do we mean by religion and spirituality? The various ways these terms have been defined are more diverse than time would allow us to review. The lack of consistent definitions of these concepts along with the intermingling of them can make it challenging to gain a coherent understanding of the literature on spirituality and religion. For the purpose of this chapter, religion and spirituality will be defined as highly related but conceptually distinct. Religion refers to the cognitive, behavioral, and systematic aspects of a person's belief system. The person's religious beliefs are based on what Frankl (2000) has termed "ultimate meaning." Spirituality refers to the transcendent and emotional qualities of life in relation to ultimate meaning (Frankl, 2000) or "whatever they may consider divine" (James, 1902/1958, p. 42). These conceptions of spirituality are similar to how Tillich (1957) defines "ultimate concern" in the context of faith. Unfortunately, the definitions used in the empirical research are not consistent between studies or with this definition. We will attempt to clarify the confusion due to altering definitions of religion and spirituality as they are encountered.

An earlier version of this chapter was published as "Selected Literature Review on Spirituality and Health/Mental Health" in *Spirituality and Psychological Health* (2005) by R. H. Cox, B. Ervin-Cox, and L. Hoffman. A special thanks to the Colorado School of Professional Psychology Press for granting permission to reprint an update of the chapter in the current volume.

The confusion among definitions continues with the concepts of physical health and psychological well-being. Fortunately, there is greater consistency with these terms in the literature. We will use the term health to refer to the various conceptions of physical health. The definitions in the mental health field are much more confusing. We use the term well-being, or psychological well-being, to refer to the various general conceptions of positive mental health. Well-being is best viewed as a multidimensional construct that includes positive affect, negative affect, and life satisfaction (Chamberlain & Zika, 1988). Within this conceptualization of well-being, the three factors are highly interrelated, yet they maintain distinctions. Psychological well-being is much more complex than simple lack of pathology. Again, the various terms referring to what we conceptualize as well-being are not consistent in the literature. We will attempt to clarify the differing usage of terms as they arise.

SPIRITUALITY AND HEALTH: SETTING THE CONTEXT

The science and art of healing is an integral part of healthcare and often has been associated with spiritual practices. Although practiced differently by different cultures and religions, the concept of healing has permeated all cultures from the beginning of humankind. The healer in some cultures is known as a faith healer. A study of the New Testament shows that Christ often ministered to the sick and the diseased. Many may well have considered him a faith healer. The disabled and sick sought out Christ for healing; therefore, it might be said that religion was a place for the sick. Matthew, a disciple of Christ, wrote, "It is not the healthy who need a doctor, but the sick" (Matthew 9:12, New International Version). This reference to healthiness refers to a conceptualization that includes mind, body, and spirit. Spirituality, as a component of belief, was paramount to the New Testament miracles and conversions. Belief is the communication that one has with the higher being. The terms *religion* and *spirituality* must, therefore, be considered carefully in that religion may well be an institutionalized function while spirituality may be the relationship one has with that higher being regardless of the religion espoused. To this end, Easterbrook (1999) suggests that belief or spirituality rather than religious practice supports better health. However, there is mixed support for this in the empirical research.

During the early twentieth century, spirituality was a controversial issue for physicians, many of whom ignored spirituality all together. However, studies in the last three decades have shown a marked interest in spirituality and health. Currently, the medical profession is increasingly acknowledging that research confirms the connection between spirituality and health. "Beginning in the 1950's, several factors saw the pendulum start to swing back in favor of a wider consideration of environmental, social, psychological and behavioral determinants of health including religious identity and practice" (Chatters, Levin, & Ellison, 1998, p. 689). Many well-respected physicians have contributed significantly with their own research, adding to research conducted by medical schools and schools of public health giving reasons to hold to the traditional view that belief—that is, a close relationship to the higher power—promotes better individual health (Benson, 1996; Christy, 1998; Easterbrook, 1999; Ellison & Levin, 1998; Faneuli, 1997).

Various medical schools and graduate programs in psychology are adding courses on spirituality to their curricula, and courses are already required in many. These are positive signs that the professions of medicine and psychology are recognizing the growing body of research indicating that spirituality has a positive effect on health (Benson, 1996; Christy, 1998; Easterbrook, 1999; Ellison & Levin, 1998).

Several books reflect the growing interest in spirituality in both the medical and psychological fields. Three prominent titles in this area are Chamberlain and Hall's (2000), *Realized Religion,* which attempts to address the effects of being religious through a selected review of the literature; Plante and Sherman's (2001) *Faith and Health,* a collection of essays that examines psychological perspectives on the relationship of faith with physical health and psychological well-being; and *Handbook of Religion and Health* by Koenig, McCullough, and Larson (2001), which is the most extensive work on religion and health to date. Koeing, McCullough, and Larson, three primary research contributors in the field, offer a comprehensive review of the literature and a discussion of the implications of their findings.

It is interesting that the *Diagnostic and Statistical Manual of Mental Disorders-IV-TR* (American Psychiatric Association, 2000) the manual used for diagnosing mental disorders, includes a code for "religious or spiritual problem," which is not classified as a disorder. This indicates that psychiatry and psychology are now considering the spiritual aspects of health to some degree.

Research psychologists have demonstrated a renewed interest in understanding the relationship between spirituality and physical health (Larson & Larson, 2003; Powell, Shahabi, & Thoresen 2003; Seeman, Dublin, & Seeman, 2003). Powell and colleagues utilized a levels-of-evidence approach in their review of literature regarding religion and spirituality's link to physical health. The levels-of-evidence approach, compared to meta-analysis, requires research to meet acceptable methodological standards in order to qualify for review. While overall the researchers judged past reviews to be overly optimistic regarding the positive relationship between religion or spirituality and physical health, they concluded that there is indeed a relationship between religion or spirituality and physical health, but that the relationship is more complex than suggested by some.

Hawks (1994), in writing about spiritual health, recognizes this importance on the gestalt and places this in the context of holistic health. Spiritual health provides the individual with meaning, a value system, and self-esteem. Emotional health allows the person to express human emotions along with the ability to give and receive love within relationships. Hawks proposes five dimensions of health: physical, intellectual, social, spiritual, and emotional. He juxtaposed his theoretical model of spirituality and holistic health with Maslow's (1998) hierarchy of needs: food and shelter, safety and security, love and acceptance, self-esteem, and self-actualization. Others have shown agreement with him—for example, Frankl's "meaning," Allport's (1958) "value system," and Maslow's "self-esteem."

Viktor Frankl (1959) revealed his depth of spiritual value in his lectures and book, *Man's Search for Meaning*. He emphasized that the desire of most people is to have a purpose and meaning to life. Frankl explains that to find the meaning of life, one must go outside of oneself and that there are three ways to do this: one may create or do a deed, one may love, or one may suffer. These are the methods by which one may fulfill the responsibility for finding the meaning in life. They are also searches for the higher spiritual purposes of life.

Clearly, religion or a belief system gives meaning to life for many individuals. Their belief system provides goals to achieve, values to satisfy, rituals to follow, a community that approves, purposes for daily living, and, in summary, something *meaningful* to accomplish. Individuals who find purpose and meaning in life through religion have a resource they can draw upon while going through life's experiences. As discussed later, it is plausible that the construct of meaning in life may be an important intervening variable between spirituality, well-being, and health.

PRAYER, RELAXATION, MEDITATION, HEALTH, AND WELL-BEING

Prayer

In a survey of Americans, Poloma and Gallup asked who prays, the forms of prayer used, and if prayer makes a difference in health and well-being (Poloma, 1993). Four types of prayer were identified: colloquial, petitionary, meditative, and ritual. According to the findings, 60 percent of those surveyed used a meditative form of prayer when praying and perceived it as an intimacy or a close relationship with God. "Prayer for healing appears to contribute to greater life satisfaction and existential well-being for those who are in poorer health but not for those in good health" (Poloma, 1993, p. 40).

Many of the persons questioned in the medical research on religion and health stated that it was religion or prayer that gave them purpose and meaning to their life (Benson, 1996). They further stated that religion or prayer offered them peace and hope when faced with life-threatening disease. Prayer, defined as communication with a higher power, was a source relied upon and that provided strength to support them through their suffering. Without prayer, their predicaments would have presumably been despair. Instead, they were able to show a positive attitude that benefited their health.

Herbert Benson (1999), a Harvard University cardiologist, in his address to the American Psychological Association, stated that persons with a spiritual or religious belief were more likely to be healed than individuals not professing to any spirituality. His early experience and research suggests that prayer has favorably influenced the health outcome of persons who pray. Benson is one of the foremost physicians of the day in the discussion on spirituality and health. The American Psychological Association, formerly not known for its emphasis on things spiritual, found Benson's session "standing room only," indicating another bellwether aspect in the consideration of spirituality and health among today's psychological community.

Benson (1996) states that individuals who continuously repeat a word and disregard intrusive thoughts experience physiological changes, such as decrease in respiration and pulse rate. These changes are the opposite of those brought on by stress. The repeating of a word is sometimes viewed as utilizing a mantra, which is important in some forms of Buddhist meditation. Many people, however, prefer to repeat a prayer from their religious tradition. This exercise has proven to be an effective therapy for the disease being treated. Benson calls this the "relaxation response" and emphasizes its calming effect on the body and mind. It appears that when belief is added to the relaxation response, the body and mind are quieted significantly more than when the relaxation response is used alone. Benson's studies suggest that the body's self-healing abilities are aided by a calm state of mind. Benson's five-year study found that patients who used meditation and felt a closeness to a higher power had more rapid recoveries and better health than those who did not make such claims. Psychologists and others trained in biofeedback and hypnosis use similar techniques to train patients to control their headaches and other stress-produced and stress-related body pains. Relaxation, meditation, yoga, hypnosis, guided imagery, and prayer have much in common.

Prayer is usually seen as part of a relationship with God and also may be a form of meditation. Research studies indicate that persons who attend worship services at least once a week and pray have better health (Benson, 1996). These studies suggest that a calm mental state influences the healing of the body. Other studies suggest that individuals who pray have lower blood pressure than those in control groups (Christy, 1998; Easterbrook, 1999).

Chamberlain and Hall (2000) distinguish between petitionary prayer and intercessory prayer in their selective review of the research. Petitionary prayer is defined as making a specific request of God. The request can be for the self or others—for example, healing physical or psychological illness. Intercessory prayer makes a request for the healing of another person. One of the more intriguing studies reviewed was conducted by Byrd (1988). This was a double blind study in which coronary patients were randomly assigned to one of two groups. The first group received intercessory prayer from a group of volunteers who had no contact with the patients. The second group was a control group. In his initial reporting of the results, Byrd indicated that the intercessory prayer had a positive effect on those being prayed for. Byrd and Sherril, in a 1995 article, reported that the prayer group had better results in 21 of 26 health-related categories. Despite the promising findings of this study, Chamberlain and Hall reported inconsistent findings in connecting intercessory prayer and petitionary prayer with better physical health.

Koenig et al. (2001) concur with the Chamberlain and Hall findings on inter-cessory prayer in their more extensive review of the literature. These authors reviewed 1997 research conducted by O'Laoire on intercessory prayer. O'Laoire looked at the effect intercessory prayer had on measures of mental health and physical health for both the person offering the prayer and the recipient of the prayer. Although no significant findings were found for the recipients of the prayers, the results did suggest that the people offering the prayers received psychological benefits.

Prayer is not always associated with better health and well-being. Koenig et al. (2001) review several research articles suggesting a negative association between ritual prayer and aspects of mental health. The relationships between other types of prayer, including intercessory and petitionary prayer, generally have inconsistent associations with mental and physical health. Similarly, Benson et al.'s (2006) review of previous studies revealed two research projects that found positive outcomes associated with intercessory prayer and two that found no significant results. Koenig et al. suggest one reason for the inconsis-tent findings between prayer and health is that people tend to increase prayer in times of trouble.

The most comprehensive study on intercessory prayer to date was conducted by Benson et al. (2006). Because of its significance, this study received much attention in the media, including the religious media. The study included a sample of over 1,800 individuals in six locations. They were divided into three groups. Two groups were uncertain whether they were receiving intercessory prayer, while one group was certain they were being prayed for. Of the uncer-tain groups, one group was being prayed for and the other was not. Contrary to previous research by Benson, this study found no positive outcomes to inter-cessory prayer and some additional complications for those who were certain they were receiving prayers.

The Benson et al. study has received its share of criticism, including a response article by Krucoff, Crater, and Lee (2006). As these authors point out, it is a plausible interpretation that telling patients that people are praying for them may illicit anxiety or the thought that they are so bad off that even the doctors are relying on prayer. Additionally, if certain usage of intercessory prayer may cause harm, then additional ethical considerations must be considered in future research.

Koenig, McCullough, and Larson's (2001) literature review suggests that people with an intrinsic faith may benefit more from their religiosity than those with extrinsic faith. Intrinsic faith, which is discussed in more detail later, is a more internalized, personal type of faith. Conversely, extrinsic faith is faith for social and other personal benefits. When applying this finding to prayer, it seems logical that people with intrinsic religiosity may benefit more from the effects of prayer than those with extrinsic religiosity. Research that controls for this confounding factor may further illuminate the relationship between prayer, mental health, and physical health.

Meditation and Mindfulness

Although meditation is less frequently associated with divine intervention or metaphysical implications, it has been purported to work in a similar manner to prayer through a connection with relaxation. For some individuals, meditation is connected to meaning in life in a manner similar to prayer. Epstein (1995), one of the leading promoters of the use of prayer in psychotherapy, dedicated much of his book *Thoughts without a Thinker: Psychotherapy from a Buddhist Perspective* to integrating meditative practices with psychotherapy.

Epstein (1995, 2006), who utilizes a variety of Buddhist practices in psychotherapy, is particularly interested in the usefulness of meditation in psychoanalytic psychotherapy. Various approaches to meditation practice can help clients become more aware of themselves, particularly their bodily experiences. This connection with increasing self-awareness makes meditation a natural integration in depth psychotherapy.

Research suggests meditation may benefit psychological health beyond the therapy room and in more ways than increasing self-awareness. The connection between meditation and relaxation appears self-evident; however, it is important for the connection to be tested through empirical investigation. Carlson, Bacaseta, and Simanton (1998) found that meditation may be useful in the treatment of anxiety disorders.

Meditation has also been purported to improve attention and concentration, which suggests its potential utility in the treatment of attention deficit hyperactive disorder. Research by Harrison, Manocha, and Rubia (2004) supports this hypothesis; however, further research is needed to explore which approaches to meditation are the most useful.

The initial research on meditation and physical health is also promising. Leserman, Stuart, Mamish, and Benson (as cited in Koenig et al., 2001) found meditation to be beneficial in treating heart disease, while Sadsuang, Chentanez, and Veluvan (as cited in Koenig et al., 2001) found meditation to increase immune functioning.

Mindfulness is a Buddhist concept often practiced in conjunction with meditation. According to Marlatt and Kristeller (1999), mindfulness is "to be fully mindful in the present moment is to be aware of the full range of experiences that exist in the here and now....Mindful awareness is based on an attitude of acceptance" (p. 68). Similar to the here-and-now focus in humanistic psychology and the idea of centering in existential-integrative therapy (Schneider & May, 1995), mindfulness emphasizes awareness of current experience.

A meta-analysis conducted by Grossman, Niemann, Schmidt, and Walach (2004) found mindfulness to be beneficial in the treatment of a wide range of psychological disorders. Similarly, Teasdale, Segal, and Williams (1995) found that mindfulness, when used with cognitive behavioral therapy, is beneficial in relapse prevention. As with meditation, mindfulness fits naturally with the psychotherapy process.

In summary, prior research on prayer, meditation, physical health, and well-being suggests the relationship between these factors can be very complex. At the current time, the research appears to more consistently support the beneficial aspects of meditation than the positive impact of prayer. This also may suggest that it is likely that meditative approaches to prayer may be more beneficial than ritualistic and intercessory prayer. Further research will need to take into account the effects of prayer and meditation over time (longitudinal studies) as well as distinguishing between various types of prayer and meditation.

SPIRITUALITY AND HEALTH

Studies from medical schools indicate that individuals who practice in mainstream religions have fewer physical disorders than the overall population (Koenig, 1999). This finding is constant even when researchers control variables such as the believers' health histories. Koenig even stated that religious belief may extend the length of our lives. Many experts in the field assert that church attendance at least once per week benefits physical health. Koenig, in another study that controlled for physical functioning and chronic illness, found older persons who regularly attended worship services had lower blood levels of interleukin-6 than their cohorts playing golf on Sunday mornings (cited in Christy, 1998; Easterbrook, 1999). The psychoneuroimmunology of this finding is staggering.

In a study by Strawbridge (1982), women who attended a worship service at least once a week lived longer, but this finding did not extend to men. Nonmainstream denominations present a different picture than individuals in mainstream denominations. It may be that the utilization of health services is significantly different for these two groups. Religious communities have differing beliefs and practices when accessing health service. For instance, some religious bodies oppose practices such as blood transfusions, organ transplants, and even basic medical care.

A Dartmouth-Hitchcock Medical Center study of 232 patients who had heart surgery found that drawing strength from religious faith was the best predictor of patient survival in the six months after surgery (cited in Christy, 1998). For those patients without religious faith, the death rate was three times greater than the rate of those who did have a belief system.

Much correlational research has been conducted on the relationship between religious involvement and mortality. McCullough, Hoyt, Larson, Koenig, and Thoresen (2000) conducted a meta-analysis of data from 42 independent sample studies exploring this relationship. They found religious involvement to be significantly associated with lower mortality, meaning that individuals who scored high in religious involvement were more often alive at follow-up than those with less religious involvement. The authors reasoned that part of the religious involvement–mortality association can be explained by the health-promotive behaviors of religious individuals.

Several factors may improve the health and well-being of individuals who regularly attend worship services. George, Ellison, and Larson (2002) suggest four psychosocial mechanisms presented in the literature as possible explanations of the health-promoting effects of religious involvement. These include health practices, social support, psychosocial resources (i.e., self-esteem and self-efficacy), and providing a sense of coherence and meaning. Some religions explicitly prescribe good health habits and strictly prohibit behavior linked to poorer health (such as use of tobacco, alcohol, or caffeine and promiscuous sexual practices). Individuals who regularly attend worship services are within a group of concerned individuals who support others when there is a need. One's local place of worship is the base for social contacts and becomes a primary support system because it not only cares for spiritual needs, but helps those who are ill or in distress. At their best, these institutions extend themselves among their members and to the community as well. This combination may extend the life span for the believer. The caring relationship also acts as therapy for the individual. A church, synagogue, or mosque provides a systematized faith and a value system that gives meaning and sense to life for the individual. Such a place of worship provides the symbols, rituals, creeds, liturgies, and formal structure in which to place the otherwise ambiguous elements of individual belief systems. Individuals benefit in their emotional, mental, and physical health as they experience acceptance, love, hope, and contentment. Regular participation in communal worship may regulate mental and physical health behavior in a way that the risk of disease is lessened (Ellison & Levin, 1998; George et al., 2002; Hawks, 1994; Larson & Larson, 1991; McGuire, 1993).

An interesting article by Rippentrop (2005) examines the cross-section of health and well-being in relationship to spirituality. Rippentrop used Medline and PsychLIT to identify a number of studies examining chronic pain and psychological variables, such as mood. In general, those engaging in spiritual practice did not receive a decrease in pain symptoms or severity but had a more positive mood, fewer instances of negative mood, and higher perceptions of social support. This suggests that spirituality, even if it does not improve physical health, may provide benefits in the patient's ability to cope with physical illness and associated pain.

Given the connection between spirituality and health shown here, physicians should advise patients of this just as they are advised of other health-supporting practices. Just as patients are asked about other habits and practices of their daily living, they should also be queried by their physicians about their spiritual practices and beliefs. This suggestion may seem uncomfortable for many in the medical profession. If so, it will certainly be intrusive to psychotherapists who consider asking about one's religion to be off limits.

Spirituality and Health in Adolescents

Minimal research has considered the relationship between religion and adolescent health. Wallace and Forman (1998) conducted a study of high school seniors using the relationship between religion and behavioral predictors of morbidity and mortality among adolescents. Religious youth were more likely to behave in healthy ways because they were less likely to use alcohol, take illegal drugs, carry weapons, and engage in fights than were their nonreligious peers. The behavior and the healthcare of adolescents during this period of life are key predictors of health in adulthood. Adolescents who engage in smoking, drug use, excessive or unsafe sexual activity, or poor dietary and physical activity are likely to continue these high-risk behaviors as adults. Adolescents who start smoking before they are 18 and continue into adulthood are prone to suffer from the three leading causes of death in adults: heart disease, strokes, and cancer. Alcohol and illicit drug use are health behaviors that cause illness and death among both adolescents and adults. Adolescents who are sexually active increase their risk for pregnancy and sexually transmitted diseases. The ramifications of unwanted pregnancies, the choices regarding abortion, and the multitudinous decisions that revolve around sexually transmitted diseases are a few of the connections between physical health and spiritual values.

American youth report high levels of religious belief and that religion is important to them (Wallace & Forman, 1998). The importance of worship attendance and spirituality for adolescent health, behavior, and health needs to be stressed among this population. Although this encouragement is typically directed toward religiosity, greater attention might need to be given to worship attendance as a preventive behavior for future health problems. This assumes that one's place of worship serves as a support group for the adolescent, encourages a life-style that aids better health, and reduces delinquent behavior patterns.

Frankel and Hewitt (1994) examined the relationship between religion and health among Canadian university students. They found that students who belonged to Christian groups on campus were healthier, more satisfied with life, and handled stress better than students who did not have such affiliation. The students affiliated with the Christian groups used the university health services less often than nonaffiliated peers.

More research must occur with this age group to add to the body of knowledge and to specific areas of adolescent spirituality, physical health, and social aspects. The research showing a positive influence for mental and physical health needs to be shared with young people to encourage them to live a healthier life-style. This research needs to find its way into the literature of adolescents, their parents, and their religious leaders and not kept within the walls of the research laboratory. Programs connecting mosques, synagogues, temples, and churches with medical and educational communities will help adolescents understand the positive rewards of being involved in the church and having a spiritual life-style.

Spirituality and Health in the Elderly

Interest in the relationship between religion and aging emerged during the 1950s. Since then, however, the amount of research has declined. This is likely due to the assumption that religion in the elderly person does not contribute to the understanding of the aging process. During the last decade, there has been a renewed interest in spirituality and health, resulting in renewed interest in the spirituality of older adults. Gerontology journals have published articles describing the religious behavior and attitudes of the elderly. There is a need to be more specific in the study of religion and how it impacts the lives of the elderly—for example, the relationship to reading scriptural texts, prayer, worship attendance, the loss of ritual, communal singing, and other specifically religious practices that frequently occur with aging.

Levin, Taylor, and Chatters (1994) considered race and gender in their research. Their findings indicated that, on the whole, women were more religious than men. Women were more likely to be church members, take part in church activities, and pray. Older persons of both African American and white ethnicity had high levels of religiosity. However, the level among African Americans was higher than among whites. Religion was an important part of their life as well as church attendance and prayer. Older African American men reported more religious participation than did older white women.

Oman and Reed (1998) found that, after five years, older persons who attended church services had lower mortality rates than those who did not attend at all. One limit to this study was its sample, which did not include persons of color. In a study of an ethnically diverse older group, Idler and Kasl (1997a) found that church attendance was not a significant predictor of health after controlling for demographics and health status.

Idler and Kasl (1997a) also considered the relationship between religion and functional disability. Their findings suggest that attendance at worship services was more important than religious involvement. They suggest that research in the experiences that individuals had—such as the music, rituals, and symbols in the services and confession and forgiveness—may be important for bodily health. Attendance may reflect the ability to participate with the group in the service rather than worshiping alone at home. For the disabled, church attendance made a positive difference in terms of well-being and social activity. This study confirms research conducted with religious and nonreligious elderly persons showing that religion improves their quality of life. In a second publication, Idler and Kasl (1997b) stated that the worship experience may aid the elderly person to transcend to a state where body affliction is less troublesome. There are indications that ability to participate in religious groups may help the elderly who have new disabilities in their recovery.

In an earlier study, Idler and Kasl (1992) addressed the relationships between religion, depression, disability, and the timing of death. The results were consistent with their later research findings that religion was a source of comfort for those with disability. Additionally, religion provided protective measures against disability and depression. Public religiosity had a stronger inverse relationship with depression and disability than did private religiosity. An interesting aspect of this study was the inclusion of the timing of death as a variable. Their results found that both Christians and Jews had fewer deaths in the month prior to religious holidays than in the month following. This suggests that meaningful religious events provide a protective measure for those who are religious.

Idler (1995) looked specifically at the spiritual aspects of religiosity in an article on nonphysical senses of self (spirituality). She reviewed three models that attempted to explain the relationship between religion and health. The first model was based of the work of Durkheim and suggested that religion, or religious activity, provided a protective buffer against health problems. The second model predicted an inverse relationship between religion and health due to people turning to religion in times of poor health. The final model predicted a complex relationship between religion and health. The results supported the third model. Idler found that disabled people were more likely to turn to religion in times of trouble but that several aspects of this religiosity were beneficial for health. Particularly, the results suggested a positive relationship between nonphysical sense of self (spirituality) and better subjective ratings of health. She explained these results suggest that, when physical health is deteriorating, individuals may benefit from focusing on the nonphysical aspects of the self that are not affected by the deteriorating physical body.

Koenig (as cited in Marwick, 1995) suggested that many of the surveys of the older population indicate that they are more religious than the younger generation. Fifty percent of the elderly attend church at least once a week. Koenig studied older people with disabling disorders such as diabetes and heart disease and developed a construct of religious coping. The study suggested that people who scored high in religious coping were less likely to become depressed. He defined religious coping as the use of prayer, Bible reading, and faith in God. Participants in the study were able to use this ability to deal with their stress.

Spirituality and Healing

It was mentioned earlier in this chapter that various cultures have had many kinds of spiritual healers through the ages. In today's world, faith healing is common to many cultures, and studies are being conducted with healers from other cultures. Targ carried out one study at California Pacific Medical Center in San Francisco (as cited in Wallis & McDowell, 1996). The study consisted of randomly selected AIDS patients. Half of them were prayed for and half were not. None knew which group they were in. Twenty faith healers were asked to participate in the study. The faith healers were not acquainted with the persons they prayed for during the study. They received photographs of the patients and their first names and were asked to pray for them at least one hour a day for a 10-week period. Targ was encouraged by the results of even this small study and thought it warranted conducting a larger study.

Krippner and Villoldo (1987) observed and describe some of the healers and their performances. The healers they interviewed were from the Philippines, Brazil, and the United States. After observing the healers and their paranormal skills, Krippner and Villoldo noted:

> It is my suspicion that much of the "healing" that occurs is "self-healing," inspired by the "healer's" pyrotechnical displays and "I guessed that even fraudulent "healers" could bring about "healing" in much the same way that a physician administers a sugar pill when the patient's complaint appears to be psychosomatic. In other words, the "placebo effect," which accounts for a sizeable proportion of "cures" in Western medicine, may also apply to both psychic and pseudopsychic "healing." (p. 232)

When talking with the authors, some of the healers stated their healing was not "psychic" but "spiritual." The authors suggested that scientific research needed to be done with appropriate experimental design and safeguards to test the truth of the healing. These authors are in agreement with others who believe that research regarding religion and health should be carried out using stronger scientific guidelines utilizing specific aspects of religious life such as prayer, faith, Bible reading, and church attendance.

Krause, Ellison, and Wulff (1998) reported an interaction between church-based emotional support and psychological well-being. The sample was comprised of clergy, elders, and lay-members of the Presbyterian Church in the United States. This is one of the few studies in the field of religion that considered the health and well-being of clergy, elders, and church leaders. The findings suggest that Presbyterian Church members believe that their participation in church activities has some effect on their well-being. The clergy reported fewer benefits than did the church members. This may be due to the fact that they do not receive the same emotional support as the members. These results suggest the church may need to find a better method of emotional support for its professional staff. Although this study was limited to the Presbyterian Church, it is likely representative of many other denominations. The clergy seem to provide acceptable emotional support to the church members; denominational leaders might find ways to offer that same support to the clergy.

Lee and Balswick (1989), in their book *Life in a Glass House: The Minister's Family in Its Unique Social Context,* review the many additional stressors that clergy must deal with in congregational life. It appears that most clergy do not look at their local church for social and emotional support. It may be that clergy will need to organize themselves to meet such needs. If spirituality has a positive relationship to health, the benefits accrued by members are not being supplied to those who supply it to others.

Health and healing is an important theme among church and religious groups in America. Many persons hold holiness, spiritual growth, salvation, emotional and physical health, and well-being as interwoven concepts. The words *healing, holiness, wholeness,* and *health* are all derivatives of the same Greek word, from which we get the concept of *holistic.* Several religious groups promoting the spiritual healing movement are eclectic in practice. They have borrowed healing practices and rituals from other cultures as well as various Western traditions. Some of these groups view medicine as inadequate and consider some social roles such as the "macho" male, the "women's place," and "successful doctor" to be among the causes of illness.

Many mainstream church denominations practice healing through anointing with oil, the laying on of hands, prayer meetings, and other rituals specifically designed for healing services. Radio and television are replete with clergy who consider themselves anointed with healing power and have amassed large followings of believers. Some extend their abilities to a handkerchief or a hand placed on the radio or television set. The impact of this phenomenon cannot be ignored when looking at the role of religious life, belief, spirituality, religious symbols, and rituals in healing.

SPIRITUALITY AND WELL-BEING

The concept of psychological well-being, as previously discussed, is one for which there is not much consensus in the mental health field. Throughout the history of mental health, there has been a much greater focus on pathology than on well-being. Often well-being has been assumed to be simply the lack of pathology. The authors have already addressed issues pertaining to the multidimensional conception of well-being that includes positive affect, negative affect, and life satisfaction.

Before discussing well-being, we need to discuss the approach to well-being taken in this chapter and its limitations. Well-being is used as a broad conceptual construct that encapsulates many other constructs, including happiness, lack of significant psychopathology, and life satisfaction. Many of the constructs used in psychological research on spirituality and well-being focus on the subconstructs, which may not utilize this same language. The discussion in this chapter will focus more on the subconstructs; however, conceptually we will point back to the larger construct of well-being.

Pargament (2002), whose research on faith and coping is reviewed below, suggested five conclusions regarding the relationship between religion and well-being based on his review of current empirical literature. First, Pargament noted some forms of religion are more helpful than others. Research is relatively consistent in support of a positive relationship between well-being and internalized, intrinsically motivated religion based on a secure relationship with God. However, religion that is imposed, unexamined, and reflective of a tenuous relationship with God is consistently negatively related to well-being. Second, Pargament presented evidence of advantages and disadvantages to controversial forms of religion. Specifically, fundamentalism was linked to increased prejudice but also to increased well-being. Pargament's third conclusion regarding the relationship between religion and well-being suggested that religion is most helpful to socially marginalized groups. This finding is likely related to the social support that comes from belonging to religious congregations and the positive benefits of participating in religious services mentioned earlier in this chapter. Fourth, religious beliefs appeared to be particularly helpful in stressful situations. Finally, Pargament noted that the efficacy of religion, in regard to well-being, is tied to the degree to which it is integrated into an individual's life. Individuals who have better-integrated religious beliefs are more likely to have greater well-being.

Koenig et al. (2001) found 100 articles that addressed the relationship of religion and well-being. Seventy-nine of the 100 articles found a positive association between religion and well-being, 13 found no relationship, 7 found a complex relationship, and 1 found a negative relationship. Koenig and colleagues pointed out that much of the research that did not find a positive relationship demonstrated poor research designs and contained small samples. This is an improvement from an earlier meta-analysis conducted by Bergin (1983), who found that 47 percent of the studies reviewed discovered a positive relationship between religion and mental health, 30 percent found no relationship, and 23 percent found a negative relationship. The different findings of these analyses may be accounted for by improvement in research methods, improved measures, and studies conducted with larger sample sizes. Additionally, Bergin's concept of mental health was broader than the conceptualization of well-being suggested by Koenig and colleagues.

Ellison (1991) looked at the relationship between religious involvement and well-being. The results indicated a positive relationship between religiosity and well-being. Several aspects of this research make it particularly interesting. The significant relationship between religion and well-being remained after controlling for a broad range of mediating variables. Ellison suggests that this indicates a directional relationship between religious belief and well-being that cannot be accounted for by the protective behavioral aspects of being religious (promoting healthy behaviors, social support, etc.). Ellison also found that spirituality may act as a buffer to stress or trauma. A final interesting aspect of this study was that, as religiosity increased with age, so did life satisfaction—but not happiness.

In a particularly well-designed study, Levin and Chatters (1998) looked at three ways to measure religion and religion's connection to health and well-being. While controlling for several potential confounding variables, they developed a structural equation model that predicted subjective religiosity, nonorganized or private religiosity, and organized religiosity would have a positive effect on health and well-being. They found a small but consistent positive relationship between religion and health and well-being. The relationship was stronger with organized religion than with subjective or private religiosity.

As discussed earlier, spirituality is a primary source from which people derive meaning for their lives. Compton (2000) found that meaning was one of the strongest predictors of various measures of well-being when compared to self-esteem, locus of control, optimism, and social support. Chamberlain and Zika (1988) found meaning to be a primary moderator in the relationship between religion and well-being for women. They used three measures of meaning, three measures of well-being, and a single measure of religiosity. They found that religion had a small, significant relationship with well-being. However, after controlling for meaning, the relationship became insignificant for two of the three measures of meaning. This suggests that meaning may be the primary means through which religion impacts well-being.

The indication that meaning is an important component of the relationship between spirituality and well-being is quite significant. It suggests that, for religion to be beneficial to individuals, it must provide some meaning for them. A research study by Hoffman and Whitmire (2002), which examined individual's response to the terrorist attacks on September 11, 2001, supports the hypothesis that meaning is an important mediator. They found that people who were able to find "meaning that went beyond the individual" showed the highest levels of stress-related growth. The research further suggested that stress-related growth was primarily associated with relationships with God and other people.

A similar study by Shaw, Joseph, and Linley (2005) supported the findings that religion and spirituality can assist people in working through traumatic events if they are able to maintain faith. They summarize their findings as follows:

> what the evidence shows is that religious and spiritual beliefs and behaviours can develop through the experience of traumatic events, that religious and spiritual beliefs can be helpful to people in their psychological recovery, and in their personal development and growth following trauma. For some, pre-existing religious and spiritual beliefs can be destroyed through the experience of trauma. (p. 6)

These studies suggest a complicated relationship between trauma, stress, spirituality, and well-being. Trauma appears to be able to challenge faith or provide a stimulus for spiritual growth. However, as Moriarty (2006) points out, traumatic events also can cause distortions in religious beliefs, thereby having a negative impact on some aspects of psychological well-being. Because the interaction between these variables is complex, it is hard to measure with traditional approaches to psychological research and also difficult for clinicians to treat without specialized training sensitive to these complex relationships.

Koenig, Kvale, and Ferrel (1988) included a measure of intrinsic religiosity when looking at the relationship between religion and well-being. This research suggested that intrinsic religiosity and organized religion have a positive relationship with well-being. Nonorganized religion was not as closely related to well-being. Intrinsic religiosity can be defined "as a meaning-endowing framework in terms of which all of life is understood" (Donahue, 1985, p. 400). Extrinsic religiosity, on the other hand, can be defined as "the religion of comfort and social convention, a self-serving, instrumental approach shaped to suit oneself" (Donahue, 1985, p. 400). Again, it can be noted that the differences between intrinsic and extrinsic religiosity are mainly in terms of the meaning dimension. Intrinsic religiosity can be seen as religion providing a meaning inherent in itself. Extrinsic religiosity may afford meaning, but it does so through associated aspects of religion instead of through religion itself.

In an investigation of well-being among three religious groups (Christian charismatic, New Age groups, and other religious groups), Glik (1990) found a positive relationship between religiosity and well-being. She predicted an inverse relationship between religiosity and well-being due to people turning to religion during times of high distress. The results partially confirmed this hypothesis. Whereas there was a positive relationship between religion and well-being in general, there was a negative relationship with certain aspects of religiosity:

> Ideational Beliefs, Mysticism, and Salience of Religion represent certain features of religiosity, lined to psychological states of healing adherents. Use of these measures provided evidence that extreme or intense religiosity may correlate negatively with some mental health indicators, thus demonstrating the differential effects that religious beliefs can have on mental well-being within different religious contexts. (Glik, 1990, p. 173)

These results allude to the importance of not consolidating all types of spirituality together into a single construct.

Spirituality and Specific Aspects of Well-Being

A generalized relationship between spirituality and psychological health is supported fairly consistently, as illustrated above. However, a more important question lies in what forms of spirituality are related to what aspects of positive *and* negative psychological health.

It is interesting to pay attention to distinctions in the various relationships between constructs within the multidimensional model of well-being. For example, Koenig, McCullough, and Larson's (2001) review of the literature shows that the connection between depression and spirituality is much less consistent than the relationship just discussed between spirituality and well-being. There may be a variety of explanations for this distinction. First, it is possible that the relationship between spirituality and depression is more complex than the relationship between spirituality and the more general construct of well-being. Second, because depression is a more precise construct than well-being, it is possible that the research has thus far been unsuccessful in teasing out the specifics of the relationship. Third, it is possible that spirituality and religion play a stronger role in promoting well-being than in protecting from pathology.

A fourth approach may suggest that religion and psychology frequently focus on different ideologies of mental health. While psychology tends to focus on the lack of symptoms and the presence of happiness, religion and spirituality stress the existential nature of all emotions. The shift to well-being (positive affect, negative affect, and life satisfaction) as the indicator of mental health represents a different paradigm than what is frequently used in psychology today. This approach implicitly states that both positive and negative emotions are part of our existential nature, which is at its core spiritual, and thus both need to be embraced. This shift in how mental health is operationally defined has important implications for future research.

Gartner (1996) reviewed the literature on religion's association to several aspects of mental and physical health. He reports that several factors tend to be positively associated with being religious, including physical health, mortality, suicide, drug use, alcohol abuse, delinquency, divorce, marital satisfaction, well-being, and depression. Several factors tend to have ambiguous or complex associations with religion, including health, anxiety, psychosis, self-esteem, sexual disorders, intelligence, and prejudice. Finally, he reports authoritarianism, dogmatism, suggestibility, dependency, self-actualization, and temporal lobe epilepsy are aspects of pathology that tend to be associated with religion.

Koenig et al. (2001) found that two religious groups are more susceptible to depression. First, those who describe themselves as nonreligious are at greater risk for depression. The second and more controversial group is those affiliated with the Jewish religion. The many attempts to explain why this population may be more prone to depression have included social, historical, and cultural explanations. Further research needs to better address these differences. However, given that much of this research has evolved over a time period in which the people of Jewish faith and cultural background have been grossly misunderstood and mistreated, it is important to be cautious about any interpretations of this faith tradition as being unhealthy. A look at the history of psychology reveals many similar interpretations that have been used to discriminate against a group of people.

Religious orientation appears to play a primary role in the relationship between religion and depression (Koenig et al., 2001; Parks & Murgatroyd, 1998). Koenig and colleagues have reported two connected trends in the literature regarding these constructs. Extrinsic religiosity appears to have an inverse relationship with depression, which suggests that people who use religion for their own self-interest or personal gain have a higher likelihood of depression. Conversely, those with intrinsic religious faith are less likely to be depressed.

In one particularly well designed study, Parks and Murgatroyd (1998) studied the relationship between spiritual orientation and depression in a sample of Korean Americans. Consistent with the trend previously noted, they found that extrinsically religious Korean Americans were more likely to be depressed. Additionally, they found that divorce, lower levels of education, and unemployment were strong predictors of depression for this population. They further discovered a strong relationship between extrinsic religiosity and depression that remained significant even after controlling for divorce, education level, and employment status. This study is particularly important because it extends findings to different cultures. Most current literature has examined samples that have been primarily white or African American.

Several studies have suggested that spirituality can protect against depression during times of increased stress (Fehring, Brennan, & Keller, 1987; Young, Cashwell, & Shcherbakova, 2000) and may even help some people grow through stressful times (Hoffman & Whitmire, 2002). Young and colleagues found that negative life experiences were associated with increases in depression and anxiety. Spirituality was a significant moderator between negative life events and depression, but not for anxiety. Thus, spirituality may help people better cope with some aspects of stressful events. Fehring and colleagues (1987) looked at depression and spiritual well-being during the transition to college. They found that the increase in depression during the transition to college was tempered by spiritual well-being. Fehring et al. used the Spiritual Well-Being Scale, which defines spiritual well-being as the cumulative scores of the existential well-being and religious well-being subscales. When taking the subscales into account, the relationship between religious well-being was no longer significant, while existential well-being remained significant. This suggests that certain aspects of spirituality provide the protective effects.

Several studies have looked at religion, loneliness, and well-being (Frankel & Hewitt, 1994; Schwab & Petersen, 1990; Stokes, 1985). Benson and Spilka (1973) found that individuals who perceive God as "angry and punishing" have negative feelings toward God and are more likely to feel lonely and have lower self-esteem. The individuals who have a positive attitude regarding God and see God as "loving and caring" are likely to have a better overall well-being and report higher self-esteem. These findings were consistent between the college population and an older adult population.

Faith and Coping

The concept of faith and coping received increased attention over the past ten years. A discussion of faith and coping adds an important, new level to the discussion thus far through its connection to both physical and mental health. Kenneth Pargament is one of the premiere leaders in research in the area of faith and coping and has strongly argued for a multidimensional approach to religious coping (Pargament, 1996; Pargament, 1997; Pargament & Ishler, 1994; Pargament & Olsen, 1992; Pargament et al., 1988; Pargament, Smith, Koenig, & Perez, 1998). Pargament et al. (1998) report a general trend that religious coping has beneficial functioning for mental and physical health. This was supported in a recent meta-analysis that revealed positive religious coping to be associated consistently with psychological health, while negative spiritual coping was associated with poorer psychological health (Ano & Vasconcellos, 2005).

This relationship, however, has often been found to be small and has been inconsistent in the research. Pargament and his colleagues argue that this is due, in part, to attempts to measure multidimensional, complex constructs in a global, unitary construct. Research in the faith and coping arena has begun to change this and move toward research that respects the complexity of these constructs. Furthermore, Pargament's arguments provide a good model to apply to other religious and mental health constructs that are not valued in their complexity.

Koenig, George, and Siegler (1988) looked at the use of coping strategies in an older adult population. They found religious coping skills to be the most frequently used of all coping skills followed by focusing attention elsewhere, "just accepting" the problem, and seeking support from family or friends. Pargament and Ishler (1994) further put the frequency of religious coping to the test. Most of the previous studies looking at the frequency of religious coping were retrospective appraisals of the frequency of religious coping skills. Pargament and Ishler looked at coping skills used during the 1990–1991 Gulf War. and found that religious coping skills were frequently used during the time of crises. Later research by Pargament et al. (1998) found that religious coping was also employed during the Oklahoma City bombings, by college students having a traumatic experience, and by hospital patients suffering from physical illness.

Religious and nonreligious coping skills do not appear to be completely independent from each other. Pargament and Ishler (1994) found a small, consistent relationship between religious and nonreligious forms of coping. This suggests that, while religious and nonreligious coping skills frequently may be used in conjunction with one another, they both contribute independently to aspects of dealing with the distress.

Research has provided conflicting results on the consistency of the use and effectiveness of coping skills across different times and situations (Maynard, Gorsuch, & Bjork, 2001; Pargament & Olsen, 1992; Schaefer & Gorsuch, 1991, 1993). Pargament et al. (1998) found that religious and nonreligious coping were both related to poorer levels of health. The authors interpreted this finding to mean that it is likely that people with poorer health are more likely to use coping skills in general, and religious coping skills in particular. The results do not necessarily indicate that religious coping negatively influences health. It does provide some initial evidence for the bidirectionality of the relationship between religion and health that will be discussed later in the chapter.

Personality variables also appear to play a role in religious coping. Different religious orientations (or motivations for religion) and different beliefs about

God influence preference for religious coping styles (Pargament & Olsen, 1992; Schaefer & Gorsuch, 1991, 1993). Pargament and Olsen (1992) looked at religious coping variables associated with intrinsic, extrinsic, and quest religious orientations. Intrinsic religiousness with a spiritual end or purpose is primarily associated with seeking God. People with this religious orientation tend to perceive negative life events as a spiritual threat, but they also see the event as an opportunity for growth. Intrinsic religiosity has been found to be associated generally with a collaborative or deferring coping style (Pargament et al., 1988; Schaefer & Gorsuch, 1991). A collaborative coping style is one in which the people see themselves as working with God. People who use a deferring coping style tend to rely on God primarily to resolve or deal with the situation.

Extrinsic religious orientation is generally associated with a self-directed coping style in which people rely solely on themselves to deal with stressful situations (Pargament et al., 1988; Schaefer & Gorsuch, 1991). Pargament and Olsen (1992) additionally found that people with this religious orientation tended to seek self-development as the end purpose of dealing with a negative life event. However, they did not see the negative life event as an opportunity to grow as did those with an intrinsic religious orientation. Extrinsic religiosity was associated with higher levels of distress. Individuals with high extrinsic religiosity were more likely to see negative life events as out of their control. Their religious coping often focused on religious action such as participating in good deeds or pleading to God for help.

The quest religious orientation was associated with viewing negative life events as having a spiritual purpose. However, this purpose was primarily searching for meaning (Pargament & Olsen, 1992). This is contrasted with intrinsically religious people, who also view these events as having a spiritual focus, but they focus on searching for God rather than meaning. People with the quest orientation's response of perceiving the negative life event as a spiritual threat and an opportunity to grow was similar to those with intrinsic religious faith. The quest orientation's religious coping was directed toward doing good deeds and voicing discontent with God.

Religious orientation has important implications for spiritual coping, well-being, and physical health as demonstrated by this review of the research and reviews conducted by others (Pargament, 2002). However, it is not the only dimensional aspect of religiosity that has implications for health and well-being. Schaefer and Gorsuch (1991) examined the influence of specific beliefs about God and their association to psychological adjustment. They found that seeing God as loving and benevolent was associated with lower levels of trait anxiety, and views of God as being impersonal and unpredictable were associated with higher levels of anxiety. Interestingly, views of God as wrathful were not significantly associated with anxiety. These results are consistent with the findings of Maynard et al. (2001), who looked at religious coping style, God-concept (cognitive view of God), and personal religious variables. They found that a person's view of God influences his or her religious coping style. Thus, religious orientation's association with well-being depend on which beliefs are intrinsically incorporated (Hathaway & Pargament, 1990). Religious orientation has earned a position of respect in the psychology of religion. However, it must not be the only multidimensional variable considered when attempting to understand the complexity of religion and spirituality.

Hathaway and Pargament (1990) examined the relationship between intrinsic religious faith, religious coping, and psychosocial competency while controlling for potential response bias. Critics have argued that religious people may tend to answer in accordance with what is deemed socially appropriate (social desirability) and may endorse religious items in a positive manner regardless of the validity of this response (indiscriminate proreligiousness). The results discovered by Hathaway and Pargament suggest that social desirability and indiscriminate proreligiousness do not contribute significant response bias to religious research. Additionally, they found the relationship between intrinsic religiosity and competency to be partially mediated by a person's religious coping style. This supports the hypotheses that the relationships between intrinsic religion, well-being, and health are partially mediated by the type of intrinsic faith.

Larson and Larson's (2003) review of the literature on spiritual/religious coping led them to conclude that there is the potential for both positive and negative effects of spiritual/religious coping. They note that studies that have investigated spiritual/religious coping and well-being suggest a large proportion of mental health clients turn to their religious/spiritual community and to their relationship with God or a higher power to help them cope with their illness. Often individuals report that relying on their spiritual or religious beliefs provided a sense of comfort, hope, belonging, and a feeling of being loved. However, Larson and Larson note that sometimes an individual's spiritual/religious beliefs led to a sense of guilt, condemnation, or abandonment. Other times individuals misuse their spirituality/religion for avoidance.

MODELS OF THE RELATIONSHIP BETWEEN SPIRITUALITY, HEALTH, AND WELL-BEING

A review of the literature of spirituality, health, and well-being reveals at least four implicit models to explain their relationship. Model 1 suggests that spirituality and religion have a positive impact on physical health as mediated by well-being. In other words, it is proposed that religion has a direct impact on improving well-being, but not on physical health. Well-being and various aspects of mental health have gained a great deal of acceptance as having a positive influence on physical health. Through improving mental health, religion may have an indirect role in improving physical health. Within this model are two variations. The first variation, represented in Figure 1, purports that spirituality's effects on well-being are moderated by certain aspects of organized religious activity (ORA) and/or nonorganized religious activity (NRA) in addition to other religious variables. It denies spirituality having any direct effects on well-being. The categories (ORA, NRA, and other religious variables) are presented as basic classifications of the various moderating aspects of religion identified by different theorists. The second variation of Model 1, represented in Figure 2, maintains that spirituality has direct, positive effects on well-being in addition to the moderating effects of the other spirituality variables. However, this model seems unlikely in light of the research in this area. Comprehensive reviews of the literature reveal that the relationship between religion and health tends to be consistent even when the relationship between religion and well-being is not (Bergin, 1983; Koenig et al., 2001; McFadden, 1995).

Model 2 suggests that religion and religious behavior have a direct relationship with physical health, but not with well-being. Health, in turn, influences well-being. Thus, this model, represented in Figure 3, suggests that religion has a positive influence on health and an indirect relationship with well-being as mediated by physical health. Spirituality's effects on health have been pro-

Figure 1
An illustration of the first variation on Model 1, which that states that spirituality's effects on well-being are moderated by certain aspects of organized religious activity (ORA) and/or nonorganized religious activity (NRA) in addition to other religious variables. The arrows indicate the direction of the suggested relationship between constructs

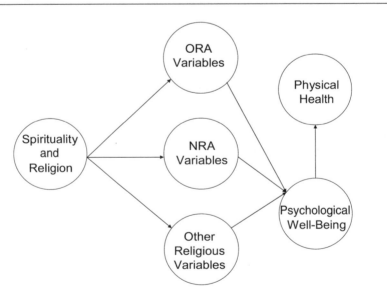

Figure 2
An illustration of the second variation on Model 1, which states that spirituality
has direct, positive effects on well-being in addition to the moderating effects
of the other spirituality variables. The only difference from the variation shown
in Figure 1 is the addition of a predicted direct effect of spirituality/religiosity
on well-being. ORA represents organized religious activity, and NRA represents
nonorganized religious activity. The arrows indicate the direction of the suggested
relationship between constructs

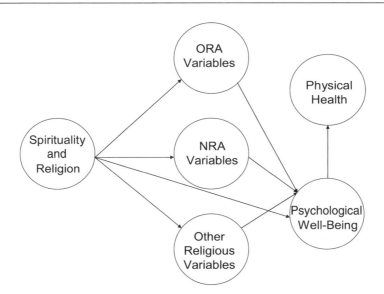

posed as being direct or moderated through other spirituality variables, as
illustrated in the first model. Levin and Chatters's (1998) structural model
provides an example of this model. A third model better represents the relationship. Model 3 proposes a complex relationship between religion, health,
and well-being. In this model, religion has direct and indirect effects on both
health and religion as well as indirect effects that may be moderated by the
other construct. This model is illustrated in Figure 4.

We propose a fourth, more complex model in which spirituality has both
direct and indirect effects on both health and well-being. Additionally, health
and well-being may directly and indirectly impact spirituality. The relationship
between physical health and well-being can better be seen in a web model in
which all constructs influence other constructs while also being influenced by
them. It would also be assumed that these relationships can be both positive
and negative at times. Model 4 is severely limited by the use of a unidimensional representation of the constructs of spirituality, health, and well-being.
This web model would be better represented by replacing the unidimensional
constructs with the more specific, discrete aspects of these constructs. However, for simplicity's sake, we illustrate the model as represented in Figure 5.

Figure 3
An illustration of Model 2, which states that religion has a positive influence on health and an indirect relationship with well-being as mediated by physical health. As with Model 2, some theorists would omit the line representing the direct effect of spirituality on health. ORA represents organized religious Activity, and NRA represents nonorganized religious activity. The arrows indicate the direction of the suggested relationship between constructs

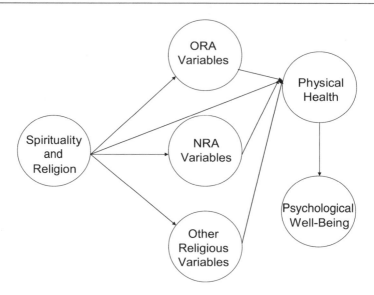

Since the original development of this model, Sperry, Hoffman, Cox, and Ervin-Cox (2006) proposed an update. The model presented above focuses on relationships between these constructs but does not address change. Sperry and colleagues propose that spirituality, or a spiritual longing, can activate a transformation process. Stated differently, spirituality can provide the impetus for making spiritual transformation, which will produce positive change outcomes in each of the constructs in the model displayed in Figure 5.

Many theorists and researchers have implied certain aspects represented as unique in the fourth model, however, few have made these assumptions implicitly known. It is important that these assumptions be made implicit in order to develop a sound theory. This theory then serves as the basis of future research models that can be tested. Koenig et al. (2001) have discussed the importance of clarifying distortions regarding the literature in this area of research. Implicitly identifying these assumptions is important in preventing and clarifying such assumptions. For example, while the bidirectional relationship between spirituality and mental health may be assumed in some research, these assumptions are made implicit. This can lead to interpretations of the literature as supporting a unidirectional relationship.

Figure 4

An illustration of Model 3, which states that religion has direct and indirect effects on both health and religion as well as indirect effects that may be moderated by the other construct. ORA represents organized religious activity, and NRA represents nonorganized religious activity. The arrows indicate the direction of the suggested relationship between constructs

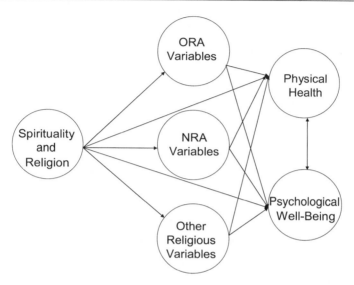

Figure 5

An illustration of Model 4, which states that spirituality has both direct and indirect effects on both health and well-being and that health and well-being may directly and indirectly impact spirituality. The relationship is assumed to be bidirectional in this model compared to the unidirectional predictions in previous models. ORA represents organized religious Activity, and NRA represents nonorganized religious activity. The arrows indicate the direction of the suggested relationship between constructs

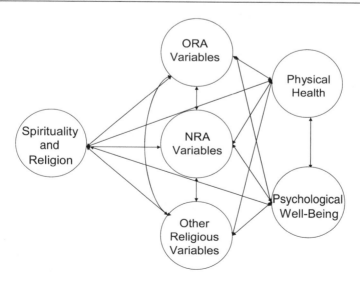

FUTURE DIRECTIONS FOR RESEARCH IN SPIRITUALITY AND HEALTH

The current research has only begun to understand the complex relationships between spirituality, health, and well-being. Given this, the most important direction for future research is developing a more comprehensive understanding of the multidimensional aspects of spirituality, health, and well-being. The complex relationships between these constructs may, at times, appear to be inconsistent or insignificant. At other times, they may appear so complex that any attempts at finding kernels of truth through research seem in vain. However, we remain optimistic that, although research will never be able to explain spirituality, we may be able to better utilize it as one of many approaches for seeking truth. More complex and rigorous research designs will be necessary to clarify the intricacies of these relationships and constructs if we are to accomplish this ambitious goal.

Religious orientation has received most of the research attention. Several important articles have reviewed research findings on religious orientation and provided a critical analysis of the construct (Donahue, 1985; Hunt & King, 1971; Kirkpatrick & Hood, 1990). Additional studies have associated intrinsic religiosity with better health and well-being outcomes than extrinsic religiosity. These findings demonstrate the importance of a multidimensional approach to religion. Religious orientation should maintain an essential place in the psychology of religion, but the manner in which it is used may need to evolve. When religious orientation is combined with measures of belief, the power of the construct may become more significant. For example, having a view of God as loving and forgiving may lack any power for a person's life if he or she is extrinsically religious. However, this same view of God will be of greater importance for a person with intrinsic faith. Religious orientation helps to clarify the understanding of how a person's belief is used in his or her life.

Koenig et al. (2001) discuss several areas of religiousness that continue to need exploration. These include religious orthodoxy, certainty of belief, religious affiliation and Christian denomination, levels of involvement in organized religion, aspects of private religiosity, subjective religiosity, religious commitment, spiritual well-being, religious and faith maturity, religious orientation, and religious coping. Several of these have been discussed in this article. The recent publication by Hill and Hood (1999), *Measures of Religiosity*, should facilitate accessibility to strong research tools.

More attention needs to be placed on translating theory and research into strategies for practice so that more people can reap the benefits from what we learn. Frequently, the only translation that occurs is through the popular media, which, as Koenig et al. (2001) point out, is not always accurate. Malony (1995) provides one of the better examples of this translation in his book entitled *The Psychology of Religion for Ministry*. This book attempts to translate a professional level of psychology in to terms usable by church and lay professionals.

CONCLUSION

The literature reviewed in this chapter demonstrates that spirituality and religion play an important role in health and well-being. In general, the majority of the research purports that spirituality and religion have a positive impact on health, though this is not always the case. It is becoming increasingly apparent that practitioners who want to take a holistic approach to treatment must consider religious and spiritual issues. Anything less is an incomplete psychology and a partial treatment. Although the current volume just scratches the surface of the literature exploring the relationship between spirituality, physical health, and well-being, many practical guides on how to integrate spirituality into practice exist (see Epstein, 1995; Leung & Hoffman, 2005; Miller, 1999; Moriarty, 2006; Richards & Bergin, 2005; Sperry & Shafranske, 2005; Tacey, 1997; 2004).

TOOL KIT FOR CHANGE

The training toolkit emphasizes the importance of the clinician's awareness of the relationship between religion/spirituality and psychological health. The several types of skills and knowledge discussed below are essential knowledge for clinicians working with religious and spiritual clients. The general skills and knowledge are important for all clinicians. The advanced skills and knowledge are important for people who specialize in working with religious and spiritual clients or who want to work more actively with religious issues in the therapy setting.

Role and Perspective of the Healthcare Professional

1. All major world religions, along with most other approaches to religiosity or spirituality, can be health-facilitating.
2. Practitioners must be aware of the potential negative influence of their own belief systems and biases toward other religious and spiritual perspectives.
3. While all practitioners should be open to exploring what spirituality means to the client, before using more active religious or spiritual interventions, practitioners should receive appropriate training and supervision.
4. Practitioners should consider ways in which religion and spirituality can be detrimental as well as beneficial. This should be explored with the client, but practitioners should avoid imposing their beliefs about what is health-facilitating and what is detrimental.
5. Consider collaboration with religious or spiritual professionals when appropriate.

Role and Perspective of the Participant

1. Religious and spiritual beliefs are an important part of health and can be included in your treatment.
2. You have the right to have your religious and spiritual beliefs respected, even if they are different from the therapist's.
3. It is important to talk about both positive and negative aspects of your beliefs.
4. You may discover new information about how your beliefs are affecting you, both positively and negatively. It is important to remain open-minded to these discoveries.
5. If you are uncomfortable sharing your beliefs, it may be beneficial to discuss this with your mental health provider.

Interconnection: The Global Perspective

1. Various religious and spiritual perspectives have different viewpoints on what it means to be healthy and the role that spirituality plays in this process.
2. Spirituality is a normal part of the individual that cannot be separated from other dimensions of the self.

REFERENCES

Allport, G. (1958). *Nature of prejudice.* Garden City, NY: Doubleday Anchor Books.

American Psychiatric Association. (2000). *Diagnostic and statistical manual of mental disorders* (Text revision, 4th ed.). Washington, DC: Author.

Ano, G. G., & Vasconcellos, E. B. (2005). Religious coping and psychological adjustment to stress: A meta-analysis. *Journal of Clinical Psychology, 61,* 461–480.

Benson, H. (1996). *Timeless healing: The power and biology of belief.* New York: Simon & Schuster.

Benson, H. (1999, August). The power and biology of belief. Paper presented at the 1999 annual convention of the American Psychological Association, Boston, MA.

Benson, H., Dusek, J. A., Sherwood, J. B., Lam, P., Bethea, C. F., Carpenter, W., et al. (2006). Study of therapeutic effects of intercessory prayer (STEP) in cardiac bypass patients: A multicenter randomized trial of uncertainty and certainty of receiving intercessory prayer. *American Heart Journal, 151,* 934–942.

Benson, P., & Spilka, B. (1973). God image as a function of self-esteem and locus of control. *Journal for the Scientific Study of Religion, 12,* 297–310.

Bergin, A. E. (1983). Religiosity and mental health: A critical reevaluation and meta-analysis. *Professional Psychology: Research and Practice, 14,* 170–184.

Byrd, R. C. (1988). Positive therapeutic effects of intercessory prayer in a coronary care unit population. *Southern Medical Journal, 81,* 826–829.

Byrd, R. C., & Sherrill, J. I. (1995). The therapeutic effects of intercessory prayer. *Journal of Christian Nursing, 12,* 21–23.

Carlson, C. R., Bacaseta, P. E., & Simanton, D. A. (1988). A controlled evaluation of devotional meditation and progressive relaxation. *Journal of Psychology and Theology, 16,* 362–368.

Chamberlain, K., & Zika, S. (1988). Religiosity, life meaning and wellbeing: Some relationships in a sample of women. *Journal for the Scientific Study of Religion, 27,* 411–420.

Chamberlain, T. J., & Hall, C. A. (2000). *Realized religion.* Philadelphia: Templeton Foundation Press.

Chatters, L. M., Levin, J. S., & Ellison, C. G. (1998). Public health and health education in faith communities. *Health Education and Behavior, 25,* 689–699.

Christy, J. H. (1998). Prayer as medicine. *Forbes, 161*(6), 136–137.

Compton, W. C. (2000). Meaningfulness as a mediator of subjective well-being. *Psychological Reports, 87,* 156–160.

Donahue, M. J. (1985). Intrinsic and extrinsic religiousness: Review and meta-analysis. *Journal of Personality and Social Psychology, 48,* 400–419.

Easterbrook, G. (1999). Faith healers. *New Republic, 221,* 20–23.

Ellison, C. G. (1991). Religious involvement and subjective well-being. *Journal of Health and Social Behavior, 32,* 80–99.

Ellison, C. G., & Levin, J. S. (1998). The religion-health connection: Evidence, theory and future directions. *Health Education & Behavior, 25,* 700–720.

Epstein, M (1995). *Thoughts without a thinker: Psychotherapy from a Buddhist perspective.* New York: Basic Books.

Epstein, M. (2006, May). *From eros to enlightenment: Desire as the subject of meditative awareness.* Keynote address presented at the Buddhism and Psychotherapy Conference, Boulder, CO.

Faneuli, N. (1997). The spirituality of wellness. *American Fitness, 15,* 42–46.

Fehring, R. J., Brennan, P. F., & Keller, M. L. (1987). Psychological and spiritual well-being in college students. *Research in Nursing and Health, 10,* 391–398.

Frankel, B. G., & Hewitt, W. E. (1994). Religion and well-being among Canadian university students: The role of faith groups on campus. *Journal for the Scientific Study of Religion, 33,* 62–73.

Frankl, V. E. (1959). *Man's search for meaning.* New York: Washington Square Press.

Frankl, V. E. (2000). *Man's search for ultimate meaning.* Cambridge, MA: Perseus.

Gartner, J. (1996). Religious commitment, mental health, and prosocial behavior: A review of the empirical literature. In E. P. Shafranske (Ed.), *Religion and the clinical practice of psychology* (pp. 187–214). Washington, DC: American Psychological Association.

George, L. K., Ellison, C. G., & Larson, D. B. (2002). Explaining the relationships between religious involvement and health. *Psychological Inquiry, 13,* 190–200.

Glik, D. C. (1990). Participation in spiritual healing, religiosity, and mental health. *Sociological Inquiry, 60,* 158–176.

Grossman, P., Niemann, L., Schmidt, S., & Walach, H. (2004). Mindfulness-based stress reduction and health benefits: A meta-analysis. *Journal of Psychosomatic Research, 57,* 35–43.

Harrison, L. J., Manocha, R, & Rubia, K. (2004). Sahaja yoga meditation as a family treatment programme for children with attention deficit-hyperactivity disorder. *Clinical Child Psychology and Psychiatry, 9,* 479–497.

Hathaway, W. L., & Pargament, K. I. (1990). Intrinsic religiousness, religious coping, and psychosocial competence: A covariance structure analysis. *Journal for the Scientific Study of Religion, 29,* 423–441.

Hawks, S. (1994). Spiritual health: Definition and theory. *Wellness Perspectives, 10,* 3–13.

Hill, P., & Hood, R. W., Jr. (Eds.). (1999). *Measures of religiosity.* Birmingham, AL: Religious Education Press.

Hoffman, L., & Whitmire, A. J. (2002, June). *The relationship between approach to coping and stress related growth in response to the events of September 11, 2001.* Poster session presented at the annual convention of the American Psychological Society, New Orleans, LA.

Hunt, R. A., & King, M. B. (1971). The intrinsic-extrinsic concept: A review and evaluation. *Journal for the Scientific Study of Religion, 10,* 339–356.

Idler, E. L. (1995). Religion, health, and nonphysical senses of self. *Social Forces, 74,* 683–704.

Idler, E. L., & Kasl, S. V. (1992). Religion, disability, depression, and the timing of death. *American Journal of Sociology, 97,* 1052–1079.

Idler, E. L., & Kasl, S. V. (1997a). Religion among disabled and nondisabled persons I: Cross sectional patterns in health practices, social activities, and well-being. *Journal of Gerontology: Social Sciences, 52B,* S294–S305.

Idler, E. L., & Kasl, S. V. (1997b). Religion among disabled and nondisabled persons II: Attendance at religious services as a predictor of the course of disability. *Journal of Gerontology: Social Sciences, 52B,* S306–S316.

James, W. (1902/1958). *The varieties of religious experience.* New York: New American Library.

Kirkpatrick, L. A., & Hood, R. W., Jr. (1990). Intrinsic-extrinsic religious orientation: The boon or bane of contemporary psychology of religion. *Journal for the Scientific Study of Religion, 29,* 442–462.

Koenig, H. G. (1999). *The healing power of faith.* New York: Simon & Schuster.

Koenig, H. G., George, L. K., & Siegler, I. C. (1988). The use of religion and other emotion regulating coping strategies among older adults. *The Gerontologist, 28,* 303–310.

Koenig, H. G., Kvale, J. N., & Ferrel, C. (1988). Religion and well-being in later life. *The Gerontologist, 28,* 18–28.

Koenig, H. G., McCullough, M. E., & Larson, D. B. (2001). *Handbook of religion and health.* New York: Oxford University Press.

Krause, N., Ellison, C. G., & Wulff, K. M. (1998). Church-based emotional support, negative interaction, and psychological well-being: Findings from a national sample of Presbyterians. *Journal for the Scientific Study of Religion, 37,* 725–741.

Krippner, S., & Villoldo, A. (1987). *The realms of healing* (3rd ed.). Berkeley, CA: Celestial Arts.

Krucoff, M. W., Crater, S. W., & Lee, K. L. (2006). From efficacy to safety concerns: A STEP forward or a step back for clinical research and intercessory prayer?: The study of therapeutic effects of prayer (STEP). *American Heart Journal, 151,* 762–764.

Larson, D., & Larson, S. (1991). Religious commitment and health: Valuing the relationship. *Second Opinion, 17,* 27–40.

Larson, D., & Larson, S. (2003). Spirituality's potential relevance to physical and emotional health: A brief review of quantitative research. *Journal of Psychology and Theology, 31,* 37–51.

Lee, C., & Balswick, J. (1989). *Life in a glass house: The minister's family in its unique social context.* Grand Rapids, MI: Zondervan.

Leung, C., & Hoffman, L. (2005). Practical applications of spirituality to the practice of psychology. In R. H. Cox, B. Ervin-Cox, & L. Hoffman (Eds.), *Spirituality and psychological health* (pp. 262–283). Colorado Springs: Colorado School of Professional Psychology Press.

Levin, J. S., & Chatters, L. M. (1998). Religion, health, and psychological well-being in older adults: Findings from three national surveys. *Journal of Aging & Health, 10,* 504–531.

Levin, J. S., Taylor, R. J., & Chatters, L. M. (1994). Race and gender differences in religiosity among older adults: Findings from four national surveys. *Journal of Gerontology: Social Sciences, 49,* S137–S145.

Malony, H. N. (1995) *The psychology of religion for ministry.* New York: Paulist Press.

Marlatt, G. A., & Kristeller, J. L. (1999). Mindfulness and meditation. In W. R. Miller (Ed.), *Integrating spirituality into treatment: Resources for practitioners* (pp. 67–84). Washington, DC: American Psychological Association.

Marwick, C. (1995). Should physicians prescribe prayer for health? Spiritual aspects of well being considered. *Journal of the American Medical Association, 273,* 1561–1562.

Maslow, A. H. (1998). *Toward a psychology of being* (3rd ed.). New York: Wiley.

Maynard, E. A., Gorsuch, R. L., & Bjork, J. P. (2001). Religious coping style, concept of God, and personal religious variables in threat, loss, and challenge situations. *Journal for the Scientific Study of Religion, 40,* 65–74.

McCullough, M. E., Hoyt, W. T., Larson, D. B., Koenig, H. G., & Thoresen, C. (2000). Religious involvement and mortality: A meta-analytic review. *Health Psychology, 19,* 211–222.

McFadden, S. H. (1995). Religion and well-being in aging persons in an aging population. *Journal of Social Issues, 51,* 161–175.

McGuire, M. B. (1993). Health and spirituality as contemporary concerns. *Annals of the American Academy of Political & Social Science, 527,* 144–154.

Miller, W. R. (Ed.). (1999). *Integrating spirituality into treatment: Resources for practitioners.* Washington, DC: American Psychological Association.

Moriarty, G. (2006). *Pastoral care of depression: Helping clients heal their relationship with God.* New York: Haworth Pastoral Press.

Oman, D., & Reed, D. (1998). Religion and mortality among the community-dwelling elderly. *American Journal of Public Health, 88,* 1469–1475.

Pargament, K. I. (1996). Religious methods of coping: Resources for the conversation and transformation of significance. In E. P. Shafranske (Ed.), *Religion and the clinical practice of psychology* (pp. 215–239). Washington, DC: American Psychological Association.

Pargament, K. I. (1997). *The psychology of religion and coping: Theory, research, practice.* New York: Guilford Press.

Pargament, K. (2002). The bitter and the sweet: An evaluation of the costs and benefits of religiousness. *Psychological Inquiry, 13,* 168–181.

Pargament, K. I., & Ishler, K. (1994). Methods of religious coping with the gulf war: Cross sectional and longitudinal analyses. *Journal for the Scientific Study of Religion, 33,* 347–361.

Pargament, K. I., Kennell, J., Hathaway, W., Grevengoed, N., Newman, J., & Jones, W. (1988). Religion and the problem solving process: Three styles of coping. *Journal for the Scientific Study of Religion, 27,* 90–104.

Pargament, K. I., & Olsen, H. (1992). God help me (II): The relationship of religious coping orientations to religious coping with negative life events. *Journal for the Scientific Study of Religion, 31,* 504–513.

Pargament, K. I., Smith, B. W., Koenig, H. G., & Perez, L. (1998). Patterns of positive and negative religious coping with major life stressors. *Journal for the Scientific Study of Religion, 37,* 710–724.

Parks, H. S., & Murgatroyd, W. (1998). Relationship between intrinsic-extrinsic religious orientation and depressive symptoms in Korean Americans. *Counseling Psychology Quarterly, 11,* 315–324.

Plante, T. G., & Sherman, A. C. (Eds.). (2001). *Faith and health: Psychological perspectives.* New York: Guilford Press.

Poloma, M. M. (1993). The effects of prayer on mental well-being. *Second Opinion, 18,* 37–51.

Powell, L. H., Shahabi, L., & Thoresen, C. E. (2003) Religion and spirituality: Linkages to physical health. *American Psychologist, 58,* 36–52.

Richards, P. S., & Bergin, A. E. (2005). *A spiritual strategy for counseling and psychotherapy* (2nd ed.). Washington, DC: American Psychological Association.

Rippentrop, E. (2005). A review of the role of religion and spirituality in chronic pain populations. *Rehabilitation Psychology, 50,* 278–284.

Schaefer, C. A., & Gorsuch, R. L. (1991). Psychological adjustment and religiousness: The multivariate belief-motivation theory of religiousness. *Journal for the Scientific Study of Religion, 30,* 448–461.

Schaefer, C. A., & Gorsuch, R. L. (1993). Situational and personal variations in religious coping. *Journal for the Scientific Study of Religion, 32,* 136–147.

Schneider, K. J., & May, R. (1995). *The psychology of existence: An integrative, clinical perspective.* New York: McGraw-Hill.

Schwab, R., & Petersen, K. U. (1990). Religiousness: Its relation to loneliness, neuroticism, and subjective well-being. *Journal for the Scientific Study of Religion, 29,* 335–345.

Seeman, T. E., Dublin, L. F., & Seeman, M. (2003). Religiosity/spirituality and health: A critical review of the evidence for biological pathways. *American Psychologist, 58,* 53–63.

Shaw, A., Joseph, S., & Linley, P. A. (2005). Religion, spirituality, and posttraumatic growth: A systematic review. *Mental Health, Religion & Culture, 8,* 1–11.

Sperry, L., Hoffman, L., Cox, R. H., & Ervin-Cox, B. (2006). *Spirituality in achieving physical and psychological health and well-being: Theory, research, and low cost interventions.* Unpublished manuscript, Boca Raton, FL.

Sperry, L., & Shafranske, E. (Eds.). (2005). *Spiritually oriented psychotherapy.* Washington, DC: American Psychological Association.

Stokes, J. P. (1985). The relation of social network and individual difference variables to loneliness. *Journal of Personality and Social Psychology, 48,* 981–990.

Strawbridge, S. (1982). Althusser's theory of ideology and Durkheim's account of religion: An examination of some striking parallels. *Sociological Review, 30,* 125–140.

Tacey, D. J. (1997). *Remaking men: Jung, spirituality and social change.* New York: Routledge.

Tacey, D. J. (2004). *The spiritual revolution: The emergence of contemporary spirituality.* New York: Brunner-Routledge.

Teasdale, J. D., Segal, Z., & Williams, J.M.G. (1995). How does cognitive therapy prevent depressive relapse and why should attentional control (mindfulness) training help? *Behavior Research and Therapy, 33,* 25–39.

Tillich, P. (1957). *The dynamics of faith.* New York: Harper & Row.

Wallace, J. M., Jr., & Forman, T. A. (1998). Religion's role in promoting health and reducing risk among American youth. *Health Education & Behavior, 25,* 721–741.

Wallis, C., & McDowell, J. (1996). Faith & healing. *Time, 147*(26), 58–63.

Young, J. S., Cashwell, C. S., & Shcherbakova, J. (2000). The moderating relationship of spirituality on negative life events and psychological adjustment. *Counseling and Values, 45,* 49–57.

Chapter Seven

THE ROLE OF CLERGY AND CHAPLAINS IN HEALTHCARE

Bruce D. Feldstein, MD, Matthew Cowden, MDiv, MFA and Jennifer Block, MA

Spirituality is intrinsic to healthcare. The diversity of today's multicultural society is reflected in the healthcare setting with patients and families of many different religious and cultural backgrounds. The Joint Commission on the Accreditation of Healthcare Organizations (JCAHO) states that patients have a fundamental right to have their cultural, psychosocial, spiritual and personal values, beliefs, and preferences respected (JCAHO, 2006). It is the role of clergy and chaplains to respond to the spiritual concerns of patients, families, and staff, not only to fulfill the JCAHO mandate, but because it is good medicine and the right thing to do.

This first section of this chapter provides a general description of the role of clergy and chaplains in healthcare, beginning with an understanding of humans as spiritual beings, the relationship between spirituality and health, and the need for spiritual care. The next three sections are written from three points of view: that of a Jewish chaplain (Feldstein), a Christian minister (Cowden), and a Buddhist chaplain (Block).

CLERGY AND CHAPLAINS AS PROVIDERS OF SPIRITUAL CARE

Humans are spiritual beings. "Regardless of culture or creed, and whether one is religious or not, humans share basic spiritual...needs for love, faith, hope, virtue and beauty...which when unfulfilled can lead to significant spiritual suffering" (Bartel, 2004, p. 188).

Spirituality can be understood as the way one finds meaning, purpose, hope, connection, and inner peace; in relationship with oneself, with others, and with the transcendent, where the transcendent can be understood in different ways—as God, the Sacred, the Divine, Higher Power, Mystery, or that which is of ultimate meaning or highest value (Feldstein, 2001; VandeCreek & Burton, 2001). Spirituality deals with questions such as: Who am I? What do I love? How shall I live, knowing I will die? What is my gift to the family of the Earth? (Muller, 1996). What is the meaning of life? What will happen to me when I die? Why is there evil in the world? Why is there suffering? (Shih & Larson, 2006). Is there a God? Who, or what, is God for me?

In this view, spirituality is inclusive of religion as well as the "existential core human dimension" (Bergman, 2004), once the identified domain of humanistic psychologies. "Many people experience spirituality through religion; some through music, art or a connection with nature. Others find it in their values and principles" (American Academy of Family Physicians, 2001). Religion can be defined as an organized system of beliefs or attitudes, moral codes and values, practices, rituals, symbols, traditions, and institutions designed to: (a) facilitate closeness to the sacred or transcendent (God, higher power, or ultimate truth/reality) and (b) foster an understanding of one's relationship and responsibility to others in living together in a community (Koenig, McCullough, & Larson, 2001; *Religion,* 2006). In the United States, most people (97%) believe in God, and a significant number actively participate in a religious tradition (Anandarajah & Hight, 2001; Thiel & Robinson, 1997).

There is evidence in the medical literature of a strong relationship between spirituality and health. Numerous studies have noted a positive relationship between religious commitment and mental and physical health, and decreased overall mortality. This is associated with increased physiological and biochemical functioning, positive health behaviors, and social and community support (Anandarajah & Hight, 2001; Koenig et al., 2001). Spirituality can help people maintain health and cope with illness, trauma, loss, and life transitions. When facing a crisis, people often turn to their spirituality as a means of coping (Pargament, 1997). Spirituality also may have a negative impact on health to the extent that it promotes unhealthy beliefs about oneself and God (such as being undeserving or having inadequate faith), thus increasing the potential for psychological distress, which negatively impacts healing and survival. Shih and Larson (2006) observe: "Religion may [also] promulgate unhealthy practices such as avoiding or substituting religious ritual for traditional medical care including surgery, antibiotics, chemotherapy, blood transfusion and immunizations" (p. 116).

As a result of illness or trauma and its treatment, including hospitalization, patients, families, and healthcare providers can experience various states of suffering (Katonah, 1985), such as alienation, anger, anxiety and fear, guilt, regret, indecision, confusion, questioning, sadness, hopelessness, despair, anguish, turmoil, violation, unfairness, and grief. They also can experience profound blessing, awe, appreciation, gratitude, vision, meaning, inspiration, a sense of connection, belonging, or new beginning.

Spiritual care involves recognizing and responding to these multiple expressions. Spiritual care is everyone's responsibility—patients, their family and friends, members of the healthcare team including hospital chaplains, as well as clergy (Mohrmann, 1995). There are many crucial moments in healthcare that call for a spiritual presence and response—a listening ear, a gentle touch, a compassionate word, and sometimes a blessing or prayer. Sometimes the physician or nurse or other healthcare providers are the ones who are available. It is not only appropriate, but sometimes necessary for them to provide a spiritual response (Feldstein, 2001). Patients often desire that their physicians address their spiritual issues and distress (Anandarajah & Hight, 2001; Shih & Larson, 2006). And yet, while spiritual care may be everyone's job, it is not everyone's primary role. Furthermore, physicians, nurses, and other healthcare providers can be overwhelmed and unprepared to respond to these needs.

In the healthcare setting, it is the primary role of the healthcare chaplain to provide for spiritual care. The role and importance of professional chaplains have been clearly delineated in an article written by representatives of the major chaplaincy organizations (VandeCreek & Burton, 2001):

- The Association of Clinical Pastoral Education
- The Association of Professional Chaplains
- The Canadian Association for Pastoral Practice and Education
- The National Association of Catholic Chaplains
- The National Association of Jewish Chaplains

Healthcare chaplains are clergy and lay professionals. They come from all faiths and provide spiritual care "in a variety of settings including: acute care, long-term care and assisted living, rehabilitation, mental health, outpatient, addiction treatment...hospice and palliative care" (VandeCreek & Burton, 2001). Chaplains also work in military, prison, business, and law enforcement settings.

Professional training for hospital chaplains usually includes clinical pastoral education (CPE). As the Association for Clinical Pastoral Education (ACPE) describes, CPE brings students and spiritual care providers of all faiths (pastors, priests, rabbis, imams, and others) into supervised encounters with persons in crisis. It was begun in the United States in 1925 as a form of clinical and theological education and takes place in the variety of settings where chaplains serve. The experiential learning that is CPE takes place through the practice of ministry and through reflection with supervisors and peers. It includes an in-depth study of "both the people who receive care as well as a study of ourselves, the givers of care" (ACPE, 2006).

Healthcare chaplains operate within the current standards of medical practice and are considered integral members of the healthcare team. Professional healthcare chaplains bring to patients, families, and staff essential interpersonal and interprofessional skills, relationships, and points of view not otherwise available in healthcare. The chaplain's role as a member of the healthcare team includes addressing traditional religious needs of patients such as prayer, worship, and rituals as well as spiritual issues relating to death, ethical consultation, patient advocacy, community outreach, crisis intervention, and advanced directives. ("The Chaplain-Physician Relationship," 1991; Flannelly, Handzo, Galek, Weaver, & Overvold, 2006; Hart & Matorin, 1997; Thiel & Robinson; 1997; VandeCreek, 1997).

In attending to patients, families, and caregivers in the healthcare setting, chaplains adapt their ministry to meet the needs of patients, families, and caregivers whose religious and cultural understandings and expectations may be different from that of the chaplain. As theologically and clinically trained clergy or laypeople, their work reflects:

- sensitivity to multicultural and multifaith realities without proselytizing
- respect for patients' spiritual or religious preferences
- understanding of the impact of illness on individuals and their caregivers
- knowledge of healthcare organizational structure and dynamics
- accountability as part of the professional patient care team
- accountability to their faith group (VandeCreek & Burton, 2001).

Spiritual care differs from counseling, psychotherapy, or advice from other professionals or friends because of its acknowledged spiritual component (Brener, 2005, p. 125). Spiritual care can be visualized as a triangular relationship between caregiver, recipient, and the transcendent. In providing spiritual care, the chaplain aims to meet the person being served in their world as it is for him or her. "Who are you? Where are you from? What are your concerns? What beliefs, values, practices, relationships and community are important to you? Who is God for you? How might I as a chaplain serve you?" By making use of basic spiritual skills of listening, assessing, accompanying, supporting, and guiding, and by using appropriate religious dialogue and ritual, the chaplain provides presence, conversation, action, and prayer to provide comfort and healing (Feldstein, 2002).

THE ROLE OF A JEWISH CHAPLAIN

In the Jewish tradition, from ancient times to the present it has been well understood that "a person's health is at least as much effected by the availability of health care and by the spiritual support provided to that person as by the direct application of medical techniques" (Dorff, 1998, p. 279).

The role of the Jewish chaplain in visiting the sick and providing spiritual care is based on Jewish teachings that have developed over the millennia, beginning with those in the Torah, the first five books of the Bible and the ultimate source of the law on which Jews rely for moral guidance (Handler, Hetherington, & Kelman, 1997). Through commentary and interpretation over time, Jewish tradition has evolved rich and practical laws and lore about the sacred religious obligation of visiting the sick. In Hebrew, a sacred religious obligation is called a *mitzvah*. The *mitzvah* of visiting the sick, of *bikur cholim*, is required of all Jews (Friedman, 2005). This *mitzvah* provides for visiting the sick of all faiths (Ozarowski, 1995, p. 33).

Jewish chaplains include rabbis, cantors, and lay professionals (National Association for Jewish Chaplains, 2006). Jewish chaplains are called on to take care of patients of all faiths as well as those who are Jewish. Like professional chaplains from all faiths, Jewish chaplains blend the general skills of spiritual care with religious and cultural understanding and practice in a way that is in keeping with: (a) the goals of medicine, to cure sometimes, to relieve often, and *to comfort always* (Kaufman, 1993) and (b) the JCAHO mandate to respect patients' cultural, psychosocial, spiritual, and personal values, beliefs, and preferences (JCAHO, 2006). This section focuses primarily on taking care of Jewish patients. In taking care of non-Jewish patients, the Jewish chaplain will provide a generalized approach that responds to the understanding and expectation of the person being served.

In many healthcare settings, such as those at Stanford University Medical Center, the majority of Jewish patients are not members of local synagogues. For those who are members, clergy from local synagogues may not be aware that their members are in the hospital or may not be available to visit them. To meet their spiritual needs and fulfill the JCAHO mandate, the Jewish community and the healthcare organization work together in different ways. A Jewish chaplain may be on the staff of the hospital's spiritual care service or part of a specialized Jewish chaplaincy program such as the Jewish Chaplaincy at Stanford University Medical Center; working in collaboration with congregational rabbis who visit their congregants, and with lay volunteers who visit the sick. A Jewish chaplain can be seen as a representative of the broader Jewish community when serving the community's ill. Where there is no Jewish chaplain on staff, Jewish spiritual care may be provided by rabbis from a local Jewish healing center, such as the Bay Area Jewish Healing Center in San Francisco, by a Jewish community chaplain sponsored by a local Jewish community federation, or by rabbis from local synagogues who make themselves available to healthcare settings for unaffiliated Jews (Bay Area Jewish Healing Center, 2006; National Center for Jewish Healing, 2006).

From the Jewish perspective, as Rabbi Jeffrey Silberman notes, the Jewish chaplain's role can be understood as "a unique combination of professional functions and leadership model rooted in Torah and rabbinic tradition. The contemporary spiritual caregiver fulfills the functions of the priest, the *chaver/* spiritual companion, the rabbi/teacher, and the prophet" (Silberman, 2005, p. 236).

In the role of priest, of *kohein,* Jewish chaplains use ritual, ceremony, and prayer to create a closer connection to personal meaning and healing, relationship with God and with Jewish community, and to help relieve the burden of guilt and regret. Prayer is an essential component of visiting the sick in Jewish tradition (for further discussion of ritual and ceremony, see Friedman, 2005). Prayer, a conversation with the divine, "uncovers the authentic inner conversation of the self and places it in dialogue with the timeless, universal conversation of the infinite. This connection can promote healing whether physical cure or the resolution of a painful situation is possible or not" (Brener, 2005, p. 125). The Jewish tradition is rich with prayers for healing such as this traditional blessing for healing, a *mi sheberach,* from a daily prayer book:

> May the One who blessed our ancestors, Abraham, Isaac and Jacob, Sarah, Rebecca, Leah and Rachel, bless ＿＿ son/daughter of ＿＿ and ＿＿ along with all the ill among us. Grant insight to those who bring healing; courage and faith to those who are sick; love and strength to us and all who love them. God, let Your spirit rest upon all who are ill and comfort them. May they and we soon know a time of complete healing, a healing of the body and a healing of the spirit, and let us say: Amen. (Handler et al., 1997, p. 51)

As spiritual companion, or *chaver,* the chaplain accompanies the patient and family on their journey of illness, offering trust, compassion, and empathy without having to fix or do something. In the role of rabbi, or teacher, the Jewish chaplain serves as religious authority and moral compass to guide patients and families through complex ethical decisions and theological questions as well as to respond to the needs and questions of patients, family members, and hospital staff. As prophet, or messenger, the Jewish chaplain acts as an advocate for the patient or as a messenger of the institution and the community—as an intermediary between patient, healthcare team, hospital, outside clergy, and the broader community—facilitating communication that may be difficult for others (Silberman, 2005).

The Jewish chaplain can assist Jewish patients with religious observance in the healthcare setting, including daily prayer following the dietary laws for keeping kosher, and the observance of Shabbat and holidays such as Rosh Hashanah, Yom Kippur, Hanukah, and Passover. For example, on Shabbat (from before sunset Friday to after sunset Saturday), the chaplain may help patients adapt Jewish practices to the hospital setting, such as candle lighting or avoiding the use of electric call buttons. They also can address religious and ethical questions concerning eating on fast days, receiving treatments derived from animals (such as pigs) that are not considered kosher, advanced directives, withdrawal of ventilator support, autopsy, organ donation, and burial (for a detailed discussion, see Dorff, 1998).

What it is like to be a chaplain can be illustrated with a personal reflection. I became a chaplain after a 19-year career as an emergency medicine physician, following an injury. Early in my chaplaincy (CPE) residency training in 1999, I came to see firsthand how being a chaplain contrasted with what I learned from being a physician, and yet was deeply consistent with one of the goals of medicine—*to comfort always.* I accompanied Father John Hester, a Catholic priest and longtime hospital chaplain, to the bedside of Emily, a 30-year-old Catholic woman with cystic fibrosis who was going to the operating room for a double lung transplant. She had requested a prayer.

Emily was sitting up and welcomed us. Father Hester joined hands with Emily's family and friends, motioning for me to join the circle. He offered an initial prayer and invited everyone to speak from their heart. One by one, Emily's brothers, sisters, mother, father, and friends spoke, telling Emily of their love and appreciation for her, and asking God to protect her. Tears flowed, including from Father Hester. "How unprofessional," I thought, seeing tears as a sign of weakness. But I was surprised. Not only were Father Hester's tears accepted by the family, they deepened their connection and appreciation of him. What I discovered was that allowing for tears required a special kind of strength and courage that permitted Father Hester to stand *with* Emily and her family in the midst of their fear, uncertainty, hope, appreciation and love, "between the medical technology and the patient, on holy ground" (Silberman, 2005, p. 241).

As patients are admitted to the hospital, they are asked if they have a religious preference. The hospital provides the hospital chaplains with a list of patients according to each patient's religious preference. Chaplains who are assigned to units—for example, the cancer unit or the intensive care unit—will see patients of all religions on that unit. As a faith-based hospital chaplain, I am responsible for visiting Jewish patients throughout the hospital.

In preparation for visiting patients, I set aside the time as sacred time and use elements of ritual and ceremony to create a separation between my everyday awareness/preoccupations and my intention to visit patients. I do this in a variety of ways, infusing everyday actions with special meaning to help prepare both my *intention* and *attention* before walking into the patient's room. I may stop in the chapel and sit; focus on my breath, breathing in that which is life-giving and letting go of that which no longer supports life; and dedicate this upcoming time, "May I be well used." As I walk down the hall, I bring awareness to each step. I feel the air against my forehead, blowing aside everyday concerns and allowing my highest and holiest self to emerge. While standing at the sink, hand washing is transformed from infection control to spiritual preparation. I feel my feet well grounded, bring awareness to my breath as I feel the water washing away preoccupations, and offer a blessing for hand washing from Jewish tradition. *Baruch atah Adonai, Eloheinu melech ha'olam, asher kidishanu b'mitzvotav, vitzivanu al netilat yadayim.* Freely translated, "Blessed are you O God, who makes us holy and invites us to join with You and walk in your ways. I lift up my hands. May I be of service." Before walking into the room, I stop and take a full and complete breath. With my awareness and intention focused, I am prepared to enter, as a visitor on behalf of community and tradition; to meet the patient and his or her family and visitors, in their world as it is for them, not where I want them to be; to provide a presence and words that may be comforting, guiding, clarifying, or empowering; to help connect the patient with his or her source of strength and faith. What matters for him or her *is* what matters for me. As I enter the room, I stop *first* and knock. I make contact first with my eyes, then with my voice, then with my touch (before extending my hand, I am aware of the practice of some orthodox Jews to not touch an adult of the opposite sex). "Hello, Mrs. Roth. My name is Bruce Feldstein. I am the Jewish chaplain at the hospital. I saw your name on our list of Jewish patients and wanted to stop by and wish you well." Thus begins the conversation.

I keep in mind that no visit is complete without a blessing or prayer. If Mrs. Roth is secular or a humanist, I may take her hand warmly and look into her eyes and tell her what I wish for her, what I hope for her, what I admire about her. If she is more familiar with Jewish tradition, I may say, "I wish you a *refuah shleymah*—a fullness of healing, a *refuat hanefesh v'refuat haguf*—a healing of your spirit and healing of your body."

Sometimes I will say, "May I offer you a blessing for healing?" If she says yes, I may offer a *mi sheberach,* a blessing for healing, introducing it in the following way:

> Mrs. Roth, I'd like to sing you a blessing for healing. Most of the words are in English and some are in Hebrew. It begins with the Hebrew words *mi sheberach,* which means a blessing for healing, from the Source of blessing; and *avoteinu* and *imoteinu,* in the name of our fathers and our mothers, may the merit of all our fathers and mothers be here to bless you. Later it asks for a *refuah shleymah. Refuah* means healing, and *shleymah* means a fullness—a fullness of healing, a complete healing of your being, of your spirit as well as your body. It says in our tradition that the healing presence of God, the *Shechinah* is present at the head of the bed of the one who is sick. So, in the presence of the *Shechinah* I would like to offer you this blessing.

At this point I always ask the patient, "Mrs. Roth, what would you like this blessing to mean for you?" I listen carefully and acknowledge her reply, recognizing that her answer is itself a prayer. I'll turn to others at the bedside, family or friends, and ask them what they would like this blessing to mean for them or for Mrs. Roth or anyone else. "Mrs. Roth, I'd like you to sit back, and receive this blessing. It is in two parts. May I take your hand?" Sitting, I take her hand and close my eyes. I pause, take a full breath, then begin the song, focusing my attention on my voice and body, on the music and words, allowing for sensations and images that arise on behalf of healing of the body and being of the one whose hand I have taken.

> *Mi sheberach avoteinu, m'kor habracha l'imoteinu:*
> May the Source of strength who blessed the ones before us
> Help us find the courage to make our lives a blessing
> And let us say: Amen.

> *Mi sheberach imoteinu, m'kor habracha l' avoteinu:*
> Bless those in need of healing with *refuah shleymah*
> The renewal of body, the renewal of spirit
> And let us say: Amen. (see Friedman, 1988)

CHRISTIAN CHAPLAINCY IN HEALTHCARE

I was sick and you visited me.

Matthew 25: 31–46

Since its origin Christianity has sought to provide well-being and quality of life to those in need of healing. Christians have not only seen it as a proper rule to live by but a fulfillment of the dictum of Jesus to serve God through serving those who are most in need (Tucker, 2002). This deep ethic of hospitality to the sick, as taught by Jesus to his earliest followers and subsequently carried on by medieval and later Christian communities, continues to be lived out in the care provided by twenty-first-century Christian clergy and chaplains.

Whether called *minister, priest, reverend,* or *chaplain,* Christian clergy have taken on the professional role of attending to the sick, as the acknowledged representatives of the community (Kirkwood, 1993). In addition, Christian laypersons also respond to the call to offer visitation and care. In healthcare settings, the Christian chaplain fulfills two primary functions: a *sacramental* role and a *pastoral* role. The chaplain adapts these roles to meet the understandings and expectation of patients and families, which may be as different as the individuals and the particular circumstances of their need for healthcare.

Sacramental Role of Christian Clergy

If a patient initiates a call for a visit by Christian clergy, it is often expected that the chaplain will provide a ritual or *sacramental* role. Especially in the case of critical illness or possible death, Christian clergy are often called to assist the suffering by providing particular rites for *initiation, reconciliation, communion,* and *healing.* These rites are called sacramental because they are believed to convey the presence of God (Tucker, 2002). Sacramental rites are generally accepted as tangible, visible expressions of God's love, acceptance, forgiveness, and favor.

The rite of initiation for Christians is baptism. The commonly accepted form among nearly all Christian denominations is for a minister to apply water to the patient while saying, "I baptize you in the name of the Father, and of the Son, and of the Holy Spirit." Baptism is understood by Christians as having an indelible quality and tends to be understood as acknowledgement of a lasting relationship with God. When this rite is called on in healthcare settings, it is usually by or for those who are close to death. While most Christian denominations believe that non-clergy members can perform the rite of baptism, there is a common understanding that the appropriate minister is the ordained clergy (*The Book of Common Prayer,* 1979).

Among the older branches of Christianity the rite of confession or reconciliation is practiced, whereby an individual may confess having made choices that were contrary to Christian teaching. A chaplain may offer a form of absolution in response to a confession with the assurance that the penitent Christian is absolved of the particular misconduct and reconciled with God (Kirkwood, 1993). Unlike baptism, this sacramental rite is typically only supplied by ordained Christian clergy and usually only one designated as a priest.

Communion is the Christian rite of ritually blessing and eating the bread and wine that represents the body of Christ. As a sacrament, bread and wine are taken by Christians as elements of the body and blood of Jesus and provide visceral assurance of the kingdom of God and for the kingdom yet to be made fully present on Earth. In a way similar to the benefits of the rite of reconciliation, participating in this sacramental meal unites Christians with Christ's salvific sacrifice (to bring salvation and redemption) and is believed to restore not only a relationship with God but a wholeness that is understood to embrace the receiver's body, mind, and spirit. Consequently, because of the all-encompassing nature of this theology, this ritual historically has been called "medicine" (Richardson, 1970). Similar to reconciliation, patients may see in the rite of communion a medicinal application for their soul that provides them assurance of God's care and relationship (Boyer, 2000). Many patients who frequently participate in this rite in their own communities will request this rite as the last meal they consume before their own death or to provide strength for their journey through pain and illness, perhaps on the eve before an important surgery.

The sacramental act of healing is attested to in Christian scripture and is closely associated with anointing of the sick with oil (*Enriching Our Worship 2*, 2000). One of the earliest Christian letters taught:

> Are any among you sick? They should call for the elders of the church and have them pray over them, anointing them with oil in the name of the Lord.
>
> James 5:14

Oil has traditionally been thought of as a carrier of healing properties. Ancient cultures used it to cover wounds to help prevent infection. The scents used to perfume oils also were believed to be curative. Christian custom has continued its use of oil, occasionally scented, and, in the advent of modern medicine, has reserved the more mystical understanding associated with the oil used for treating the sick. It is usually blessed or prayed over by an ordained clergy person whose ordained capacity is thought, by some Christians, to impart a holiness or healing capacity to the oil to be used.

The other traditional association with this rite is the use of the chaplain's hands in applying the oil (*The Book of Common Prayer*, 1979). Touching a sick patient as a therapeutic intervention emerged from the practices of early Christians, following the example of Jesus as healer. They understood healing through touch as evidence of God's care, even and especially for those who suffer the most. Although employed to varying degrees in Christian denominations throughout the centuries, today when a chaplain offers a rite of healing or if it is a requested rite for a patient, the chaplain is often asked to touch the patient, regardless of whether oil is being applied. This is typically referred to as a "laying on of hands." An alternative is for the chaplain to lift up his or her hands over the patient or in the patient's direction while offering a prayer for the patient's well-being.

Expectations vary, for both clergy and patients, about the effects such healing rites provide. There is occasionally a strong expectation that a chaplain's hands, prayers, or oil will provide miraculous healing beyond contemporary medical expectations and the current understanding of the physical laws of nature. Christian scriptures are filled with descriptions of miraculous healing and promises that the followers of Christ will be capable of performing similar miracles. Specifically praying for miracles in healthcare settings by Christian clergy and chaplains may have Christian theological precedence but is usually not the most helpful intervention with patients and families. Some fields of science are beginning to support the belief that some Christians have about the efficacy of prayer; some studies include claims of miraculous recoveries that seem to defy the laws of current science (Dossey, 1996). Such studies are not to be ignored. The primary concern, however, is that when a chaplain specifically prays for a miracle that later proves unfulfilled, this tends to complicate the grief and anxiety that a patient or family is experiencing. Theological explanations for specifically asked-for healing prayers that then appear to resolve as unfulfilled range from simply ignoring any connection to the prayer to blaming the faith or belief of the patient, a family member, or the chaplain. Such anxiety then forms a new presenting issue that may be related to deeper psychological and social issues for the patient's friends and family members. To continue toward health in the bodies and minds of patients and all those connected, Christian chaplains typically pray for "God's will to be done" while offering hope of healing and the assurance that God cares for them even in their suffering.

Finally, the sacramental rites that Christian chaplains provide in healthcare settings can sometimes be reduced to a functionary role by patients, families, hospital staff, and even by the chaplains themselves. Such a functionary role sometimes misses the relationship with the Christian belief in God's care or the community of believers on whom Jesus called. As noted, clergy, too, are prone to fall into a functionary role, dispensing prayers or communion, rather than focusing on the relationship or the quality of life such sacraments might provide. Calling for a sacramental rite may not necessarily mean that the patient is seeking a deeper relationship with either God or the Christian community; rather the patient may simply be seeking a private resolution to a specific fear. For the patient, the chaplain may be seen as a functionary means to an end without any need or request for further interaction. While this may not be an entirely theologically correct interpretation of Christian sacraments, this functionary role is appropriate in some cases. Sensitive chaplains learn when it is appropriate to simply fill a functionary role and when a patient or family may be calling on a deeper relationship with either God or the representative from the Christian community that the chaplain embodies. When that deeper relationship is sought, it is then the *pastoral* role of a Christian chaplain that is brought forth.

Pastoral Chaplaincy

In healthcare settings, when a Christian chaplain's personhood becomes the vehicle for a patient's relationship with God, or the chaplain's empathy offers validation for suffering, or their role or presence provides some healing to the patient, then the pastoral, or spiritual, role of the chaplain is most evident. The pastoral role of the chaplain is emerging as the primary understanding of the role of Christian clergy in healthcare today. Many contemporary Christian chaplains see the traditional sacramental rites as secondary to the pastoral responsibility (Lester, 1995). Sacraments are generally a means to a deeper relationship with God and one another through the role and person of the chaplain. The sacramental events provided by Christian clergy in healthcare settings are left aside if they appear to be inappropriate for the situation or relationships found among the patient and families, particularly with non-Christian patients. The pastoral role, or spiritual care function, emphasizes the relationships that are discovered or that emerge in chaplaincy interactions. With the pastoral relationship as his or her primary role, the chaplain incorporates deep listening skills, empathy, and validation for the patient's experiences.

In emphasizing this pastoral relationship, Christian clergy are often more self-disclosing with patients and families, offering story or conversation elements from their own life events and experiences. This usually increases the possibility of the chaplain's involvement in the life of the patient or with those who are close to the patient. Occasionally the chaplain takes on the role of advocate for the patient or family in a healthcare setting but usually does not go beyond the limits of his or her expertise.

Whereas the sacramental role provides the Christian patient with a transcendental focus on God or Jesus Christ with its immanent vehicles (bread, water, oil), the pastoral role is an immanent experience through the person and personality of the chaplain. In place of imparting sacraments to assure a patient of God's presence, the conversation and relationship with the chaplain becomes the source for seeking or identifying it.

This listening and reflecting by a chaplain may, however, transcend his or her immediate personhood and provide pastoral support through the chaplain's representative role in the wider community. This might occur through the chaplain's teaching or informing patients about how their suffering may be viewed by the community of faith or assuring them that the wider community is holding them in prayer. Again, the pastoral role continues to emphasize relationship, but here that relationship is widened to include the broader system of the Christian community or the community at large. In this case, Christian scriptures can supply the content of a conversation in a pastoral relationship. Sometimes biblical verses are applied in a routine way, being methodically called upon to apply to a given situation, but more often quotations from scriptural passages tend to emerge more organically from the listening and reflecting pastoral relationship. Whether routine or organic, however, Christian clergy can provide scripture for framing suffering, allowing for a patient or family to contextualize their experiences. Quoting sacred scripture or stories from the Bible, however, is not usually intended to warrant or justify suffering, nor is it usually used as a description of a particular sin that is being connected to suffering, although this can occur. Some branches of Christianity do interpret scripture in this way, and this use of scripture has been common enough in the history of the church. This is not, however, the prevailing theological use of scripture today.

Currently, scripture is most often applied pastorally by establishing a precedent, or a historical and spiritual antecedent to the patient's current condition. It provides for a larger relationship with the Christian community or with God. By using evidence from scripture, assurance is provided that the patient is not alone, that they are a part of a system of relationships that includes God—most often in the person of Jesus Christ—and the Christian community. This assurance includes the healing comfort that God cares for them despite any wrongdoings and is with them even in their deepest pain. As I heard one chaplain sum this up with an adult patient at a large urban hospital, "The scriptures all point to the fact that no matter what we are going through, *God is with us, God is for us.*"

Prayer is another essential way that chaplains provide reassurance, connection, relationship, and healing. These prayers for the sick are from *The Book of Common Prayer* (1979).

For Recovery from Sickness

O God, the strength of the weak and the comfort of sufferers:
Mercifully accept our prayers, and grant to your servant *N.*
the help of your power, that his sickness may be turned into
health, and our sorrow into joy; through Jesus Christ our Lord. Amen.

For a Sick Child

Heavenly Father, watch with us over your child *N.*, and grant
that he may be restored to that perfect health which it is
yours alone to give; through Jesus Christ our Lord. Amen.

For Doctors and Nurses

Sanctify, O Lord, those whom you have called to the study
and practice of the arts of healing, and to the prevention of
disease and pain. Strengthen them by your life-giving Spirit,
that by their ministries the health of the community may be
promoted and your creation glorified; through Jesus Christ our Lord. Amen.

A chaplain's pastoral role embodies both the personhood of the chaplain as well as the larger Christian community's relationship with this God who is "for us." Because the chaplain's pastoral role emphasizes the relationships that emerge, perhaps the most important statement that patients could say is, "The chaplain is with us, the chaplain is for us."

TOWARD A DEFINITION OF BUDDHIST CHAPLAINCY

Buddhist chaplaincy is in the formative stage as a modern-day discipline and profession; at the intersection of Buddhism, chaplaincy, and health-care as Buddhist chaplains join chaplains from other faith traditions in the healthcare setting. In this section I propose, in broad brushstrokes, what it means to me to be a Buddhist chaplain.

The seeds of Buddhist chaplaincy as a vocation begin with the Buddha. The three most common causes of people needing healthcare today—old age, sickness, and death—were the same that inspired the Buddha to reach beyond the familiar to greater truth and happiness. In doing so, he eventually found a path to peace in the midst of all that is difficult, uncomfortable, and confounding. Reaching out to the men and women in his community who were seeking ways to alleviate their pain, he offered care through careful guidance and a myriad of teachings. In essence, the Buddha was a chaplain—or rather, Buddhist chaplains who comfort others are walking in the footsteps of the Buddha.

For 2,500 years, Buddhists have contemplated sickness, old age, and death to find an end to suffering. Buddhist chaplains continue this practice in hospitals, hospices, and other healthcare facilities, helping people to reduce their pain and skillfully deal with what is happening to them, in the moment.

In a classically Buddhist sense, there is not a lot of emphasis on hope or intercession from an outside source or deity, but more on how to use one's intelligence and basic goodness to be skillful and more at ease in the middle of what is difficult. Although there are denominations or currents in Buddhism that seek guidance from Lord Buddha, in the most classic rendition of Buddhist history, the Buddha did not teach for or against "the gods," but only that extreme attachment or aversion to them was problematic. So one is free to choose, and obliged to choose wisely.

Everyone needs encouragement, assistance, and direction on their life's journey. The role of a Buddhist chaplain is to accompany individuals as their awakening and freedom from suffering unfolds. This may mean simply being a good listener or an encouraging companion, an intelligent guide, or a piercing truthteller. Overall, the purpose of a Buddhist chaplain is to alleviate suffering in its many forms: physical pain, difficult emotions, and confusing or disturbing thoughts such as agony, fear, anger, guilt, depression, loneliness, and grief.

All of the teachings of the Buddha can be summed up by the phrase: Nothing whatsoever should be clung to as *me* or *mine*. Interventions of chaplains exist to serve this goal, to aid in this realization, by either describing the situation or providing a skillful means to perceive it. *To cling to nothing* is a guide to the proper relationship to experience, as well as a statement of the way things are when the goal is reached. All difficult situations can be improved by applying intelligent perspective and loosening one's tight grasp on how things have always been, or should be right now. This means any of us can work internally with our suffering to change it for the better, even if what is happening outside of us does not change.

According to Buddhist tradition, in the latter part of the sixth century B.C.E., Siddhartha Gautama wandered through northern India. Local villagers became curious about his uniquely radiant character and asked, "Are you a celestial being or a god? Are you a man?" To these questions he replied, "I am none of these. I am awake." He then became known as the Buddha, which literally means the Awakened One. What does it mean to be awake? In the Buddhist tradition, it is taught that the answer to this question is found through deep insight into the interdependent nature of the world as we experience it. When we look at the world, we do not see things as they are, but rather through the lens of our individual hopes, fears, and dreams. The Buddha pointed to this lens as the root of suffering and taught that we each have the potential to awaken from what is imaginary to what is real.

The connecting theme of this approach as a chaplain is *the possibility of awakening,* as understood from Buddhist teaching. Our deepest desire is to have a sense of belonging, and when we are able to recognize ourselves in others, we can then care for them in a fundamentally different way. The function of the various approaches and interventions is to offer tools that will enable people to open their hearts and minds so that they may develop greater awareness of their true nature and, from that awakening, truly heal and transform.

Although the Buddha neither taught about higher powers nor denied their existence, many Buddhists acknowledge a universal life force. Humans are both unique selves and part of this great universal life force—but if we overidentify with who we are or what we believe, we suffer. Our tendency is to embrace one thing as right/pleasing and its opposite as wrong/unsatisfactory. Making such dualistic distinctions is natural to the human mind, and it serves people on many practical levels. However, clinging to or aversion toward dualistic categories causes more suffering than benefit. A middle path between dualistic opposites offers peace and freedom; the Buddha called this the *middle way.*

According to Buddhist teaching, suffering arises from ignorance of interconnectedness and change and bondage to dualistic thinking. Every aspect of creation is a process of becoming, into new, transformed states. Things fall apart and come together, fall apart again and come together again. If we clearly and deeply see that all objects and mind states are impermanent and without selfhood, we see that there is nothing worth clinging to, and when we stop clinging to (or averting from) things as they are, we experience liberation from suffering. Our very perceptions can change, and everything can appear in a new and fresh light, leading to a more wakeful and skillful way of life.

With time, reflection, and compassion, Buddhist chaplains help people realize that there is beauty and safety in change. One can learn to dwell peacefully in things as they are and develop an unconditional openness to whatever arises, is born, and/or dies—within the self, others, and all of creation. We become increasingly aware of our true nature: wisdom and compassion. Realizing compassion and wisdom in one's life is awakening, a change of perception—like suddenly seeing a three-dimensional object where previously one could only see it as flat. Wisdom means seeing creation and oneself as they are through the practice of mindful, nonjudgmental attention to ordinary experience. Compassion can be defined as liberation from the illusion of separateness. A heart can be broken open to compassion through suffering as well as through love. One experiences compassion as a great affection for creation as manifest in the self, others, and the nonhuman world. This is experienced as an urge to embrace the world. Compassion enhances our appreciation for things and assures us that we are embraced by a wider community, not forsaken as isolated individuals.

This healing process is not something mysterious. Awakening to one's true nature is available anywhere and everywhere, at all times. It exists within all phenomena, right here and now. It is a matter of removing the layers of our own projections that obscure the pure vision of reality. However, to wake up is not necessarily easy. We must first realize that we are asleep. Next, we need to identify what keeps us asleep, start to take it apart, and keep working at dismantling it until it no longer functions. The good news is that as soon as we make an effort to wake up, we begin to open up to how things actually are. We experience what we have suppressed or avoided and what we have ignored or overlooked.

Over time, one can develop an unconditional openness to whatever happens, arises, is born, and/or dies within oneself, others, and all of life. Buddhist chaplains are motivated by lovingkindness, an opening of the heart through spiritual practice, and are characterized by love for, compassion toward, equanimity among, and sympathetic joy for others. Buddhist chaplains do not serve as intermediaries or authorities per se, but as capable, steady companions who have investigated suffering through their own life experiences. So from their spiritual practice, Buddhist chaplains learn to lend patients their spirit and stability of mind for the possibility for their own healing, awakening, and transformation. Specifically, spiritual support from a Buddhist perspective can be defined as:

- Willingness to bear witness
- Willingness to help others discover their own truth
- Willingness to sit and listen to stories that have meaning and value
- Helping another face life directly
- Welcoming paradox and ambiguity into care—and trusting these will emerge into some degree of awakening
- Creating opportunity for people to awaken to their true nature

As a Buddhist chaplain, I serve others in realizing that most of life's events are not solely within human control, but rather are within the control of something greater than us. Simple yet profound, life-changing universal truths are discovered or remembered to help people experience the deepest, authentic peace and satisfaction—a heart and mind relaxed and open to what is. Buddhist spiritual care means helping people access the stillness, clarity, and love existing within our hearts. I have a sense of accomplishment or success when a patient begins to allow room for all of everything to happen: room for grief, for relief, for misery, for joy. Gone is the sense of separation, of internal nothingness, or of not being quite present. This is what I call the mystery of spirituality and healing.

CONCLUSION: ON HOLY GROUND

Hospital chaplains and clergy of all faiths help fulfill an essential dimension of caring and healing not otherwise available in healthcare. They stand on holy ground between patients and the healthcare system, on behalf of so much that is often overlooked in healthcare—meaning, comfort, coping, healing, relationship, love, hope, dignity, peace, justice, community, and mystery.

Chaplains and clergy are often asked, "How can you do this work? It must be so hard!" What Rabbi Amy Eilberg says in response to this applies not only for chaplains, but for healthcare providers as well.

> We walk amid a great deal of sadness, grief and fear. We regularly encounter the face of injustice and we frequently find ourselves in the midst of trauma and conflict. It is indeed a heavy burden to carry. This demands a great deal of us. It calls on the best of our capacity for compassion. It requires us to be courageous and wise, generous and unwavering. It requires a complex dance of giving and limit-setting, of opening the heart and of clear boundaries. We regularly come face-to-face with our own mortality....
>
> Nevertheless, this work also gives us great gifts: We witness much holiness and beauty. We have the privilege of being invited into the most sacred and intimate moments of another's life. We encounter extraordinary acts of love and devotion, of trust and courage. Our days contain many moments of awe. (Eilberg, 2005, p. 396)

TOOL KIT FOR CHANGE

Role and Perspective of the Healthcare Professional

1. To address a patient's spirituality helps fulfill the goals of medicine. Doing so can bring satisfaction to you as well as meaning and comfort to your patient.
2. In preparing to see a patient, it is important to stop and prepare one's intention as well as one's attention—to remind yourself of your aim and let go of distractions and preoccupations. This can be accomplished through actions such as focused breathing while hand washing.
3. Meet patients in their world as it is for them. Respect cultural and religious differences. It is unethical to proselytize. Consider offering a simple blessing with

each patient using phrases such as: What I wish for you is….What I hope for you is….What I admire about you is….

4. Consider consultation with or referral to a chaplain or clergy for spiritual issues when *you are uncomfortable,* there is spiritual distress, the spiritual issues are complex, when addressing these *particular* issues will take *much* more time than the allotted appointment time (Shih & Larson, 2006), and in decision-making situations involving advanced directives, do-not-resuscitate orders, and ethical and religious directives. Create a network for spiritual consultation and support, for your patients and for yourself. Chaplains can work with patients of different faith traditions and make connections to specific traditions. Establish a relationship with your healthcare organization's chaplain and/or relationships through a local ministerial association or spiritual care department of a local hospital or with students of a local religious educational facility (Shih & Larson, 2006).

Role and Perspective of the Patient

1. The interruption of illness and hospitalization can be a pivotal point in one's life. For some it can open a window into meaning, leading to personal transformation and growth. It is useful to pay attention to one's hopes, dreams, yearnings, and urges that may point toward understanding and new beginnings. For others it can be a period marked by rhetorical questioning and resentment.
2. Spirituality helps one maintain health and cope with illness, trauma, loss, and life transition by integrating body, mind, and spirit. Spiritual care can facilitate coping as well as growth and transformation.
3. Chaplains are trained to accompany patients and families along the journey of illness as they encounter spiritual questions and experiences.
4. Patients have the right to make decisions that reflect their personal, cultural, spiritual, and religious values. This includes refusing treatment as well as requesting treatments. Patients have the right to involve family members and friends in their decision making as well. Chaplains and patient advocates are available to ensure that a patient's rights are respected.

Interconnection: The Global Perspective

1. Humans are spiritual beings, concerned with matters of love, faith, hope, meaning, purpose, virtue, and beauty. There is a strong relationship between spirituality and health. Attention to spirituality and what matters most is not just a good idea; it is essential for health and healing.
2. Spirituality is intrinsic to healthcare. Spiritual care is everyone's responsibility—the patient and his or her family and friends; healthcare staff, including physicians, nurses, therapists, and chaplains; and clergy.
3. Healthcare "institutions that ignore the spiritual dimension…increase their risk of becoming only 'biological garages where dysfunctional human parts are repaired or replaced.' Such 'prisons of technical mercy' obscure the integrity and scope of persons" (VandeCreek & Burton, 2001, Section I, paragraph 4).

REFERENCES

American Academy of Family Physicians. (2001). *Spirituality and health.* Retrieved October 8, 2006, from http://familydoctor.org/650.xml.

Anandarajah, G., & Hight, E. (2001). Spirituality and medical practice: Using the HOPE questions as a practical tool for spiritual assessment. *American Family Physician* *63*(1), 81–89.

Association for Clinical Pastoral Education. (2006). *Mission statement.* Retrieved October 8, 2006, from http://www.acpe.edu.

Bartel, M. (2004). What is spiritual? What is spiritual suffering? *Journal of Pastoral Care & Counseling, 58*(3), 187–201.

Bay Area Jewish Healing Center. (2006). *Our mission.* Retrieved October 30, 2006, from http://www.jewishhealingcenter.org/bajhc-about-2004.htm.

Bergman, L. (2004). Defining spirituality: Multiple uses and murky meanings of an incredibly popular term. *Journal of Pastoral Care & Counseling, 58*(3), 157–167.

The book of common prayer and administration of the sacraments and other rites and ceremonies of the church. (1979). New York: Church.

Boyer, M. (2000). *Meditations for ministers.* Chicago: ACTA.

Brener, A. (2005). Prayer and presence. In D. A. Friedman (Ed.), *Jewish pastoral care: A practical handbook from traditional and contemporary sources* (2nd ed.). Woodstock, VT: Jewish Lights.

The chaplain-physician relationship [Special issue]. (1991). *Journal of Health Care Chaplaincy, 3*(2).

Dorff, E. N. (1998). *Matters of life and death: A Jewish approach to modern medical ethics.* Philadelphia: Jewish Publication Society.

Dossey, L. (1996). *Prayer is good medicine, how to reap the healing benefits of prayer.* New York: HarperCollins.

Eilberg, A. (2005). Walking in the valley of the shadow: Caring of the dying and their loved ones. In D. A. Friedman (Ed.), *Jewish pastoral care: A practical handbook from traditional and contemporary sources* (2nd ed.). Woodstock, VT: Jewish Lights.

Enriching our worship 2: Ministry with the sick or dying, burial of a child. (2000). New York: Church.

Feldstein, B. (2001). Toward meaning. *Journal of the American Medical Association, 296*(11), 1291–1292.

Feldstein, B. (2002). *Guidelines for spiritual care of Jewish patients and families in the hospital.* Unpublished manuscript, Jewish Chaplaincy at Stanford University Medical Center, Stanford Hospital & Clinics, Stanford, CA.

Flannelly, K., Handzo, G., Galek, K., Weaver, A., & Overvold, J. (2006). A national survey of hospital directors' views about the importance of various chaplain roles: Differences among disciplines and types of hospitals. *Journal of Pastoral Care & Counseling, 60*(3), 213–225.

Friedman, D. L. (1988). *Mi sheberach.* Sounds Write Productions (ASCAP).

Friedman, D. A. (Ed.). (2005). *Jewish pastoral care: A practical handbook from traditional and contemporary sources* (2nd ed.). Woodstock, VT: Jewish Lights.

Handler, J., Hetherington K., & Kelman, S. (1997). *Give me your hand. Traditional and practical guidance on visiting the sick* (2nd ed.). Albany, CA: EKS.

Hart, C., & Matorin, S. (1997). Collaboration between hospital social workers and pastoral care to help families cope with serious illness and grief. *Psychiatric Services, 48*(12), 1549–1552.

Joint Commission on Accreditation of Healthcare Organizations. (2006). *Joint commission 2006 requirements related to the provision of culturally and linguistically appropriate health care.* Retrieved October 22, 2006, from http://www.jointcommission.org/NR/rdonlyres/1401C2EF-62F0–4715-B28A-7CE7F0F20E2D/0/hlc_jc_stds.pdf.

Katonah, J. (1985). Hospitalization: A rite of passage. In L. E. Holst (Ed.), *Hospital ministry: The role of the chaplain today* (pp. 55–67). New York: Crossroad.

Kaufman, S. (1993). *The healer's tale.* Madison: University of Wisconsin Press.

Kirkwood, N. A. (1993). *A hospital handbook on multiculturalism and religion.* Harrisburg, PA: Morehouse.

Koenig, H., McCullough, M., & Larson, D. (2001). Definitions. *Handbook of religion and health* (pp. 17–23). Oxford, England: Oxford University Press.

Lester, A. D. (1995) *Hope in pastoral care and counseling.* Louisville, KY: Westminster John Knox Press.

Mohrmann, M. E. (1995). *Medicine as ministry: Reflections on suffering, ethics, and hope.* Cleveland, OH: Pilgrim Press.

Muller, W. (1996). *How then shall we live?* New York: Bantam Books.

National Association for Jewish Chaplains. (2006). *About us.* Retrieved October 30, 2006, from http://www.najc.org.

National Center for Jewish Healing. (2006). *About Jewish healing.* Retrieved October 31, 2006, from http://www.jewishhealing.org.

Ozarowski, J. (1995) *To walk in God's ways. Jewish pastoral perspectives on illness and bereavement.* Northvale, NJ: Jason Aronson.

Pargament, K. (1997). *The psychology of religion and coping: Theory, research, practice.* New York: Guilford Press.

Religion. (2006). *Wikipedia.* Retrieved November 26, 2006, from http://en.wikipedia.org/wiki/Religion.

Richardson, C. C. (1970). *Early Christian fathers.* New York: Macmillan.

Shih, K., & Larson, D. (2006). Religion and spirituality. In M. Micozzi (Ed.), *Complementary and integrative medicine in cancer care and prevention: Foundations and evidence-based interventions* (pp. 95–119). New York: Springer.

Silberman, J. (2005). Jewish spiritual care in the acute care hospital. In D. A. Friedman (Ed.), *Jewish pastoral care: A practical handbook from traditional and contemporary sources* (2nd ed.). Woodstock, VT: Jewish Lights.

Thiel, M., & Robinson, M. (1997). Physicians' collaboration with chaplains: Difficulties and benefits. *Journal of Clinical Ethics, 8*(1), 94–103.

Tucker, K.B.W. (2002). Liturgical ministry to the sick. *The New Westminster Dictionary of Liturgy and Worship* (pp. 436–438). Louisville, KY: Westminster John Knox Press.

VandeCreek, L. (1997). Collaboration between nurses and chaplains for spiritual caregiving. *Seminars in Oncology Nursing, 13*(4), 279–280.

VandeCreek, L., & Burton, L. (Eds.). (2001). *Professional chaplaincy: Its role and importance in healthcare.* Retrieved October 8, 2006, from http://www.healthcarechaplaincy.org/publications/publications/white_paper_05.22.01/02.html.

Chapter Eight

THE ART AND SCIENCE OF MEDITATION

Shauna L. Shapiro, PhD and Roger Walsh, MD, PhD

Meditation has been practiced in many forms in many cultures over many centuries. It has been practiced for at least three thousand years since the dawn of Indian yoga and is a central discipline at the contemplative core of all of the world's great religions. It is most often associated with the Indian traditions of yoga and Buddhism but has also been crucial to the Chinese Taoist and neo-Confucian traditions. The great monotheisms—Judaism, Christianity, and Islam—have also offered a variety of meditative techniques, although they never obtained the popularity and centrality accorded them in India.

THE PERENNIAL PHILOSOPHY

The importance accorded meditation by the perennial philosophy—the common core of wisdom and worldview that lies at the heart of all of the great religions—is based on three crucial assumptions that speak to the most vital aspects of our nature and potential as human beings. Yet, with the exception of transpersonal and integral psychologies, these assumptions lie outside most mainstream Western psychology and thought.

Portions of this chapter have been presented elsewhere and most especially in Shapiro, S. L., & Walsh, R. (2003). An analysis of recent meditation research. *Humanistic Psychologist*, *31*(2–3), 86–114.

1. Our usual, psychological state is suboptimal and immature.

   William James provided a pithy and poetic summary, stating that "most people live, whether physically, intellectually or morally, in a very restricted circle of their potential being. They make use of a very small portion of their possible consciousness. We all have reservoirs of life to draw upon, of which we do not dream."

2. Higher states and stages are available as developmental potentials.

   What we call normality and have regarded as the ceiling of human possibilities increasingly looks like a form of arbitrary, culturally determined, developmental arrest (Walsh & Vaughan, 1993; 2000). Mainstream developmental psychology is coming to a similar conclusion. Beyond Piaget's formal operational thinking lies postformal operational cognition; beyond Kohlberg's conventional morality are postconventional stages; beyond Fowler's synthetic-conventional faith lie conjunctive and universalizing faith; beyond Maslow's self-esteem needs await self-actualization and self-transcendence; and beyond Loevinger's conformist ego lie the possibilities of the autonomous and integrated ego (Fowler, 1981; Kohlberg, 1981; Loevinger, 1997; Maslow, 1971; Wilber, 2000). In short, beyond conventional, personal stages of development await postconventional, transpersonal stages and potentials.

3. Psychological development to transpersonal states and stages can be catalyzed by a variety of psychological and spiritual practices.

   Indeed, the contemplative core of the world's religions consists of a set of practices to do just this. Comparison across traditions suggests that there are seven practices that are widely regarded as central and essential for effective transpersonal development: an ethical life-style, redirecting motivation, transforming emotions, training attention, refining awareness, fostering wisdom, and practicing service to others (Walsh, 1999). Contemplative traditions posit that meditation is crucial to this developmental process because it facilitates several of these processes.

DEFINING MEDITATION

For all of the above reasons, meditation is of great interest to transpersonal and integral researchers. This leads to the important question, "what is meditation?" Meditation can be defined as a family of practices that train attention and awareness, usually with the aim of fostering psychological and spiritual well-being and maturity. Meditation does this by training and bringing mental processes under greater voluntary control and directing them in beneficial ways. This control is used to cultivate specific mental qualities such as concentration and calm and emotions such as joy, love, and compassion. Through greater awareness, a clearer understanding of oneself and one's relationship to the world develops. Additionally, it is held that a deeper and more accurate knowledge of consciousness and reality manifests.

A common division is into concentration and awareness types of meditation. Concentration practices attempt to focus awareness on a single object such as the breath or a mantra (internal sound). By contrast, awareness practices allow attention to move to a variety of objects and investigate them all.

Contemplative traditions posit that, through the process of meditation, physical, psychological and spiritual health are cultivated. Contemporary research offers preliminary yet growing support for some of these claims. Below, we briefly summarize the general findings of studies that have examined the effects of meditation on reducing physical and psychological symptoms. We then review recent studies that explore the effects of meditation on psychological and transpersonal health as well as on its physiological correlates.

FOUNDATIONAL RESEARCH STUDIES

Researchers primarily have examined meditation's effects as a self-regulation strategy for stress management and symptom reduction. Over the past three decades, considerable research has examined the psychological and physiological effects of meditation (for reviews, see Murphy, Donovan, & Taylor, 1997; Shapiro & Walsh, 1984; West, 1987). Meditative practices are now utilized in a variety of healthcare settings. This is understandable because research suggests that meditation may be an effective intervention for cardiovascular disease (Zamarra, Schneider, Besseghini, Robinson, & Salerno, 1996); chronic pain (Kabat-Zinn, 1982); anxiety and panic disorder (Edwards, 1991; Miller, Fletcher, & Kabat-Zinn, 1995); substance abuse (Gelderloos, Walton, Orme-Johnson, & Alexander, 1991); dermatological disorders (Kabat-Zinn et al., 1998); reduction of psychological distress and symptoms of distress for cancer patients (Speca, Carlson, Goodey, & Angen, 2000); and reduction of medical symptoms in clinical and nonclinical populations (Kabat-Zinn, Lipworth, & Burney, 1985;Williams, Kolar, Reger, & Pearson, 2001).

Few researchers have examined meditation's original purpose as a self-liberation strategy to enhance qualities such as compassion, understanding, and wisdom. However, a small number of pioneering studies provide a valuable foundation. These studies suggest meditation can produce improvements in self-actualization (Alexander, Rainforth, & Gelderloos, 1991); empathy (Lesh, 1970; Shapiro, Schwartz, & Bonner, 1998); sense of coherence and stress-hardiness (Kabat-Zinn & Skillings, 1989; Tate, 1994), happiness (Smith, Compton, & West, 1995), increased autonomy and independence (Penner, Zingle, Dyck, & Truch, 1974); a positive sense of control (Astin, 1997); increased moral maturity (Nidich, Ryncarz, Abrams, Orme-Johnson, & Wallace, 1983); and spirituality (Shapiro et al., 1998). Positive behavioral effects include heightened perception (visual sensitivity, auditory acuity);

improvements in reaction time and responsive motor skill; increased field independence; and increased concentration and attention (see Murphy et al., 1997). In addition, meditation appears to result in improvements in aspects of intelligence, school grades, learning ability, and short- and long-term recall (see Cranson et al., 1991; Dillbeck, Assimakis, & Raimondi, 1986) and some forms of creativity (Cowger & Torrance, 1982).

These pioneering studies are not without limitations, and several caveats should be noted. Many of these studies do not demonstrate rigorous research design (including lack of randomization, lack of follow-up, and imprecise measurement of constructs) and sometimes are based on small samples. Researchers often failed to report what type of meditation technique was taught or the length and intensity of the practice. Also, several of the studies retrospectively compare meditators to control subjects, which yields useful correlational but no causal inferences. Furthermore, most meditation research is derived from relative beginners of meditation practice.

Despite these limitations, the studies provided a solid beginning upon which recent research has been building. We review a sample of recent, well-designed studies on the effects of meditation on variables important in the field of transpersonal psychology.

ANALYSIS OF RECENT RESEARCH

Psychological Findings

Cognition and Creativity

Three recent studies by So and Orme-Johnson (2001) examined the effects of transcendental meditation (TM) on cognition. One hundred fifty-four Chinese high school students were randomized into a TM group or a napping group. The TM technique and napping were practiced for approximately 20 minutes twice a day. At six-month follow-up, the TM group demonstrated significantly increased practical intelligence, field independence, creativity, and speed of information processing, as well as significantly decreased anxiety compared to the control group. The authors suggest that these findings indicate that TM's effects extend beyond those of ordinary rest.

The findings of this study were replicated in a sample of 118 junior high Chinese students who were randomly assigned to a TM group, a contemplative meditation group, or a no treatment control group. All students practiced their respective meditation techniques for 20 minutes twice a day. At six-month follow-up, the TM group showed improvement on creativity, anxiety, information processing time, and practical intelligence as compared to the contemplation group. The contemplation group improved on information processing time as compared to the control group.

These general findings were replicated in a third study examining the effects of TM compared to a no-treatment control group on 99 male vocational students from Taiwan. At 12-month follow up, the TM group significantly increased practical intelligence, field independence, whole-brained creativity, and speed of information processing and significantly decreased anxiety as compared to the control group. In summarizing the implications of these three studies, the authors suggest that the findings strongly support the hypothesis that TM improves performance on a number of cognitive and affective measures.

Attention and Concentration

To examine the effects of meditation on attention, Valentine and Sweet (1999) conducted an elegant study design, which incorporated type of meditation (concentration vs. mindfulness), length of practice (long-term meditators > 25 months, short-term meditators < 24 months), and expectancy effects (expected vs. unexpected stimuli). Participants consisted of 24 controls, 5 short-term concentrative meditators, 4 short-term mindfulness meditators, 6 long-term concentrative meditators, and 4 long-term mindfulness meditators. A measure of sustained attention was employed with all participants. The meditation group was tested following their usual meditation practice. Results demonstrated that meditators' attention and accuracy was greater than the control subjects'. Further, long-term meditators demonstrated better attention processes than short-term meditators.

There were no differences in performance between concentrative and mindfulness meditators when the stimulus was expected. However, when the stimulus was unexpected, mindfulness meditators were superior to concentrative meditators. The authors suggest that these differences are due to the fact that, in concentration meditation, attention is focused on an expected stimulus. Therefore, attention is impaired when the stimulus is unexpected. Conversely, in mindfulness meditation, attention is evenly distributed and therefore no stimulus or set of stimuli becomes more salient than others. Despite the thoughtful design of the study, limitations exist, and therefore results should be interpreted cautiously. First, there was no measurement of individual differences (e.g., education level, socioeconomic status) between groups, and therefore the differential performance in attention cannot be solely attributed to meditation. Second, the meditators practiced their respective meditation before the attentional testing; therefore, the data do not represent persistent or general effects of the practice of meditation. For example, perhaps attention/concentration is increased immediately after a meditation session but not continually throughout the day. A final limitation of this study is the small sample size.

Interpersonal Relationships

Meditative practices for cultivation of love, compassion, empathetic joy, and equanimity have a long tradition in the meditative disciplines (Walsh, 1999). Most notable are the Brahma Vihara practices (Kornfield, 1993; Salzberg, 1995). A recent study (Carson, Carson, Gil, & Baucom, 2004) incorporated the meditative practice of metta—or lovingkindness, one of the Brahma Vihara meditations—into a mindfulness-based intervention for couples. Forty-four couples that were in well adjusted relationships and had been married an average of 11 years were randomly assigned to a waiting-list control group or a meditation intervention group. The program consisted of eight two-and-a-half-hour sessions and a six-hour retreat. In addition to components modeled on the Mindfulness-Based Stress Reduction Program (Kabat-Zinn, 1990), a number of elements related to enhancing the relationship were added, including lovingkindness meditation (Kornfield 1993; Salzberg, 1995); partner yoga exercises, focused application of mindfulness to relationship issues, and group discussions. Results demonstrated that the couples in the meditation intervention significantly improved relationship satisfaction as well as relatedness to and acceptance of the partner. In addition, individuals reported significant increases in optimism, engagement in exciting self-expanding activities, spirituality, and relaxation. Interestingly, increases in engagement in exciting self-expanding activities significantly mediated improvements in relationship quality (Carson et al., 2006).

Carson et al.'s (2006) study supports earlier research that compared the effects of Zen breath meditation to relaxation on college adjustment (Tloczynski and Tantriella 1998). Seventy-five undergraduates, matched on initial anxiety, were randomized into meditation, relaxation, and control groups. The students received one hour of instruction in either technique and were instructed to practice it once daily for at least 20 minutes. Interestingly, after six weeks, interpersonal problem scores significantly decreased only in the meditation group. However, anxiety and depression scores significantly decreased in both meditation and relaxation groups as compared to the control group.

Prevention

In a multicenter randomized clinical trial, the effects of mindfulness-based cognitive therapy (MBCT) were evaluated for recovered patients with recurrent depression. The aim of this study was to determine whether the meditation-based intervention could help prevent relapse of major depression. One hundred forty-five patients who were currently in recovery or remission for major depressive disorder were randomized to continue with treatment as usual (TAU), or, in addition, to receive MBCT. The group intervention consisted of eight weekly two-hour sessions and four monthly booster sessions. Relapse or recurrence of major depression was assessed over a 60-week period.

Findings indicated that, for patients with recurrent major depression who had three or more episodes, MBCT approximately halved rates of relapse and recurrence during the follow-up period compared with patients who continued TAU. The absence of a comparison group limits the value of this study, because cognitive therapy by itself has been shown to reduce depression relapse rates. However, the study offers a promising avenue for future relapse prevention meditation research.

Another innovative use of meditation for prevention is mindfulness-based relapse prevention (MBRP), a synthesis of relapse prevention and mindfulness meditation for addictive behaviors. The aim of MBRP is to help prevent relapse of substance abuse by developing awareness and acceptance of thoughts, feelings, and sensations and to utilize mindfulness in the face of high-risk situations (Witkiewitz, Marlatt, & Walker, 2004).

Antidepressants and Meditation

Depression is a common and sometimes serious disorder that can certainly affect meditators. Yet meditators may be resistant to using antidepressants for several reasons: they may believe that they should be able to heal themselves with spiritual practices alone, that drugs are "unspiritual," and that drugs may impair their meditation. Yet no data are available on drug effects in this population, despite the fact that, because of their introspective skills, meditators might be uniquely valuable informants about drug effects.

In a recent study, meditators filled out surveys on their observations of the effects of antidepressants on their daily and retreat meditation experience (Bitner, Hillman, Victor, & Walsh, 2002). As anticipated, respondents reported reduced negative emotions and enhanced positive ones. They also reported greater energy, calm, clarity, concentration, equanimity, motivation, and self-esteem. In short, contrary to widespread fears in the meditation community, the responses were surprisingly positive. However, this conclusion must be qualified by several study limitations. Subjects were self-selected, data were subjective and retrospective, and drug type and dosage varied. Despite these limitations, the findings are encouraging to meditators who may need antidepressant therapy.

Informal Practice: Assessment during Daily Life

Very little research has been devoted to examining the effects of practicing meditation throughout the moment-to-moment experience of daily life (informal practice). This topic of research is crucial, because the goal of meditation is not simply to alter one's state of consciousness during formal meditation practice, but to learn to bring this quality of awareness to each experience of one's life. Easterlin and Cardena (1999) evaluated the effects of Vipassana meditation in the daily lives of beginning and advanced meditators. Participants consisted of 43 meditators—19 beginners and 24 advanced meditators—who responded to daily random pager signals containing questions related to awareness, acceptance, affect, and cognitive style. Relative to the beginners, the advanced meditators reported greater awareness, positive mood, greater acceptance, lower anxiety levels, lower stress, and a healthier sense of control.

A more recent study of the effects of mindfulness meditation on women with breast cancer found that informal practice was significantly related to enhanced sleep quality (Shapiro, Figueredo, Bootzin, Lopez, Figueredo, & Schwartz, 2003)

Long-Term Retreats

Page et al. (1997) performed a largely exploratory qualitative analysis of the written self-perceptions of retreat participants after a six-month period of isolation and silent meditation during the third year of a four-year Tibetan Buddhist retreat. Retreat participants were 46 self-reported Tibetan Buddhists from internationally distributed locations. Three independent raters categorized the subjects' written responses into smaller units of independently meaningful content, divided them into "internal" or "external" categories, and then grouped internal units into emergent themes.

Five themes of internal self-perception were identified: (1) happiness/ satisfaction, (2) struggle leading to insight, (3) practice/meditation, (4) sense of time, and (5) goals/expectations. Women tended to write more about satisfaction, while men wrote more about struggle leading to insight. Sense of time was reported to be absent or distorted, and future goals tended to be generalized toward maintaining the conscious self-awareness acquired during isolation. These preliminary findings suggest that a long-term retreat, including six months of isolation, may enhance personal awareness to a level that supports increased life satisfaction. And yet these findings should be considered with caution. Only 23 of 46 original participants remained by the third year of the retreat, an attrition rate that could signify a high potential for self-selection bias in terms of motivation, happiness, and expectation. With such a unique population, more comprehensive measures, quantitative analysis, and a more developed and delineated description of self-awareness would be of great benefit.

Synesthesia

Synesthesia is cross-modality perception in which stimuli in one sense modality such as sound are also experienced in other modalities, such as sight, touch, or taste. It is considered to be a rare, innate, uncultivatable ability (one per several thousand people), yet surveys of meditators suggest otherwise. In a recent study by Walsh (2002), three groups of Buddhist meditators (Tibetan Buddhist retreat participants, medical students and physicians, and meditation teachers) and a comparison group of medical students were surveyed by questionnaire, and two raters analyzed responses. Among retreat participants, 35 percent of respondents described synesthesia, and they had almost twice as much meditation experience as those who did not experience synesthesia. In the medical and teacher groups, 63 percent and 86 percent, respectively, met criteria for synesthesia, compared to only 9 percent of the nonmeditating comparison group. The presence of synesthesia correlated significantly with amount of meditation experience as measured by both years of practice and total time spent in retreat. This study is limited by small sample sizes. However, its findings, which are consistent with other perceptual studies, suggest that meditation can significantly enhance perceptual sensitivity and abilities.

Self-Concept

Using a cross-section study design, Haimerl and Valentine (2001), investigated the effect of Buddhist meditation on intrapersonal (self-directedness), interpersonal (cooperativeness), and transpersonal (self-transcendence) levels of the self-concept. Subjects included prospective meditators ($n = 28$) with no experience, beginners ($n = 58$) with less than 2 years of experience, and advanced meditators ($n = 73$) with more than two years of experience. Advanced meditators scored significantly higher than prospective meditators on all three subscales; advanced meditators scored significantly higher than beginners on the interpersonal subscale; and beginners scored significantly higher than prospective meditators on the transpersonal subscale. Only the advanced meditators scored higher on the transpersonal than on the intrapersonal subscale. The authors concluded that scores on the intrapersonal, interpersonal, and transpersonal levels were a positive function of meditation experience, suggesting that progress in Buddhist meditation leads to significant growth in these components of personality.

Empathy

All schools of meditation have emphasized concern for the condition of others and an intention to "promote an empathy with created things that leads toward oneness with them" (Murphy et al., 1997, p. 82).

A randomized controlled study Shapiro, Schwartz, and Bonner (1998) examined the effects of a mindfulness meditation–based program on 78 medical and premedical students. Results indicated increased levels of empathy and decreased levels of anxiety and depression in the meditation group as compared to the wait-list control group. Furthermore, these results held during the students' stressful exam period. The findings were replicated when participants in the wait-list control group received the mindfulness intervention.

The findings of this study are supported by a recent study examining the effects of mindfulness-based stress reduction (MBSR) on counseling psychology students' empathy. Participants in the eight-week MBSR course demonstrated significant increases in empathic concern for others as compared to a matched control group (Shapiro, Brown, & Biegle, 2006). Further, increases in mindfulness as measured by the Mindful Attention and Awareness Scale (Brown & Ryan, 2003) predicted increases in empathy. This is one of the first studies to demonstrate that MBSR leads to mindfulness and that mindfulness is a significant predictor of outcome.

Spirituality

In the study by Carson and colleagues (2006), the couples who received the mindfulness meditation relationship enhancement intervention reported significantly more spirituality than the control group. This supports earlier findings that MBSR intervention significantly increased spiritual experience in medical students as compared to wait-list control subjects. These results were replicated when the control group received the same mindfulness intervention. Further, Astin (1997) demonstrated significant increases in spiritual experience in a randomized controlled study comparing a mindfulness meditation intervention to a control group of undergraduate students.

Self-Compassion

Self-compassion is defined as being kind and understanding toward oneself in instances of pain or failure rather than being harshly self-critical; perceiving one's experiences as part of the larger human experience rather than seeing them as isolating; and holding painful thoughts and feelings in balanced awareness rather than overidentifying with them (Neff, 2006). Two recent studies have found that mindfulness meditation-based intervention significantly increases self-compassion (Shapiro et al, 2005; Shapiro et al, 2006). In the first study...The second study was a matched controlled design examining the effects of MBSR for counseling psychology students.

Interestingly, a recent study found that self-compassion, is significantly predictive of other positive psychological variables including wisdom, personal initiative, curiosity and exploration, happiness, optimism, and positive affect (Neff, Rude, & Kirkpatrick, in press). Further, self-compassion remained a significant predictor of psychological health after controlling for shared variance with positive affect and personality.

PHYSIOLOGICAL CORRELATES OF MEDITATION

As Ryff and Singer (1998) aptly point out, "human wellness is at once about the mind and the body and their interconnections" (p. 2). Although the implications of the physiological correlates of meditation are as yet unclear, it seems likely that some of the changes represent "physiological substrates of flourishing" (Ryff & Singer, 1998, p. 2).

Improvements in immune system functioning or reversal of immune suppression may be an important marker of such physiological substrates of health and well-being. For example, Davidson and colleagues (2003) found a greater increase in influenza antibodies among participants receiving an mindfulness-based stress reduction intervention than among control subjects. Similarly, in cancer patients, meditation practice had a number of effects on immune parameters that are consistent with a shift to a more normal profile (Carlson, Speca, Patel, & Goodey (2004)).

Another widely reported positive physiological effect of meditation is relaxation. A state of physiological rest is indicated by changes on a number of parameters, including reduced respiration rate and plasma lactate levels and increased skin resistance. Statistical meta-analysis showed that changes in these particular variables are consistent across studies (Dillbeck & Orme-Johnson, 1987) and twice as large as those associated with eyes-closed rest. Also, consistent with increased calm are declines in blood cortisol and lactates (Jevning, Wilson, & Davidson, 1978) and more stable phasic skin resistance (Alexander et al., 1991).

Although associated with physiological rest, there are several indicators that meditation simultaneously facilitates heightened alertness (Wallace, 1986). These changes are marked by increased cerebral blood flow; enhanced alpha and theta EEG power and coherence in the frontal and central regions of the brain; marked increased in plasma arginine vasopressin; faster H-reflex recovery; and shorter latencies of auditory evoked potential (e.g., O'Halloran, Jevning, Wilson, Skowsky, & Alexander, 1985; Orme-Johnson & Haynes, 1981; Wallace, 1986).

Research explicitly comparing meditation and relaxation confirms that they are physiologically distinct. Dunn, Hartigan, and Mikulas (1999) compared concentration meditation versus mindfulness meditation versus a relaxation control condition. When collapsing mindfulness and concentration meditations into one group, results indicated that the EEGs of meditators were different from the EEGs of relaxed participants. The authors interpret the results as indicating that meditations produce different cortical patterns relative to relaxation. Differences were also found between concentration and mindfulness states.

Another indication of physiological flourishing comes from recent research indicating that meditation practice may enhance the left-to-right ratio of activation of the prefrontal cortex, which has been linked to positive emotions and mental health (Davidson et al., 2003). Participants in an eight-week MBSR program demonstrated increases in left frontal EEG activation as compared to a control group (Davidson et al., 2003). These findings provide physiological evidence of meditation's ability to change the structure of the brain.

Further data providing structural evidence that meditation experience affects plasticity come from a recent study examining the effects of mindfulness meditation practice on changes in the brain's physical structure (Lazar et al., 2005). Magnetic resonance imaging was used to assess cortical thickness in 20 participants with extensive mindfulness practice. Brain regions associated with attention, interoception, and sensory processing—including the prefrontal cortex and right anterior insula—were thicker in meditation participants than they were in the matched control subjects. These data provide preliminary evidence that meditation contributes to the development of the physiological structures that support intelligence.

In conclusion, physiology studies constitute a valuable direction for future research. However, they are limited by the resolution of current techniques and our inadequate understanding of neural pathways and brain function. Consequently, we can draw only limited conclusions about the precise relationships between the subtle subjective shifts induced by meditation and their neural substrates. For critical reviews of this issue and of the new field of neurotheology, see Groopman (2001) and Wilber (2000a).

DISCUSSION

As the above findings make clear, meditation has the potential to enhance physiological, psychological, and transpersonal well-being on a wide variety of measures. However, for research to continue to refine and expand our knowledge of meditation and its effects, it is essential to develop broader paradigms for the field, which include specific directions for future studies. Below we discuss potential directions for the field, beginning with a theoretical orientation and concluding with specific suggestions for future study designs.

The Importance of Developing Big Maps

On the theoretical side, it is crucial that meditation research be held within a sufficiently encompassing and comprehensive conceptual framework. Because meditation is intrinsically subjective, introspective, and induces transpersonal experiences, states, and stages, much that is crucial to it lies outside current mainstream maps and models. For example, introspective approaches and transpersonal experiences and stages are currently suspect in mainstream psychology—although they are rapidly gaining respect (Varela & Shear, 1999). Sufficiently comprehensive maps would encompass these and include both ontological and developmental dimensions.

On the ontological side, such maps must include both subjective and objective domains. This seems simple and obvious enough. And yet the reigning paradigm within science is a generally unquestioned materialism—sometimes called scientific materialism—which often reduces subjective experience to mere neural fireworks. Yet materialism has gaping holes, the mind-body problem remains utterly unsolved, and some notables such as John Eccles think it may be insoluble (Griffin, 1998; Popper & Eccles, 1997). However, many scientists are somewhat philosophically naive, so scientific materialism and reductionism continue.

In some ways this is not surprising, because several additional forces favor this reductionism. The scientific enterprise, with its focus on observable, measurable data, emphasizes objective phenomena and tends to make such things seem more real than subjective experiences. A further factor favoring materialism and reductionism is scientism. This is the pseudo philosophy that science is the best or only means of acquiring valid information. A final factor may be the lack of deep meditative experience among researchers, a point we will return to later in the chapter.

One nonreductionistic ontological map that is currently exciting considerable interest is Ken Wilber's (2000c) four-quadrant model. Wilber creates four quadrants by dividing reality into subjective and objective domains and these into individual and collective domains. The resulting four quadrants are individual-subjective, collective-subjective (cultural), individual-objective (behavioral), and collective-objective (societal). A comprehensive approach to meditation research will consider all four quadrants (for one possible meditation research program using Wilber's model, see Wilber & Walsh, 2002).

In the developmental domain, an adequate map will necessarily include transpersonal, postconventional stages. These are "higher" stages that emerge after the conventional ones, in which the sense of identity extends beyond (trans) the individual person and personality to encompass wider aspects of humankind, life, psyche, and cosmos. They include, for example, many of the classical contemplative mystical stages, as well as stages described by transpersonal theorists such as Grof, Washburn, and Wilber (Grof, 1998; Walsh & Vaughan, 1993; Wilber, 2000). The inclusion of these transpersonal stages requires only a minor expansion of mainstream psychology, because, as previously discussed, developmental researchers increasingly recognize three major stages: prepersonal, personal, and transpersonal or preconventional, conventional, and postconventional (Wilber, 2000).

The failure to recognize transpersonal stages results in several problems. The first is what Ken Wilber (1999) has discussed as the pre/trans fallacy. This is the confusion of prepersonal states and stages with transpersonal ones. For example, when pathological regressions such as psychosis are mistaken for spiritual openings, or, conversely, when genuinely transpersonal experiences, such as peak experiences, are dismissed as prepersonal, borderline pathology.

The second problem that follows from this fallacy is the pathologizing of meditative experiences. Clinicians unaware of transpersonal possibilities can easily misdiagnose powerful, transpersonal meditation experiences as pathological. Transpersonal progressions are then dismissed as prepersonal regression, and the results to clients can be devastating (Grof & Grof, 1990; Walsh & Vaughan, 1993).

Another risk of not acknowledging transpersonal stages is not as clinically dangerous, but is perhaps just as theoretically and societally tragic. This is the overlooking of what are most central and crucial in meditative disciplines: higher states, stages, and capacities. This results in a tragically constricted view of human nature and possibilities. As Gordon Allport (1964, 27–44) put it, "By their own theories of human nature, psychologists have the power of elevating or degrading that same nature. Debasing assumptions debase human beings; generous assumptions exalt them." Meditation researchers have the privilege of introducing more generous assumptions into psychology and thereby exalting humans. To do this may well require comprehensive theories that include at least the four quadrants as well as transpersonal states and stages (Wilber, 2000; Wilber & Walsh, 2002).

Suggestions for Future Research

The results of past research are qualified by their limitations in methodology. We suggest the following 10 criteria to ensure future rigorous designs:

1. Differentiation between types of meditation. There are many types of meditation. This is crucial to recognize for theoretical, practical, and research reasons. Yet researchers often implicitly assume that different meditations have equivalent effects. This is an assumption to be empirically tested. Most likely, different techniques have overlapping, but by no means equal, effects. In general, we anticipate that there will be both general and specific effects of different types of meditation. Many meditations may foster psychological and spiritual well-being and development on multiple dimensions. However, specific meditations may also produce very specific effects (e.g., Tibetan dreams yoga for developing lucid dreams and a variety of practices that cultivate emotions of love or compassion). Therefore, it is essential that researchers clearly define the type of meditation being studied.
2. Temporal effects. Frequency and duration of meditation practice must be recorded (e.g., in meditation journals) to determine whether more meditation induces greater effects, and, if so, is the relationship linear, curvilinear, or some other pattern.
3. Follow-up assessment. Follow-up should include long-term as well as short-term assessment.
4. Inclusion of experienced meditators. Researchers should include long-term, experienced meditators as well as beginning meditators. Also, when matching control subjects to long-term meditators in retrospective studies, in addition to age, gender, and education, it would be important to consider matching subjects on the dimension of an alternative attentional practice (e.g., playing a musical instrument).
5. Component analysis. Meditation is a multifaceted process with multiple potentially potent components. These range from nonspecific factors such as belief and

expectancy through postural, somatic, attentional, cognitive, and other factors. Research can attempt to differentiate the effects and interactions of various components. This is a kind of component analysis.

6. Examination of interaction effects. The practice of meditation may interact with a variety of relevant psychological, spiritual, and clinical factors. Factors of current interest include other health and self-management strategies and especially psychotherapy.

7. Mediating variables. Development of subjective and objective measures will help to determine the mediating variables that account for the most variance in predicting change.

8. Qualitative data. The subtlety and depth of meditation experiences do not easily lend themselves to quantification. Further, the interplay between subjective and objective is essential to understanding meditation. Qualitative data provide a means to access the subjective experience of the meditator.

9. Expanding the paradigm from pathology to positivity and the transpersonal. Most meditation research has used the traditional biomedical paradigm in which the focus is on symptom reduction. Future research could expand this model by examining the effects of meditation on problem prevention and health enhancement and on variables consistent with the classical goals of meditation, such as the development of exceptional maturity, love and compassion, and life-styles of service and generosity.

10. The value of practice. Several lines of evidence suggest that personal practice of meditation may enhance one's understanding of meditative and transpersonal experiences, states, and stages. This is a specific example of a general principle. Without direct experience, concepts (and especially transpersonal concepts) remain devoid of experiential grounding. Without this grounding, we lack the capacity to comprehend the deeper grades of significance of phenomena (Schumacher, 1977). As philosopher Philip Novak (1989, p. 67) pointed out, in meditation the "deepest insights are available to the intellect, and powerfully so, but it is only when those insights are discovered and absorbed by a psyche made especially keen and receptive by long coursing in meditative discipline, that they begin to find their fullest realization and effectiveness." Good books for beginners include Bodian (1999) and Tart (2001).

Therefore, for research to progress, optimally it may be helpful for researchers to have a personal meditation practice, similar to the anthropological view that one must be a participant observer. Without direct practice and experience, we may be blind to the deeper grades of significance of meditation experiences and blind to our own blindness.

CONCLUSION

During the past four decades, research in meditation has developed a strong foundation, demonstrating significant psychological, physiological, and therapeutic effects. As discussed above, we suggest 10 specific recommendations, which may help the field continue to progress. The exploration of meditation requires great sensitivity and a range of methodological lenses. Future research will benefit by looking through all of them, thereby illuminating the richness and complexity of meditation.

TOOL KIT FOR CHANGE

Role and Perspective of the Healthcare Professional

1. Meditation offers a rich and complex field of study. Over the past 40 years, several hundred research studies have demonstrated numerous significant findings, including changes in psychological, physiological, and transpersonal realms.
2. Meditation can be defined as a family of practices that train attention and awareness, usually with the aim of fostering psychological and spiritual well-being and maturity. Meditation does this by training and bringing mental processes under greater voluntary control and directing them in beneficial ways.
3. Meditation can be used by healthcare professionals for both self-care and care of clients.

Role and Perspective of the Participant

1. Meditation can have significant beneficial effects on a patient's well-being, both physical and mental. These benefits include enhanced immune functioning, decreases in anxiety and depression, and increases in positive qualities such as joy and compassion.
2. A patient must be willing to put the time into meditation practice, because it requires a strong intention to practice.
3. Through the practice of meditation, the patient gains greater awareness, and a clearer understanding of oneself and one's relationship to the world develops.

Interconnection: The Global Perspective

1. Meditation has the potential to enhance physiological, psychological, and transpersonal well-being.
2. Research will continue to refine and expand our knowledge of meditation and its effects; however, it is essential to develop broader paradigms for the field, which include specific directions for future studies.
3. The exploration of meditation requires great sensitivity and a range of methodological lenses. Future research will benefit by looking through all of them, thereby illuminating the richness and complexity of meditation.

REFERENCES

Alexander, C., Rainforth, M., & Gelderloos, P. (1991). Transcendental meditation, self-actualization and psychological health: A conceptual overview and statistical meta-analysis. *Journal of Social Behavior and Personality, 6,* 189–249.

Allport, G. (1964). The fruits of eclecticism: Bitter or sweet? *Acta Psychologica, 23,* 27–44.

Andresen, J. (2002). Meditation meets behavioral medicine: The story of experimental research on meditation. *Journal of Consciousness Studies, 7,*(11–12), 17–74.

Astin, J. A. (1997). Stress reduction through mindfulness meditation: Effects on psychological symptomatology, sense of control, and spiritual experiences. *Psychotherapy & Psychosomatics, 66,* 97–106.

Bitner, R., Hillman, L., Victor, B., & Walsh, R. (2002). *Effects of antidepressants on and observed through the practice of meditation.* Unpublished manuscript. Irvine, CA.

Bodian, S. (1999). *Meditation for dummies.* Foster City, CA: IDG Books.

Brown, K. W. and Ryan, R. M. (2003). The benefits of being present: The role of mindfulness in psychological well-being. *Journal of Personality and Social Psychology, 84,* 822–848.

Carlson, L. E., Speca, M., Patel, K. D., & Goodey, E. (2004). Mindfulness-based stress reduction in relation to quality of life, mood, symptoms of stress and levels of cortisol, dehydroepiandrostrone-sulfate (DHEAS) and melatonin in breast and prostate cancer outpatients. *Psychoneuroendocrinology, 29,* 448–474.

Carson J., Carson, K., Gil, K., & Baucom, D. (2004). Mindfulness based relationship enhancement. *Behavior Therapy, 35,* 471–494.

Cowger, E. L., & Torrance, E. P. (1982). Further examination of the quality changes in creative functioning resulting from meditation (Zazen) training. *Creative Child and Adult Quarterly, 7*(4), 211–217.

Cranson, R. W., Orme-Johnson, D. W., Gackenbach, J., Dillbeck, M. C., Jones, C. H., & Alexander, C. N. (1991). Transcendental meditation and improved performance on intelligence-related measures: A longitudinal study. *Personality & Individual Differences, 12*(10), 1105–1116.

Davidson, R. J., Kabat-Zinn, J., et al. (2003). Alterations in brain and immune function produced by mindfulness meditation. *Psychosomatic Medicine, 65,* 564–570.

Dillbeck, M. C., Assimakis, P. D., & Raimondi, D. (1986). Longitudinal effects of the transcendental meditation and TM-Sidhi program on cognitive ability and cognitive style. *Perceptual Motor Skills, 62*(3), 731–738.

Dillbeck, M. C., & Orme-Johnson, D. W. (1987). Physiological differences between transcendental meditation and rest. *American Psychologist, 42*(9), 879–881.

Dunn, B. R., Hartigan, J. A., & Mikulas, W. L. (1999). Concentration and mindfulness meditations: Unique forms of consciousness? *Applied Psychophysiology and Biofeedback, 24,* 147–164.

Easterlin, B. L., & Cardena, E. (1999). Cognitive and emotional differences between short- and long-term Vipassana meditators. *Imagination, Cognition & Personality, 18*(1), 68–81.

Edwards, D. L. (1991). A meta-analysis of the effects of meditation and hypnosis on measures of anxiety. *Dissertation Abstracts International, 52*(2-B), 1039–1040.

Fowler, J. (1981). *Stages of faith: The psychology of human development and the quest for meaning.* San Francisco: Harper & Row.

Gelderloos, P., Walton, K., Orme-Johnson, D., & Alexander, C. (1991). Effectiveness of the transcendental meditation program in preventing and treating substance misuse: A review. *International Journal of the Addictions, 26*(3), 293–325.

Griffin, D. (1998). *Unsnarling the world knot: Consciousness, freedom, and the mind-body problem.* Berkeley: University of California Press.

Grof, C., & Grof, S. (1990). *The stormy search for self: Understanding spiritual emergence.* Los Angeles: Tarcher.

Grof, S. (1998). *The cosmic game.* Albany: State University of New York Press.

Groopman, J. (2001, September 17). God on the brain: The curious coupling of science and religion. *The New Yorker,* 165–168.

Haimerl, C. J., & Valentine, E. (2001). The effect of contemplative practice on interpersonal, and transpersonal dimensions of the self-concept. *Journal of Transpersonal Psychology, 33*(1), 37–52.

Huxley, A. (1945). *The perennial philosophy.* New York: Harper & Row.

Jevning, R., Wilson, A. F., & Davidson, J. M. (1978). Adrenocortical activity during meditation. *Hormones and Behavior, 10*(1), 54–60.

Kabat-Zinn, J. (1982). An outpatient program in behavioral medicine for chronic pain patients based on the practice of mindfulness meditation: Theoretical considerations and preliminary results. *General Hospital Psychiatry, 4,* 33–47.

Kabat-Zinn, J. (1990). *Full catastrophe living.* New York: Delacorte Press.

Kabat-Zinn, J., Lipworth, L., & Burney, R. (1985). The clinical use of mindfulness meditation for the self-regulation of chronic pain. *Journal of Behavioral Medicine, 8,* 163–190.

Kabat-Zinn, J., & Skillings, A. (1989, March). *Sense of coherence and stress hardiness as predictors and measure of outcome of a stress reduction program.* Paper presented at the Society of Behavioral Medicine conference, San Francisco, CA.

Kabat-Zinn, J., Wheeler, E., Light, T., Skillings, A., Scharf, M. J., Cropley, T. G., et al. (1998). Influence of mindfulness meditation–based stress reduction intervention on rates of skin clearing in patients with moderate to severe psoriasis undergoing phototherapy (UVB) and photochemotherapy (PUVA). *Psychosomatic Medicine, 60*(5), 625–632.

Kohlberg, L. (1981). *Essays on moral development: Vol. I. The philosophy of moral development.* New York: Harper & Row.

Kornfield, J. (1993). Even the best meditators have old wounds to heal: Combining meditation and psychotherapy. In R. Walsh & F. Vaughan (Eds.), *Paths beyond ego* (pp. 67–68). New York: Tarcher/Putnam.

Lazar S. W., Kerr, C., Wasserman, R. H., Gray, J. R., Greve, D., Treadway, M. T., et al. (2005). Meditation experience is associated with increased cortical thickness. *NeuroReport, 16,* 1893–1897.

Lesh, T. (1970). Zen meditation and the development of empathy in counselors. *Journal of Humanistic Psychology, 10*(1), 39–74.

Loevinger, J. (1997). Stages of personality development. In R. Hogan, J. Johnson, & S. Briggs (Eds.), *Handbook of personality psychology* (pp. 199–208). San Diego, CA: Academic Press.

Maslow, A. (1971). *The farther reaches of human nature.* New York: Viking.

Miller, J., Fletcher, K., & Kabat-Zinn, J. (1995). Three-year follow-up and clinical implications of a mindfulness-based intervention in the treatment of anxiety disorders. *General Hospital Psychiatry, 17,* 192–200.

Murphy, M., Donovan, S., & Taylor, E. (1997). *The physical and psychological effects of meditation: A review of contemporary research with a comprehensive bibliography* (2nd ed.). Petaluma, CA: Institute of Noetic Sciences.

Neff, K. D., Rude, S. S., & Kirkpatrick, K. L. (in press). A comparison of self-compassion and other constructs related to healthy psychological functioning. *Journal of Research in Personality.*

Nidich, S. I., Ryncarz, R. A., Abrams, A. I., Orme-Johnson, D. W., & Wallace, R. K. (1983). Kohlbergian cosmic perspective responses, EEG coherence, and the TM and TM-Sidhi program. *Journal of Moral Education, 12,* 166–173.

Novak, P. (1989). Buddhist meditation and the great chain of being: Some misgivings. *Listening, 24*(1), 67–78.

O'Halloran, J. P., Jevning, R. A., Wilson, A. F., Skowsky, R., & Alexander, C. N. (1985). Hormonal control in a state of decreased activation: Potentiation of arginine vasopressin secretion. *Physiology and Behavior, 35,* 591–595.

Orme-Johnson, D. W., & Haynes, C. T. (1981). EEG phase coherence, pure consciousness, and TM-Sidhi experiences. *International Journal of Neuroscience, 13,* 211–217.

Page, R. C., McAuliffe, E., Weiss, J., Ugyan, J., Stowers-Wright, L., & MacLachlan, M. (1997). Self-awareness of participants in a long-term Tibetan Buddhist retreat. *Journal of Transpersonal Psychology, 29,* 85–98.

Penner, W. J., Zingle, H. W., Dyck, R., & Truch, S. (1974). Does an in-depth transcendental meditation course effect change in the personalities of the participants? *Western Psychologist, 4,* 104–111.

Popper, K., & Eccles, J. (1977). *The self and its brain: An argument for interactionism.* Heidelberg, Germany: Springer-Verlag.

Ryff, C. D. & Singer, B. (1998). Human health: New directions for the next millennium. *Psychological Inquiry, 9*(1), 69–85.

Salzberg, S. (1995). *Lovingkindness.* Boston: Shambala.

Schumacher, E. (1977). *A guide for the perplexed.* New York: Harper & Row.

Shapiro, D., & Walsh, R. (Eds.). (1984). *Meditation: Classic and contemporary perspectives.* New York: Aldine.

Shapiro, S. L., Bootzin, R., Lopez, A. M., Figueredo, A. J., & Schwartz, G. (2003). The efficacy of mindfulness-based stress reduction in the treatment of sleep disturbance in women with breast cancer: An exploratory study. *Journal of Psychosomatic Research, 1,* 1–7.

Shapiro, S. L., Brown, K. W., & Biegle, G. (2006, March). Cultivating empathy and well being in counseling psychology students. Paper presented at the Mindfulness in Medicine, Health Care and Society fourth annual conference, Worcester, MA.

Shapiro, S. L., Schwartz, G.E.R., & Bonner, G. (1998). The effects of mindfulness-based stress reduction on medical and pre-medical students. *Journal of Behavioral Medicine, 21,* 581–599.

Smith, W. P., Compton, W. C., & West, W. B. (1995). Meditation as an adjunct to a happiness enhancement program. *Journal of Clinical Psychology, 51*(2), 269–273.

So, K., & Orme-Johnson, D. (2001). Three randomized experiments on the longitudinal effects of the transcendental meditation technique on cognition. *Intelligence, 29*(5), 419–440.

Speca, M., Carlson, L., Goodey, E., & Angen, M. (2000). A randomized wait-list controlled clinical trial: The effect of a mindfulness meditation-based stress reduction program on mood and symptoms of stress in cancer outpatients. *Psychosomatic Medicine, 62,* 613–622.

Tart, C. (2001). *Mind science.* Novato, CA. Wisdom Editions.

Tate, D. B. (1994). Mindfulness meditation group training: Effects on medical and psychological symptoms and positive psychological characteristics. *Dissertation Abstracts International, 55*(55-B), 2018.

Tloczynski, J., & Tantriella, M. (1998). A comparison of the effects of Zen breath meditation or relaxation on college adjustment. *Psychologia: An International Journal of Psychology in the Orient, 41*(1), 32–43.

Valentine, E. R., & Sweet, P.L.G. (1999). Meditation and attention: A comparison of the effects of concentrative and mindfulness meditation on sustained attention. *Mental Health, Religion and Culture, 2,* 59–70.

Varela, F., & Shear, J. (Eds.). (1999). The view from within. *Journal of Consciousness Studies 6*(2), 69–95.

Wallace, R. K. (1986). *The Maharishi technology of the unified field: The neurophysiology of enlightenment.* Fairfield, IA: MIU Neuroscience Press.

Walsh, R. (1999). *Essential spirituality: The seven central practices.* New York: Wiley.

Walsh, R. (2002). *Can synesthesia be cultivated?: Suggestions from surveys of meditators.* Unpublished manuscript, Irvine, CA.

Walsh, R., & Vaughan, F. E. (1993). *Paths beyond ego: The transpersonal vision.* New York: Tarcher/Putnam.

West, M. (Ed.). (1987). *The psychology of meditation.* Oxford, England: Clarendon Press.

Wilber, K. (2000). *Integral psychology: Consciousness, spirit, psychology, therapy.* Boston: Shambala.

Wilber K., & Walsh, R. (2002). An integral approach to consciousness research: A proposal for integrating first, second and third person approaches to consciousness. In M. Velmans (Ed.), *Investigating phenomenal consciousness.* Amsterdam: John Benjamins.

Williams, A., Kolar, M. M., Reger, B. E., & Pearson, J. C. (2001). Evaluation of a wellness-based mindfulness stress reduction intervention: A controlled trial. *American Journal of Health Promotion, 15*(6), 422–432.

Witkiewitz, K., Marlatt, G. A., & Walker, D. D. (in press). Mindfulness-based relapse prevention for alcohol use disorders: The meditative tortoise wins the race. *Journal of Cognitive Psychotherapy.*

Zamarra, J. W., Schneider, R. H., Besseghini, I., Robinson, D. K., & Salerno, J. W. (1996). Usefulness of the transcendental meditation program in the treatment of patients with coronary artery disease. *American Journal of Cardiology, 77,* 867–870.

Chapter Nine

PRAYER AND INTENTION IN DISTANT HEALING: ASSESSING THE EVIDENCE

Marilyn Schlitz, PhD, and Dean Radin, PhD

The authors would like to thank Jenny Mathew, Charlene Farrell, and Cassandra Vieten for their help on the production of this chapter.

INTRODUCTION

Throughout history and in almost all cultures, people have claimed they were healed by another person's caring intention or will (Whitmont, 1993). From botanicas in Mexico, to street markets in Senegal, the desert of the Kalahari, healing shrines in Japan, and suburban neighborhoods in the United States, we find settings in which people attempt to help others by consciously intending their well-being, even at a distance (Schlitz & Braud, 1997a).

Distant healing intention is often associated with the religious practice of prayer, and rituals for fostering such intentions can be found in all the major religions. Some individuals spend their lives in contemplative prayer, such as Carmelite nuns, and some monks and nuns devote a substantial proportion of their prayers to requests for healing. For example, the Unity Church has offered prayers on behalf of anyone who requests it, 24 hours a day and 365 days a year, for over a century. In Jerusalem, an Internet prayer service allows people around the globe to request prayer at the Wailing Wall. During the holy month of Ramadan, millions of Moslems gather at Mecca to engage in group prayer several times each day.

In contemporary U.S. culture it is difficult to determine the precise prevalence of the use of distant healing intention as a complementary and alternative medicine (CAM) therapy, not because it is rarely used but because it is so popular that surveys have had to focus on finding the exceptions. We do know that distant intention is the most common healing practice used outside of conventional medicine. In a recent survey of adult Americans, conducted by the Centers for Disease Control and Prevention's National Center for Health Statistics, of the top five most popular CAM healing practices, three involved prayer and spirituality (Barnes, Powell-Griner, McFann & Nahin, 2004), the most popular CAM practice was prayer for self, and the third most popular was prayer for others.

An earlier national survey found that 82 percent of Americans believed in the healing power of prayer, and 64 percent felt that physicians should pray with patients who request it (Wallis, 1996b). Another survey found that 19 percent of cancer patients reported that they augmented their conventional medical care with prayer or spiritual healing (Cassileth, 1984). And a survey of American Cancer Society support groups for women with breast cancer showed that 88 percent found spiritual or religious practice to be important in coping with their illness (Johnson & Spilka, 1991), although the extent to which specific prayers or intentions of healing were part of their activities was not clear. In acute illnesses, such as cardiac events, these numbers are higher. For example, Saudia, Kinney, Brown, and Young-Ward (1991) found that 96 percent of patients stated that they prayed for their health before undergoing surgery. Some 33 percent of Hispanic patients with AIDS reportedly sought such prayer assistance (Suarez, 1996). And in the United Kingdom, there are more distant healers (approximately 14,000) than therapists from any other branch of CAM (Astin, Harkness, & Ernst, 2000), indicating the widespread practice and use of distant healing.

Among medical professionals, the concepts of spiritual healing, energy healing, and prayer are slowly gaining acceptance as well. In a 1996 survey of northern California physicians (Wallis, 1996b), 13 percent of practitioners reported using or recommending prayer or religious healing as an adjunct to conventional interventions. Therapeutic touch, which can be performed at a distance, is used by nurses in at least 80 hospitals in the United States (Maxwell, 1996) and has been taught to more than 43,000 healthcare professionals (Krieger, 1979). Among the lay public, Reiki International, the largest training organization for "subtle-energy healing," reports having certified more than 500,000 practitioners worldwide. While Reiki healing is frequently performed through physical contact, it is also regularly practiced over distances of thousands of miles (Schlitz & Braud, 1985).

Many terms have been used to describe intentional interventions. They include intercessory prayer, spiritual healing, nondirected prayer, intentionality, energy healing, shamanic healing, nonlocal healing, noncontact therapeutic touch, and level III Reiki. Each of these modalities describes a particular theoretical, cultural, and pragmatic approach toward mediating a healing or biological change through mental intention of one person toward another (Schlitz & Braud, 1997a). Those who engage in distant healing often share the conviction that their process involves contact with an ineffable spiritual realm.

While many patients and healthcare providers regard intention and prayer as vitally important, what support is there that distant intention extends beyond mundane psychological and sociological explanations? From a psychological perspective, all forms of intentional therapy may be thought of as employing a simple coping mechanism in the face of uncertainty or dire need. In addition, the concept that prayer for self promotes healing is no longer considered radical because of the growing literature on the salutary effects of meditation and placebo and, perhaps more importantly, the plausibility of psychoneuroimmunological models of self-regulation (Kiecolt-Glaser, McGuire, Robles, & Glaser, 2002).

Likewise, prayer for others is understandable as a practical coping mechanism, but the idea that it might be efficacious remains controversial. Distant healing effects are considered scientifically doubtful because the term *distant* in this context means shielded from all known causal interactions (Sloan & Ramakrishnan, 2005; Wallis, 1996a). Science is slowly coming to grips with the concept of "spooky action at a distance" in fundamental physics (Walach, 2005), but so far the idea that nonlocal effects might also be important in the behavior of living systems evokes as much scorn as it does interest. Because the mechanisms underlying distant healing are unknown, most experiments studying the hypothesized effects have been concerned with the more straightforward empirical question: Does it work?

THE SCIENCE OF DISTANT HEALING

Distant healing intention (DHI) may be defined as "a compassionate mental act intended to improve the health and well-being of another person at a distance" (Sicher, Targ, Moore, & Smith, 1998). The fundamental assumption in DHI is that the intentions of one person can affect the physiological state of another person who is distant from the healer.

Over the past half-century, researchers have developed techniques for measuring possible distant healing effects on living systems (Benor, 1993; Dossey, 1993; May & Vilenskaya, 1994; Schlitz et al., 2003; Schmidt, Schneider, Utts, & Walach, 2004; Solfvin, 1984). The goal of these experiments has been to see whether an individual's intentions can produce a measurable response in a distant living system. The best experiments have employed rigorously controlled designs that rule out all known conventional sources of influence, including environmental factors, physical manipulations, suggestion, and expectancy (Schlitz et al., 2003).

A relatively small but compelling body of experimental literature supports the DHI effect in organisms ranging from bacteria (Nash, 1982) to laboratory animals (Snel, van der Sijde, & Wiegant, 1995) to randomized clinical trials with human patients (Byrd, 1988; Sicher et al., 1998). As of 1992, at least 131 controlled DHI studies had been published, of which 56 found a statistically significant effect (Benor, 1992). More recent reviews of subsets of these experiments continue to show positive trends (Astin et al., 2000; Schmidt et al., 2004). We will review a few of these experiments to illustrate the research and its relevance to assessing the plausibility of genuine distant healing.

DISTANT HEALING INTENTIONS IN A BASIC SCIENCE PARADIGM

Numerous studies have addressed the question of whether physiological measures—specifically autonomic nervous system activity in humans—might be susceptible to distant intentions. In the majority of these experiments, electrodermal activity (EDA) was used as the physiological measure. EDA provides a sensitive, noninvasive measure of the degree of activation in the autonomic nervous system.

Beginning in the 1970s, Braud and Schlitz conducted a series of experiments in which skin conductance was measured in the target person (a "receiver"), while a "sender" in an isolated, distant room attempted to interact with him or her by means of calming or activating thoughts, images, or intentions (Braud & Schlitz, 1983; Schlitz & Braud, 1997a; Schlitz & LaBerge, 1997). In these studies, the sender's intentions were not necessarily aimed toward distant *healing*, but the experimental task was consistent with a distant mental influence as proposed by DHI.

In 2004, psychologist Stefan Schmidt and his colleagues from the University of Freiburg Hospital, Germany, published a meta-analysis of these EDA-based experiments in the *British Journal of Psychology* (Schmidt et al., 2004). Schmidt's team found 40 experiments conducted between 1977 and 2000. Overall the results were in favor of replicable DHI-like interactions ($p < 0.001$, Cohen's d weighted effect size $d = 0.11$). The possibility of inflated statistical results due to selective reporting practices was investigated, and no such biases were found. In addition, no significant relationships were found between experimental methods and the resulting outcomes, so the results were not explainable as design flaws. In a second set of EDA-based experiments focusing on an effect conceptually similar to distant intention, namely "the sense of being stared at" (over closed circuit television to avoid sensory interactions), Schmidt's team found 15 experiments conducted between 1989 and 1998. The meta-analysis again found a significant overall effect ($p = 0.01$, Cohen's $d = 0.13$), no evidence of selective reporting biases, and no relationship between study quality and outcome. In discussing their findings, Schmidt's group noted that, "because of the unconventional claim of the studies under research, we always chose a more conservative strategy whenever such a decision had to be made." They concluded that, for both classes of experiments, "There is a small, but significant effect. This result corresponds to the recent findings of studies on distant healing and the 'feeling of being stared at.' Therefore, the existence of some anomaly related to distant intentions cannot be ruled out."

With decades of repeatable, statistically significant findings reported from different laboratories, confidence is increasing that DHI effects are real. The absolute magnitude of the effects observed in the laboratory is small, but this is true for many other medically relevant effects. For example, a major clinical study on the use of aspirin to prevent second heart attacks was stopped early because researchers decided it was unethical to withhold the drug from the control group given its observed, positive effects. The effect size for the aspirin effect was 0.03—nearly four times smaller than the equivalent distant intention effect size of 0.11 (Schlitz & Braud, 1997b).

A recent experiment attempted to build a bridge between basic science investigations of distant healing using healthy volunteers and clinical studies on distant healing under conditions of genuine need (Radin et al., in press). The study investigated what would happen when the powerful motivations associated with clinical trials of DHI were combined with the controlled context and objective measures offered by laboratory protocols. It also explored the role of training in potentially modulating DHI effects. In the "trained group," the sender of distant healing (the healthy partner) attended a day-long training program involving discussion and practice of a secular DHI technique based on the Tibetan Buddhism practice of Tonglen meditation, Judeo-Christian forms of meditation, and therapeutic touch.

After attending the training session and practicing the DHI meditation daily for three months, each healthy partner and his or her spouse or friend undergoing treatment for cancer were tested in the laboratory. In a wait group condition, the couple was tested before the healthy partner attended the training. A third control group condition consisted of healthy couples who received no training. The results of this experiment showed that the overall effect size for the motivated condition was 0.74, nearly 7 times larger than the earlier DHI meta-analytic estimate of 0.11, and over 24 times larger than the aspirin study mentioned above. This suggests that distant healing practiced with very high motivation and training may be far more robust than previously observed in laboratory studies.

DHI IN CLINICAL STUDIES: ADDRESSING THE "SO WHAT?" QUESTION

Although there appears to be evidence to support proof of principal for the hypothesis that the intentions of one person have a measurable effect on the biology of another living system, we are still left with the question: Does DHI have clinical relevance? Can focused intention affect the course of healing within real patient populations? To date, only a small number of scientific studies have directly addressed this important question. So far, these clinical studies provide conflicting evidence that DHI can improve medically relevant outcomes in people suffering from conditions including arthritis, cardiac problems, hernia surgery, and AIDS. Interpretation of these clinical studies is complicated by lack of homogeneity in patient populations, lack of control and documentation of current medications, lack of consistency in healer background and intervention (Sicher, Targ and Smith, 1998), and uncertainty about the role of patient expectancies and belief in DHI outcomes. However, this is not to say that there is no evidence. The majority of randomized, double-blind investigations to date support the clinical efficacy of DHI (Roberts, Ahmed, & Hall, 2000; Schlitz & Lewis, 1996). In a systematic review published in the *Annals of Internal Medicine,* John Astin and colleagues (2000) found that 57 percent (13 of 23) of the published randomized, controlled clinical trials (RCTs) on DHI showed a positive treatment effect in a wide range of human populations, including both genders and a wide range of ages and ethnicities. As noted by Astin and colleagues (2000, p. 910):

> We believe that additional studies of distant healing that address the methodological issues outlined above are now called for to help resolve some of the discrepant findings in the literature and shed further light on the potential efficacy of these approaches.

Clinical trials of DHI were initiated in a seminal study by cardiologist Randolph C. Byrd (1988). In the 1980s, Byrd, then a cardiologist at San Francisco General Hospital, conducted an RCT to assess the effects of intercessory prayer on health outcomes in 393 patients admitted to the coronary care unit. Patients were randomly assigned to a prayed-for group or a control group; both groups underwent comparable conventional medical treatment. The healers Byrd chose were people with an active Christian life manifested by daily devotional prayer and an active fellowship with a local church. Each person prayed daily that the cardiac patients would achieve specific outcomes, including rapid recovery, prevention of complications and death, and any other areas they believed helpful to the patient.

The study results showed that members of the group receiving healing prayer were five times less likely to require antibiotics and three times less likely to develop pulmonary edema compared to the control group. In addition, fewer among them died compared to the control group, and none of the prayed-for group required endotracheal intubation, while 12 in the control group did.

These results were intriguing, but the study was not without problems. Byrd did not assess the psychological health of those entering the study;

thus, it is possible that the treated and control groups differed in this regard. Nevertheless, the results of this experiment have been quoted from pulpits to podiums and hailed enthusiastically as proof that prayer really works.

Given the scientific, social, and possible spiritual relevance of Byrd's findings, it is surprising that it took another dozen years for other researchers to conduct a more rigorously controlled replication. Finally, Harris and colleagues (1999), working with 999 patients admitted to a hospital coronary care unit, found that the medical course of his patients was better in those who were prayed for than in the control group. Harris's study, unlike Byrd's, used distant healers from a variety of Christian traditions (35 percent were listed as nondenominational, 27 percent Episcopalian, and the remainder were either Protestant or Roman Catholic). Harris also chose a more global score to assess the outcome of prayer on coronary recovery. Like Byrd, Harris concluded that his patients significantly benefited from the intercessory prayer they received.

Together, these two studies provided preliminary evidence that the intention of people engaged in healing prayer can affect the physical well-being of people at a distance. A few years after the Harris study, another study of DHI was reported in the *Western Journal of Medicine* by Fred Sicher and his colleagues (1998). These observations included a small pilot and a larger confirmation study involving the effects of intercessory (petitionary) prayer on patients with advanced AIDS. Their choice of healers was interesting. Because it is not known whether one form of distant healing is more effective than another, Sicher incorporated a wide range of self-identified healing practitioners, representing many different healing, spiritual, and religious traditions. They reasoned that by combining DHI efforts they would be more likely to see a positive effect rather than relying on a fortuitous choice of one particular practice that might be effective. Healers received a photograph of their patient, his or her last name and first initial, and sometimes the T-cell count (an index of immune system functioning). The healers provided DHI to each patient for seven days, and at six months the prayed-for patients had acquired significantly fewer new AIDS-defining illnesses, had lower illness severity, fewer doctor visits, fewer hospitalizations, fewer days of hospitalizations, and improved mood as compared to the control patients. These were highly significant outcomes, given that AIDS at the time of this study had a grim prognosis and no effective treatments.

After the systematic review by Astin et al. was completed, an additional three DHI RCTs have been published; none found significant evidence for a DHI effect. In the first, an NIH-funded clinical trial initiated by Elisabeth Targ and others at California Pacific Medical Center (later completed by John Astin), distant prayer had no effect on outcomes for AIDS patients. However, there was a surprising outcome: the treated patients correctly guessed that they were assigned to the treatment group to a highly statistically significant degree, unlike the control patients, who guessed at chance. This suggests that the treated patients accurately sensed the healers' distant intentions, but those perceptions did not correlate with medically relevant outcomes. This finding is consistent with laboratory DHI studies, which also indicate that one person's intentions can influence the nervous system of a distant person, without implying a healing effect.

The second DHI study was conducted under the direction of cardiologist Mitchell Krucoff of Duke University Medical Center. Earlier in his career, Dr. Krucoff was a volunteer in a spiritually based hospital in an ashram in rural India. There he observed that, despite sometimes primitive facilities (it was the only place he had ever seen bare feet in an operating room) and poor prognoses, patients appeared relaxed and calm, filled with a sense of well-being. He wondered what created the "healing space" he had experienced? Could the same atmosphere in the ashram's hospital be translated into a state-of-the-art hospital in the United States, and would the combination of modern medical care and attention to spiritual well-being help patients more than standard medical care alone?

To test these questions, Krucoff conducted a pilot project on 150 cardiology patients scheduled for angioplasty at the Durham Veterans Affairs Medical Center from April 1997 to April 1998. Before the procedure, each patient was randomly assigned to either standard care or to an intervention involving guided imagery, stress relaxation, healing touch—all performed at patients' bedsides—or to intercessory prayer, which was distributed among prayer groups including Buddhists, Roman Catholics, Moravians, Jews, Baptists, and the Unity School of Christianity. The results showed that all of the interventions were helpful, and patients in the prayer group did the best (Krucoff, Crater, & Green, 2001). However, a larger and more recent follow-up study involving 748 cardiac patients (Krucoff et al., 2005) found no overall result on the primary study outcome. A surprisingly strong effect was observed in one condition in which a group of people were assigned to pray for the prayers. This potential additive or "booster" effect leaves researchers intrigued despite the failure of the primary outcome to support the DHI hypothesis.

In the third recent clinical study involving cardiac patients, conducted by Herbert Benson and his colleagues (2006) at Harvard Medical School, a group who received intercessory prayer without knowing that they were in the treatment group showed no improvement. But the group who did know that they were the object of distant prayer showed results that were significantly *worse* than the control group. This new experimental condition, which combines expectation plus DHI, had not been studied before, and it implies that, under some conditions, knowledge of receiving prayer may have a detrimental effect. Some researchers speculate that this might have occurred because patients with such knowledge may have feared that they were receiving prayer because their health had a particularly poor prognosis.

Based on all clinical trials conducted so far, we are left with more questions than answers. Should we conclude that DHI does not influence healing based on recent experiments that failed to show an effect? Or should the weight of all published clinical and experimental studies influence our decision in a more positive direction? Should we conclude from the Harvard study that knowing someone is praying for us might cause harm? Does it make sense that DHI can be effective independent of any personal relationship between the person who prays and the person who is prayed for?

Researchers are faced with these and other challenges in designing and establishing scientific protocols to objectively measure whether a particular medical problem may be helped by prayer or intention. Some of the most significant and still unresolved experimental questions include what type of prayer to use, how often to pray, how to describe what healers did so that others may reproduce the results, and how to match the belief systems of the patient with that of the healer. Investigators also face sociological constraints from both scientists and theists, neither of whom wants this research to take place at all. The former assert that prayer is nonscientific, and the latter maintain that testing prayer is blasphemous.

None of the clinical trials conducted so far has made use of what scientists call "ecological validity." This means the trials were not designed to model what happens in real life, where people often know the person for whom they are praying and with whom they have a meaningful relationship. In the Harvard study, for example, prayer groups were instructed for the sake of standardization to use a pre-scripted prayer that was different from what the prayers used in their normal practice. So the Harvard experiment did not really test what the healers claimed works for them. In addition, in most of the clinical studies, the investigators were tightly focused on medical outcomes, and hardly any attention was paid to the inner experiences of the healers and the patients.

THEORETICAL CONTEXT FOR DISTANT HEALING

One of the primary reasons that mainstream science and medical researchers doubt that distant healing is effective is that it seems to violate what might be called folklore physics—the physics of everyday experience. Sloan and Ramakrishnan (2005) assert that: "Nothing in our contemporary scientific views of the universe or consciousness can account for how the 'healing intentions' or prayers of distant intercessors could possibly influence the [physiology] of patients even nearby let alone at a great distance" (pp. 1769–1770).

But is it true that nothing in science suggests the presence of connections between apparently isolated objects? Quantum entanglement, a far from common sense effect predicted by quantum theory—described by Einstein as "spooky action at a distance" and later demonstrated as fact in the laboratory (Walach, 2005)—shows that, under certain conditions, particles that interact remain instantaneously connected after they separate, regardless of distance in space or time. If this property is truly as fundamental as it appears to be, then in principle everything in the universe might be entangled to some degree (Radin, 2006). Everyday objects do not appear to show such entanglements, and there are arguments why quantum entanglement would be difficult to sustain at the human scale.

But one cannot help wondering, what if this concept *did* apply to humans. Between an indifferent, unmotivated couple, entanglements between their minds and bodies may be difficult to detect. But in a highly motivated couple, such as a dedicated healer and a patient in great need, the underlying correlations might become more evident. Such a relational model is appealing because it does not require anything (force, energy, or signals) to pass between the healer and the patient. Instead, it postulates a physical correlation that is always present between people (and everything else) due to the "nonlocal threads" from which the fabric of reality is woven (Radin, 2006; Walach, 2005).

COMMON ELEMENTS ACROSS HEALING PRACTICES

Many spiritual practitioners maintain that anyone can be a healer. All that is required is a compassionate heart. At the other end of the spectrum, some traditions believe that only a special few have the gift of healing. Meanwhile, research by Elisabeth Targ and others suggests that most people have inherent healing capacities but that special training, motivation, and practice are required to bring these gifts to fruition. In our studies of healing practices across many traditions, we have found a few common guidelines. These include:

Set an intention: Bring one's awareness, with purpose and a sense of efficacy, toward a healing response in the distant person.

Focus attention: Cultivate a state of concentration on the intention. For healing, this requires a mind focused on the act of intending a healing outcome.

Cultivate love and compassion: Compassion is one person's selfless love and care for another's suffering. Experience a sense of connection to others.

Suspend disbelief: Confidence and openness to the healing method is associated with the ability to give and receive distant healing.

Take time: Professional healers often set aside at least an hour a day to provide healing intention.

CONCLUSION

Surveys consistently show that distant healing intention (in a secular sense) and prayer (in a religious sense) are very commonly used. The question is whether these practices and beliefs are efficacious beyond acting as psychological coping strategies. We have addressed this question by splitting the relevant evidence into basic science, which seeks a proof-of-principle answer, and clinical research, which seeks to understand possible applications. The answer to the first question appears to be yes. The laboratory studies have been successfully replicated by numerous researchers around the world, and meta-analyses continue to provide significant evidence for these effects.

The answer to the second question—do these influences produce medically efficacious outcomes?—is more complex. Overall, the clinical trials suggest that DHI occasionally improves some patients' health under some circumstances. However, the effects are not easy to reproduce, and they appear to interact strongly with many factors that are difficult to control. These include variables such as who is praying, for what exactly are they praying, how did they pray, what is their usual mode or style of prayer, what are the relationships among the healers, the patients, and the investigators, and so on. Dozens of such factors make studying the effects of intention on healing exceptionally challenging.

In her book, *Kitchen Table Wisdom,* oncologist Rachel Remen observes, "An unanswered question is a fine traveling companion. It sharpens your eye for the road." DHI researchers have discovered over the last few decades that their collective eyes are becoming increasingly sharpened. What we've learned so far is that there is something interesting about the role of distant intention in healing, and that this something appears to be highly sensitive to the questions being asked about it. Undoubtedly, as new questions are posed, surprising new answers will patiently await us.

TOOL KIT FOR CHANGE

Role and Perspective of the Healthcare Professional

1. Prayer and compassionate intention are vital aspects of many patients' practice. As such, it is important for healthcare professionals to have knowledge and sensitivity about what is known about these modalities.
2. Many patients today want their practitioners to pray with them; an informed opinion on the role of prayer in healing is vital to effective communication and increased compliance.
3. Attending to their own spiritual care is an important part of health professional wellness.

Role and Perspective of the Participant

1. One way in which patients take an active role in their management of pain or suffering is the use of compassionate intention and prayer for self and others.

2. Distant healing is a sought-after form of healing intervention by many patients and has been shown to reduce stress and anxiety.
3. Data from laboratory studies support the usefulness of distant healing as a component of an integral program—one with which patients can be actively involved.

Interconnection: The Global Perspective

1. Prayer and healing are part of a worldview that includes dimensions that are not included in standard medical education.
2. Gaining knowledge of other worldviews is useful for enhanced communication between patients, health professionals, and the family and society in which they live.

REFERENCES

Astin, J. A., Harkness, E., & Ernst, E. (2000). The efficacy of "distant healing": A systematic review of randomized trials. *Annals of Internal Medicine, 132*(11), 903–910.

Barnes, P. M., Powell-Griner, E., McFann, K., & Nahin, R. L. (2004). *Complementary and alternative medicine use among adults* (Advance Data Report #343). Bethesda, MD: National Center for Complementary and Alternative Medicine.

Benor, D. J. (1992). *Healing research, Vol. 1.* In (Vol. Chapters 1–2). Deddington, United Kingdom: Helix Editions.

Benor, D. J. (1993). *Healing research: Holistic medicine and spiritual healing.* Munich, Germany: Helix Verlag.

Benson, H., Dusek, J. A., Sherwood, J. B., Lam, P., Bethea, C. F., Carpenter, W., et al. (2006). Study of the therapeutic effects of intercessory prayer (STEP) in cardiac bypass patients: A multicenter randomized trial of uncertainty and certainty of receiving intercessory prayer. *American Heart Journal, 151*(4), 934–942.

Braud, W., & Schlitz, M. (1983). Psychokinetic influence on electrodermal activity. *Journal of Parapsychology, 47,* 95–119.

Byrd, R. C. (1988). Positive therapeutic effects of intercessory prayer in a coronary care unit population. *Southern Medical Journal, 81*(7), 826–829.

Cassileth, B. R. (1984). Contemporary unorthodox treatment in cancer medicine. *Annals of Internal Medicine, 101,* 105–112.

Dossey, L. (1993). *Healing words: The power of prayer and the practice of medicine.* San Francisco: Harper.

Harris, W. S., Gowda, M., Kolb, J. W., Strachacz, C. P., Vacek, J. L., Jones, P. G., et al. (1999). A randomized, controlled trial of the effects of remote intercessory prayer on outcomes in patients admitted to the coronary care unit. *Archives of Internal Medicine, 159*(19), 2273–2278.

Johnson, S. C., & Spilka, B. (1991). Coping with breast cancer: The roles of clergy and faith. *Journal of Religion and Health, 30,* 21–33.

Kiecolt-Glaser, J., McGuire, L., Robles, T., & Glaser, R. (2002). Psychoneuroimmunology and psychosomatic medicine: Back to the future. *Psychomatic Medicine, 64,* 15–28.

Krieger, D. (1979). *The therapeutic touch: How to use your hands to help or heal.* Englewood Cliffs, NJ: Prentice-Hall.

Krucoff, M., Crater, S., Gallup, D., Blankenship, J., Cuffe, M., Guarneri, M., et al. (2005). Music, imagery, touch, and prayer as adjuncts to interventional cardiac care: The monitoring and actualisation of noetic trainings (mantra) II randomised study. *Lancet, 366*(9481), 211–217.

Krucoff, M., Crater, S., & Green, C. (2001). Integrative noetic therapies as adjuncts to percutaneous intervention during unstable coronary syndromes: Monitoring and actualization of noetic training (mantra) feasibility pilot. *American Heart Journal, 142*(5), 760–767.

Maxwell, J. (1996). Nursing's new age? *Christianity Today, 40*(3), 96–99.

May, E., & Vilenskaya, L. (1994). Some aspects of parapsychological research in the former Soviet Union. *Subtle Energies, 3,* 1–24.

Nash, C. B. (1982). ESP of present and future targets. *Journal of the Society for Psychical Research, 51*(792), 374–377.

Radin, D. I. (2006). *Entangled minds: Extrasensory experiences in a quantum reality.* New York: Simon & Schuster.

Radin, D. I., Stone, J., Levine, E., Eskandarnejad, S., Schlitz, M., Kozak, L., et al. (in press). Effects of motivated distant intention on electrodermal activity. *Explore: The Journal of Science and Healing.*

Roberts, L., Ahmed, I., & Hall, S. (2000). Intercessory prayer for the alleviation of ill health. *Cochrane Database Systematic Reviews, 2.*

Saudia, T. L., Kinney, M. R., Brown, K. C., & Young-Ward, L. (1991). Health locus of control and helpfulness of prayer. *Heart Lung, 20*(1), 60–65.

Schlitz, M., & Braud, W. (1985). Reiki plus natural healing: An ethnographic and experimental study. *Psi Research, 4,* 100–123.

Schlitz, M., & Braud, W. (1997a). Distant intentionality and healing: Assessing the evidence. *Alternative Therapies in Health and Medicine, 3*(6), 62–73.

Schlitz, M. J., & Braud, W. G. (1997b). Distant intentionality and healing: Assessing the evidence. *Alternative Therapies, 3*(6), 62–73.

Schlitz, M. J., & LaBerge, S. (1997). Covert observation increases skin conductance in subjects unaware of when they are being observed: A replication. *Journal of Parapsychology, 61,* 185–196.

Schlitz, M., Lewis N. (1996). The healing powers of prayer. *Noetic Sciences Review,* Summer, 29–33.

Schlitz, M., Radin, D., Malle, B. F., Schmidt, S., Utts, J., & Yount, G. L. (2003). Distant healing intention: Definitions and evolving guidelines for laboratory studies. *Alternative Therapies in Health and Medicine, 9*(Suppl. 3), A31–A43.

Schmidt, S., Schneider, R., Utts, J., & Walach, H. (2004). Distant intentionality and the feeling of being stared at. *British Journal of Psychology, 95,* 235–247.

Sicher, F., Targ, E., Moore, D., & Smith, H. S. (1998). A randomized double-blind study of the effect of distant healing in a population with advanced aids. Report of a small scale study. *Western Journal of Medicine, 169*(6), 356–363.

Sloan, R., & Ramakrishnan, R. (2005). The mantra II study. *Lancet, 366,* 1769–1770.

Snel, F.W.J.J., van der Sijde, P. C., & Wiegant, F.A.C. (1995). Cognitive styles of believers and disbelievers in paranormal phenomena. *Journal of the Society for Psychical Research, 60*(839), 251–257.

Solfvin, J. (1984). Mental healing. In S. Krippner (Ed.), *Advances in Parapsychological Research, 4,* 31–63.

Suarez, M. (1996). Use of folk healing practices by HIV-infected hispanics living in the United States. *AIDS Care, 8*(6), 685–690.

Walach, H. (2005). Generalized entanglement: A new theoretical model for understanding the effects of complementary and alternative medicine. *Journal of Alternative and Complementary Medicine, 11*(3), 549–559.

Wallis, C. (1996a). Faith and healing. *Time/CNN poll,* 58–64.

Wallis, C. (1996b, June 24). Faith and healing. *Time,* 58–64.

Whitmont, E. C. (1993). *The alchemy of healing.* Berkeley, CA: North Atlantic.

Chapter Ten

YOGA AND MIND-BODY MEDICINE

Eleanor Criswell, EdD

Enlightenment means recovering our true identity as the Self, or Spirit. This magnifi-
cent inner event spells the end of all our suffering and confusion. It means coming home.

—Georg Feuerstein

Millions of people in the East and West have made yoga part of their lives.
Some of these have chosen to do so because of media exposure, word-of-mouth
recommendations, or research findings. Many of them were encouraged to
take a yoga class by their physicians or other healthcare providers. This is the
natural evolution of mind-body medicine. People are spontaneously practicing preventive medicine using an ancient mind-body integration technique:
yoga. The deliberate inclusion of yoga in mind-body medicine is a more recent
development. Individuals, professionals, and institutions are beginning to
bring yoga into medical treatment or ongoing health maintenance programs.
Yoga is the embodiment of mind-body medicine. Because yoga is a mind-
body medicine and has much to offer medical endeavors, it is valuable to look
at what yoga is and how it works; its history, science, and psychophysiology;
contemporary approaches to yoga; yoga research and education; goals and
outcomes, health benefits, and the psychospiritual dimension of yoga; indications and contraindications for yoga; yoga therapy; and future directions for
yoga in mind-body medicine.

Mind-body medicine may be as old as human existence. Archeologists have
found evidence of shamanic methods as far back as 20,000 years ago (Achterberg,
1985). The use of mind-body practices to alter oneself and the impact of the

environment are probably much older. This desire to control oneself and one's environment is a natural human tendency, as seen in the behavior of children in the early stages of cognitive development. Folk healing methods using imagination and ritual have been found across time and throughout the world. Contemporary mind-body medicine has developed within the last 40 years. Eastern and Western physical, psychological, and spiritual methods have been combined with modern medicine to form mind-body medicine. Yoga, an ancient mind-body discipline, has a great deal to offer the development of contemporary mind-body medicine.

WHAT IS YOGA?

Yoga comes from a Sanskrit word. It is derived from the root *yuj*, meaning to yoke, harness, or unite (Feuerstein, 1997b). Unification or reunification of the self with the universal self is its goal. There are two approaches to unification: dualistic (yoga) and nondualistic (Advaita Vedanta). The dualistic approach refers to the perceived separation of humans from the All of existence and the need to move toward a state of union through various yoga practices. The nondualistic approach sees humans as already in a state of union and needing only to remember that state. From the dualistic perspective, yoga also means the reunification of the person—mentally, physically, emotionally, and spiritually. Ultimately, yoga refers to the reunification of humankind with the universe or cosmic consciousness or Absolute. A psychospiritual technology (Feuerstein, 1998), yoga is the discipline and training of the human's embodied being toward what it is capable of becoming. Yoga provides physical and mental training to further refine the unified mind-body. It includes the perspective of the mind-body as an integrated whole.

The principles of yoga posit that the body must be trained before it is possible to train the mind. The goal of training the mind is to make it one-pointed or focused. When the mind remains focused on a meditation target long enough, the experience of samadhi occurs. Samadhi is the union of the meditator with the object of meditation. There are several levels of unification. The first level of unification is that of the mind and body. Then the practitioner achieves unification with other aspects of existence. Union with the All of existence, cosmic consciousness, or Brahman is the ultimate state of unification. Few people achieve this ultimate state of union.

HISTORY OF YOGA

Yoga is a 5,000-year-old discipline. Its history can be divided into preclassical, classical, postclassical, and contemporary. Classical yoga refers to the yoga codified by Patanjali circa 200 B.C. (Prabhavananda & Isherwood,

1953). Classical yoga (Raja or Ashtanga) has eight limbs or categories of practices: (1) yamas; (2) niyamas; (3) asanas; (4) pranayama; (5) pratyahara; (6) concentration; (7) meditation; and (8) unification or samadhi. Classical yoga begins with an ethical system: the yamas and niyamas. These are rules for behavior. The yamas or abstentions include non-injury, truthfulness, non-theft, spiritual conduct, and non-greed. The niyamas—or observances—include cleanliness, contentment, austerity, self-study, and attentiveness to God or the All of existence. The asanas are the movements and postures of yoga. Patanjali describes a simple set of postures in his *Yoga Sutras*, mainly devoted to meditation. Pranayama includes breathing exercises that focus on the redirection of the flow of prana, the primal energy. Pratyahara encourages relaxation and sense withdrawal or redirection of consciousness. In concentration, attention is fixed on the selected focus; meditation is the nonverbal dialogue or interchange between the meditator and his or her focus of meditation; and samadhi is the meditator's absorption into the object of meditation, a temporary or more permanent state of union. The meditator ceases to have a separate sense of self. Classical yoga is a valuable contribution to mind-body medicine.

CONTEMPORARY APPROACHES TO YOGA

Because there are many approaches to yoga, there is a yoga for everyone who practices it. No two people can duplicate the yogic orientation exactly. Yoga—classic, contemporary, eclectic—takes many forms. Some students work with a guru; some students learn on their own. It is important to find the way that most suits one's inner being. (In more a collectivistic culture, such as India, the connection with a guru is highly valued; in the United States, a more individualistic culture, students tend to be more autonomous, studying with a variety of teachers.)

Hatha, Raja, Jnana, Karma, Mantra, Bhakti, and Purna (Integral) are some of the well-known approaches to yoga. Hatha yoga emphasizes physical discipline. Raja yoga uses mental discipline. Jnana yoga, the yoga of knowledge, focuses on discriminating knowledge as the yogic way. Selfless service and action in the world is the way of Karma yoga. The use of sacred sounds and thoughts is the way of Mantra yoga. Bhakti yoga is the way of universal love and devotion. Bhakti yoga practices include chanting, singing, and dancing. Purna yoga or Integral yoga is a synthesis of all the yogas and included social service. All yogas endeavor to regain the sense of union with the ground of Being (Atman rejoined with Brahman).

Currently, the most popular type of yoga in the United States is Hatha yoga, which emphasizes physical postures (asanas) and breath control (pranayama). It may include some meditation, but the main emphasis is on the person's physical development. Eighty-four or 84,000 (some yogis have estimated that there are 84 postures; others estimate 84,000) postures have been created over the millennia. How those postures are achieved varies from teacher to teacher and lineage to lineage. Contemporary yogas from the Hatha yoga tradition include Ananda yoga (from Paramahansa Yogananda's teachings and developed by Swami Kriyananda), Ashtanga yoga (K. Pattabhi Jois), Bikram yoga (Bikram Choudhury), Hidden Language yoga (Swami Sivananda Radha), Integral yoga (Swami Satchidananda), Iyengar yoga (developed by B.K.S. Iyengar), Kundalini yoga (Yogi Bajan), Kripalu yoga (developed by Yogi Amrit Desai and inspired by Kripalvananda), Sivananda yoga (Swami Vishnudevananda), Viniyoga (begun by Shri Krishnamacharya and carried forward by T.K.V. Desikachar, his son), Somatic yoga (a combination of Raja and Hatha yoga developed by Eleanor Criswell), and others (Feuerstein, 1999).

Haridas Chaudhuri (1975) says that "the ultimate goal of all of the above self-disciplines is blissful union with the Self in its transcendental dimension of oneness with timeless Being" (p. 236). These yogas are different in their approaches, but they all move toward self-realization and ego-transcendence. Moving beyond development of the self to the use of the self in society is Chaudhuri's conception of Integral yoga, which blends transcendence and participation in the world. Chaudhuri describes samadhi as "the experience of freedom, immortality, transcendence of subject-object dichotomy, inexpressible bliss, limitless expansion of consciousness" (p. 246). A brief period of inaction follows self-realization. This is followed by a new kind of action. This action is empowered by Being-energy, which is used along the lines of destiny or dharma. Chaudhuri says that "the unmistakable mark of this authentic self-realization [the individual's] would be his egoless dedication to cosmic welfare" (p. 252).

Yoga is especially suited to mind-body medicine, because, in yoga, the mind-body duality has never existed (Chaudhuri, 1975). Yoga sees both the mind and body as having evolved or manifested out of Prakriti, the primordial energy. The environment and the mind-body evolved from the same source, and a continuity exists in all forms of existence. A part of the continuity is the atman or self as pure consciousness. This is the view of the Samkhya metaphysical system—the philosophical foundation of yoga psychology.

HOW YOGA WORKS

How does yoga contribute to so many positive changes, including health and wellness? Because yoga helps the practitioner move toward homeostasis, various medical conditions caused or exacerbated by psychophysiological

imbalances are modified. For example, yoga provides stimulation for the following physiological systems:

A. Central nervous system: meditative practices and all yogic practices
B. Sensory systems:
   1. Visual: eye exercises, visual meditation targets, internal visual experiences
   2. Auditory: chants, internal sounds, Indian music
   3. Olfactory: incense, perfumes and essential oils, flowers
   4. Gustatory: special candies, foods, and spices
   5. Tactile: textures and massage
C. Vestibular system: balancing and inverted postures
D. Respiratory system: breathing and breath-holding patterns
E. Cardiovascular system: various practices in combination
F. Somatic nervous system (neuromuscular system): active and static asanas (postures)
G. Gastrointestinal system: fasting and special dietary recommendations
H. Autonomic nervous system (sympathetic and parasympathetic nervous system):
   all yoga practices (Criswell, 1989).

PSYCHOPHYSIOLOGY OF YOGA

To get maximum benefit from yoga practices, it is valuable to know how they
work psychophysiologically. Psychophysiology is the study of the physiological
effects of psychological and other experiences. Psychophysiological changes are
measured by electronic devices (such as biofeedback equipment), biochemical
testing, behavioral measures, functional magnetic resonance imaging (fMRI),
and others. These measures are looked at in the context of psychophysiological
baselines before and after yoga practice. The neurophysiology of humans can
be divided into the central nervous system (brain and spinal cord) and peripheral nervous system (autonomic and somatic nervous systems). The autonomic
nervous system is divided into the sympathetic nervous system (fight, flight,
or freeze) and the parasympathetic nervous system (rest, maintenance, and
repair). Using biofeedback and physiological monitoring equipment, the
central nervous system can be measured by the electroencephalograph. Electrodermal activity (formerly galvanic skin response) is a direct measure of
sympathetic nervous system activity. Eccrine gland secretions of the hands,
produced by the sympathetic nervous system, can be used to conduct a mild
electrical current. Moist hands conduct a mild electrical current put out by the
equipment more readily. The skin temperature recording and hand warming is
an indirect measure of parasympathetic nervous system activity. The somatic
nervous system (musculoskeletal system) is measured by the electromyograph.
Respiration can be measured using a respiration strain gauge. (Inhalation is a
sympathetic nervous system event; exhalation is a parasympathetic nervous

system event). Heart rate can be measured using a photoplethysmograph. These modalities are measured by computerized psychophysiological monitoring systems.

Yoga is a practice in self-regulation. The physiological systems function in their habitual ways, at habitual levels, using brain stem areas such as the medulla. When a person decides to engage in a yoga practice—for example, an asana—nonvoluntary motor activity is replaced with voluntary motor activity. This shifts the level of control of the muscles from the brain stem motor tracts to the voluntary motor cortex. The voluntary motor cortex has a map (the motor homunculus) of the opposite half of the body. For example, the right hemisphere holds the map of the left side of the body. One half of the body is mapped upside down on each hemisphere. Approximately one-third of the homunculus is devoted to the face, mouth, and tongue; one-third is devoted to the hand; and the remaining third is devoted to the rest of the body. In front of the primary motor cortex is the premotor cortex. A portion of that area, the supplementary motor cortex, has a map of the entire body on each hemisphere. The supplementary motor cortex is the area that "lights up" during positron emission tomography (PET) measures taken while the person visualizes movement. As the yoga practitioner voluntarily contracts certain muscles to accomplish the posture, the neurons of the voluntary motor cortex send a volley of action potentials down their axons to excite the motor units (neuron and all its muscle fibers) to cause a contraction of the muscle fibers. The transmitter substance that is secreted by the alpha motor neurons is acetylcholine. Acetylcholinesterase stops the process at the synapse.

The contracted muscles are called agonists; their opposing muscles are called antagonists. The contracting muscles are engaged in a concentric contraction; the opposing muscles are engaged in eccentric contractions (lengthening contractions). The eccentric contractions allow for a controlled movement into the yoga position. As the posture is held for a period of time, the areas of the motor cortex involved in maintaining the posture continue to be stimulated. As the yoga practitioner comes slowly out of the posture, the motor cortex sends impulses to the spinal cord segment for the muscles that were contracted to inhibit the firing of the motor units. This allows the muscles to gradually relax. It also allows the motor cortex to reset the resting tonus of the muscles.

Some approaches to yoga emphasize stretching. This is a misunderstanding of the meaning of yoga. Yoga is not about stretching; it is about union. If the intention is to stretch the muscle, part of the body will be stabilized and other parts of the body will pull against the stabilized area. This has the effect of stretching the contracted muscle. There are receptors in the muscle (neuromuscular spindles) that are sensitive to stretch. When they are stretched, they send a message back to the spinal cord to excite the motor units causing the muscle to return to its original contraction level. Sometimes this recontraction becomes a muscle spasm. This is a spinal cord event, a temporary relaxation at best.

Accomplished yogis probably do their yoga with greater central brain organization than the average yoga student. For example, as they begin a posture, they neurologically create a good motor plan. Motor planning uses the association cortex and limbic system. From there, the plan is translated into programs and subprograms using the primary motor cortex, basal ganglia, cerebellum, and brain stem. Finally, the programs are executed at the spinal cord level. With central organization of the posture, the brain lengthens the opposing muscle (antagonist) before the contraction of the agonist. Then the primary motor cortex sends impulses to inhibit the motor units and, therefore, lengthen the contracted muscle. For example, while doing the shoulderstand, the neck is in anterior flexion, the elbows are bent, the hands are supporting the back, and the legs are extended toward the ceiling. The anterior muscles of the neck are contracted, and the posterior muscles of the neck are lengthened. The slow movements of yoga enable the practitioner to use the voluntary motor cortex, which is the only part of the motor system that can inhibit the output to the muscles. This inhibition is what allows the muscles to relax.

Sensory feedback from the yoga movements before, during, and after the posture is received by the sensory cortex. The sensory feedback lets the brain know what is taking place in the body. The sensory homunculus (sensory cortex), similar to that of the motor cortex, receives information about various aspects of the movement from the opposite side of the body. The sensory cortex receives information from the neuromuscular spindles (length and speed of lengthening of the muscle) and Golgi tendon organs (force of the contracted muscle), slow cutaneous and fast cutaneous adaptation, and joint receptors. The sensory feedback facilitates the movement. This feedback completes the sensory-motor loop.

Other yoga practices have a similar effect: Involuntary functions, such as respiration, are voluntarily controlled for a period of time. This enables the yoga practitioner to re-establish a relaxed and comfortable functioning of the system. Meditation is accomplished by stimulating areas of the brain that process sensory input (meditation target) while inhibiting other areas of the brain. For example, a visual meditation target, such as a mandala or other object, stimulates the visual system. Auditory meditation targets, such as chanting or quiet music, stimulate the auditory system. The brain is entrained by the repeated stimulation of the same or adjacent areas.

Other areas of the brain are inhibited, becoming quieter and more synchronized. The synchronized brain wave that is produced is called alpha (8 to 12 cycles per second or Hertz) and sometimes theta (4 to 7 Hz). Brain waves are a comparison across time of the electrical potential difference between two electrodes placed on the scalp. The electrical activity measured from the scalp reflects the cortical activity of the brain beneath the electrodes (Criswell, 1995).

YOGA RESEARCH

Thousands of years of careful and systematic exploration led to the practical science of yoga. The early science of yoga used the process of observation, hypotheses, and experimental testing. The testing was experiential. Empirical in the original sense of the word, the development of yoga was based on immediate experience. The principles and practices of yoga were tested pragmatically. "If individuals and small groups had similar experiences with certain recommended practices, if the effects were repeated generation after generation, if isolated practitioners reported similar results, then the knowledge could be said to have been validated empirically through experience" (Criswell & Patel, 2003, p. 206). As a science, yoga most nearly paralleled Western science from the time of Aristotle to the middle of the nineteenth century. The mind-body split was contributed by the French philosopher René Descartes to Western science in the sixteenth century. Coming from a different cultural tradition, yoga did not suffer from the Cartesian legacy. With the founding of the first laboratory devoted to the scientific study of yoga in Kaivalyadhama at Lonavola, Poona, India, in the 1920s, yoga entered the era of modern science (Funderburk, 1977).

Yoga research is conducted all over the world, but especially in India. Yoga research methodologies have varied over time and in various cultural contexts. Nearly 30 years ago in *Science Studies Yoga* (1977), James Funderburk gathered all the contemporary yoga research. The studies collected explored the third (asana), fourth (pranayama), and seventh (meditation) limbs of Raja yoga. The areas of research include the following:

- *Asana:* EMG (electromyographic or muscle activity) studies, measures of flexibility, pressure changes in internal cavities, and the effect of breath
- *Pranayama* (respiratory responses): nostril dominance, respiratory pattern (breath rate, breath holding time, respiratory amplitude), air movement (tidal volume, minute ventilation, vital capacity), gaseous transfer
- Circulatory response to Hatha yoga: cardiovascular efficiency, blood-flow alterations, heart rate, heart control, blood pressure, blood composition
- Endocrine and nervous system responses: secretory products, autonomic nervous system balance, electroencephalographic (EEG) changes
- *Meditation:* muscular system responses during meditation, circulatory system responses during and after meditation, respiratory effects, endocrine and nervous system responses to meditation (EEG during meditation) (Criswell & Patel, 2003, p. 211).

A particularly significant area of contemporary yoga research concerns the psychophysiological effects of yoga. The International Association of Yoga Therapists maintains a data base of research concerning the psychophysiological effects of yoga practices (Lamb, 2004). The field of psychophysiology has enabled the physiological monitoring (EEG, electrocardiogram, electromyogram, respiration, etc.) of yogic practices. Monitoring meditation and other yogic practices with fMRI, PET, and other brain imaging techniques shows areas of the brain involved in these practices.

Since 1977, yoga research throughout the world has continued to explore areas similar to those outlined by Funderburk (1977). The findings are comparable. Physiologists, medical researchers, and psychologists are exploring the physical and mental effects of yoga using contemporary scientific methods. Psychophysiological research into the effects of yoga is particularly important. There are two sources of evidence for the psychophysiological effects of yoga: research using yoga practices (such as the research conducted at the Vivekananda Kendra Yoga Research Foundation in India and at the All-India Institute of Medical Sciences) and from the research findings from other fields—physiology, biochemistry, kinesiology, psychophysiology, psychology, and medicine. These findings help shed light on the reported effects of yoga practices. A phenomenological analysis from a psychophysiological perspective of yoga practices can serve as the basis for further controlled studies.

Yoga research has been published in many journals such as the *Journal of the International Association of Yoga Therapists, International Journal of Psychophysiology, Indian Heart Journal, Indian Journal of Medical Research, Indian Journal of Physiology and Pharmacology, Journal of Psychosomatic Research, Neurology India, Psychophysiology, Psychosomatic Medicine,* and *Yoga-Mimamsa.*

YOGA EDUCATION

Historically, yoga was passed down from teacher to student on an individual basis. Contemporary yoga classes teach yogic practices at different levels of difficulty to groups of students. Yogic training and development usually occur in an educational rather than therapeutic context. An accomplished teacher usually guides the student or students. Finding a qualified yoga teacher is important. (See Yoga Alliance—www.yogaalliance.org—to check the credentials of yoga teachers or the International Association of Yoga Therapists—www. IAYT.org. The events that occur in yoga classes are supervised by the teacher. Yoga does not work from a pathological model: The growth and development of the student is the focus. In some yoga classes, the teaching begins with where the student is and unfolds as the student progresses. Yoga training seen from this perspective has great benefits. The teacher works to develop the student's potential rather than beginning with the student's deficiencies.

GOALS AND OUTCOMES OF YOGA

The goals or outcomes of yoga include the following: peace of mind; increased will and motivation; increased capacity to love; increased intelligence; enhanced psychic faculties; better concentration; control of emotions; bodily health, suppleness, beauty, and longevity; and prevention and removal of psychosomatic dangers and troubles (Wood, 1962). Although mind-body medicine is particularly concerned with the health benefits of yoga, the other outcomes of yoga also have health benefits.

The goals or outcomes of yoga can be explored from the perspective of mind-body medicine. Each goal or claim will be examined to reveal the relationship between it and mind-body medicine. Each one will be expanded to show the reality behind the goal or claim. Although yoga encourages a non–goal-oriented approach, it is valuable to be aware of the possible outcomes to allow for their unfolding without interfering with them. The yoga practitioner is encouraged to notice but remain unattached to the outcomes.

Although the final goal of yoga is union with cosmic consciousness, ultimate reality, and the Absolute, these intermediary goals or gains are possible:

Peace of mind. Through yoga practice, including meditation, comes a gradual balancing of physiological systems. The practitioner begins to create a calm mind. Relaxation leads to a shift toward parasympathetic nervous system dominance. The parasympathetic nervous system includes activation of the brain's anterior hypothalamus. Milder emotions are increased.

Will and motivation. With yoga practice, there are changes in intentions and motivations. Of the various theories of motivation, the one that is most relevant to the exploration of yoga has to do with the activation and arousal of the organism by the reticular activating system. Sometimes noticed during sustained yoga practice are increased motivation, the capacity to set goals, and move toward actualizing them. Motivation and compliance with recommendations are very important in mind-body medicine.

Love. The yoga practitioner sometimes notices an increased capacity to love. The practitioner notices this with regard to special persons in his or her life or toward people in general. There may be increased feelings of love toward the environment and objects in the environment. There may be an increased love of life. The practitioner may notice an increased capacity to love him- or herself. Research conducted by the Heart Math Institute indicates that heart rate variability, considered an index of health, is enhanced by entertaining loving feelings. Heart rate variability is said to enhance physiological coherence (Childre & Martin, 1999).

The shift toward the parasympathetic nervous system dominance that is encouraged by yoga practice is accompanied by changes in neurochemistry, which leads to pleasant emotions. The yoga practitioner may experience decreased ego boundaries and increased feelings of merging with persons or objects. There is the feeling of kinship and awareness of the beauty inherent in the person or object. Feelings of gratitude may accompany this state.

Increased intelligence. Intelligence is essentially the ability to function effectively in the world. Yoga practitioners report an increase in effective intelligence. Yoga practices provide physiological experiences that increase circulation to the brain. Concentration exercises increase the effective use of mental capacity.

Psychic faculties. For a thousands of years, practitioners of yoga have reported psychic experiences (siddhis or psi). The experiences reported by practitioners and observers range from telepathic to psychokinetic. Dramatic changes in psychic abilities do not usually happen during yoga development, but the yoga student may experience those at the lower end of the continuum. These experience include "increased empathic responses to other people, increased feelings of understanding what other people are thinking, or the increased feeling for the flow of events before they happen" (Criswell, 1989). Native American healing practices and healers from other traditions report that healing is fostered by altered states of consciousness with experiences suggestive of psi.

Concentration. In Western culture and educational systems, very little is done to teach concentration or attention. Learning how to focus one's mind is a valuable experience. Concentration skills—physiological and psychological—are fostered by yoga practice. Concentration is an important part of mind-body medical practices.

Control of emotions. Some people try to learn how to experience their emotions more intensely and authentically, to be more in touch with their feelings. Being able to control emotions is important in many contexts. To reduce irritation and anger, to maintain peace of mind, and to spend more time in a happy state facilitates one's health and the health and happiness of others. Yoga aids the control of emotions through a shift to the parasympathetic nervous system dominant state. The role of emotional expression and positive emotions in health and healing is increasingly recognized in correlational studies.

Bodily health, suppleness, beauty, and longevity. Many yoga practitioners report a change in their general state of health. They notice this in the "decrease in the number and incidences of illness during any given period of time" (Criswell, 1989, p. 14). This is probably due to the enhanced immune system functioning that has been reported in meditation studies. This enhanced immune system function persists as long as there is regular yoga practice. An increase in suppleness (flexibility) follows sustained yoga practice. This flexibility is noticed during postures and with other activities of daily living. If yoga practice is stopped, there is a decrease in flexibility. When yoga practice begins again, there is a return to the postures again and the previous suppleness. Through yoga practice, weight normalization may occur.

It has been reported that yoga practice leads to increased longevity. Indra Devi, once a famous Hollywood yogini, is a prime example of someone who lived to over a hundred and continued to teach yoga in her ashram in South America. It is has been observed that advanced "yogis do gain longevity, but that they then choose the times of their deaths, when they choose to go into samadhi or mahasamadhi" (Criswell, 1989). The yoga practitioner can be expected to live out his or her life with greater health, mobility, and an enhanced quality of life. It is said that yoga practice retards the effects of aging. It seems that long-time yoga practitioners do behave with more youthful vigor.

Prevention and removal of psychosomatic problems. Psychosomatic diseases are physical complaints that originate from a psychological or emotional cause. The patient's behavior or psychological state impacts over time on the physiological state. Psychosomatic complaints include asthma, various kinds of headaches, gastrointestinal difficulties, and hypertension. Many of these complaints include a reaction to long-term stress. Yoga enables the practitioner to shift toward parasympathetic nervous system dominance, the maintenance and repair system. The shift from a stress state to one of relaxation is the outcome. With yoga practice, there develops an easier return to homeostasis following stress. Therefore, the practitioner is less likely to stay in a prolonged stress state that may lead to psychosomatic complaints. Yoga practice allows the practitioner to maintain a state of bodily health, which tends to prevent psychosomatic difficulties. Through yoga practice, existing psychosomatic complaints are resolved or managed.

HEALTH BENEFITS OF YOGA

The health benefits of yoga include enhanced immune system function with a decrease in the number and length of illnesses; increased flexibility and enhanced balance; a decrease in psychosomatic symptoms with fewer asthma episodes, headache reduction (in terms of frequency, intensity, and duration), lower risk of hypertension, diabetes (reduction in blood sugar level), cardiac issues; and enhanced healing and decreased stress response with a move from sympathetic nervous system dominance toward parasympathetic nervous system dominance and homeostasis.

INDICATIONS FOR YOGA IN MIND-BODY MEDICINE

Yoga would be indicated for a patient in whom the presenting complaints are related to psychosomatic illnesses, health recovery, and coping with chronic medical conditions. It would also be useful in a preventive medicine, health maintenance context and for successful aging. It is useful when stress is a factor. Yoga has been beneficial in the management of such conditions as arthritis, asthma, back pain, cancer care, chronic fatigue syndrome, diabetes, cardiac conditions, headaches, hypertension, insomnia, irritable bowel syndrome, multiple sclerosis, Parkinson's disease, repetitive strain injury, sciatica, pregnancy, and many others. Yoga is a key component in Dean Ornish's (1990) well-known program for reversing heart disease. Psychological conditions benefited by yoga have included anxiety, depression, eating disorders, phobias, and stress management. The patient must be receptive to yoga to receive maximum benefits.

CONTRAINDICATIONS FOR YOGA IN MIND-BODY MEDICINE

Yoga practice is not always indicated for a given individual. The conditions under which yoga would not be indicated are called contraindications. Several factors—such as the type and level of difficulty of the yoga class—need to be taken into consideration when referring a patient for a yoga class or yoga therapy. Yoga may affect the patient's psychophysiology, and the particular presenting complaint of the patient needs to be considered in this regard. Ongoing medications may need to be altered in light of the new physiological state. For example, decreased stress lowers blood sugar levels. Therefore, the patient's insulin prescription may need to be regulated. The physician needs to monitor the physiological changes regarding maintenance medications. Medicine and other recommendations need to be monitored because of the physiological changes that might accompany yoga practice.

It is important to remember the dangers of yoga practice listed by Haridas Chaudhuri (1975): (1) extreme introversion; (2) spiritual hedonism or gluttony; (3) regression; (4) emotional fixation on the guru; and (5) self-mutilation.

Complications from other medical complaints need to be considered—for example, blood pressure considerations may preclude some yoga postures. Psychological factors such as depression, dissociative tendencies, and others may need to be taken into consideration by the psychologist or counselor who is working with the yoga student.

YOGA THERAPY

Yoga therapy originated in India. Indian gurus (spiritual teachers) frequently were reported to engage in healing practices or to have healing effects. Yoga therapy as a specific discipline uses yoga practices to benefit physiological and psychological issues. Yoga therapy usually takes place in a one-on-one setting but also can be conducted in a group setting or class. The therapeutic use of yoga concerns medical complaints such as hypertension, asthma, diabetes, musculoskeletal pains (e.g., back pain), dealing with chronic illnesses, and stress management. Psychological complaints may include anxieties, phobias, and stress responses.

Definitions of Yoga Therapy

The International Association of Yoga Therapists (IAYT) is working to develop a shared definition of yoga therapy. Meanwhile, it has published on its Web site (www.iayt.org) several definitions developed by significant contributors to the field. Georg Feuerstein, noted yoga scholar, says that "yoga therapy aims at the holistic treatment of various kinds of psychological or somatic dysfunctions ranging from back problems to emotional distress. Both approaches, however, share an understanding of the human being as an integrated body-mind system, which can function optimally only when there is a state of dynamic balance." Richard Miller, cofounder of IAYT and a renowned Advaita yoga teacher, says that "yoga therapy may be defined as the application of yogic principles to a particular person with the objective of achieving a particular spiritual, psychological, or physiological goal." Finally, Judith Hanson Lasater—physical therapist, well-known yoga teacher, and cofounder of the *Yoga Journal*—says that yoga therapy is "the use of the techniques of Yoga to create, stimulate, and maintain an optimum state of physical, emotional, mental, and spiritual health."

Approaches to Yoga Therapy

Approaches to yoga therapy include those found in India, the United States, and elsewhere. Yoga therapy in India may be conducted in an institute (such as the Yoga Institute, Santa Cruz (E) in Mumbai), in an ashram, in clinical contexts, or by a trained practitioner in a particular yoga tradition. It is frequently part of Ayurvedic medical treatment. In the West, yoga therapy is conducted in clinical contexts or by yoga therapists working independently. Many of these approaches have evolved training programs. Some of the yoga therapy training programs in the United States include: the Yoga Therapy Certification program at Loyola Marymount University, Los Angeles (Chris Chapple and Larry Payne); Structural Yoga Therapy (Mukunda Stiles); Phoenix Rising Yoga Therapy (Michael Lee); Integrative Yoga Therapy (Joseph LePage); and American Viniyoga Institute (Gary Kraftsow). Other yoga therapies practiced in the United States include Iyengar Yoga Therapy and Kundalini Yoga Therapy.

Trained and certified yoga therapists can provide yoga therapy. Currently, they are certified by their training programs. The IAYT maintains a list of qualified yoga therapists. Standards for the training of yoga therapists are being developed by IAYT in cooperation with the various yoga therapy training programs.

The current board of IAYT—John Kepner, executive director; Veronica Zador, president; Eleanor Criswell, secretary/treasurer; and Janice Gates, member-at-large—is overseeing that process.

A Typical Yoga Therapy Session

The typical yoga therapy session begins with an assessment that gathers information about the client's presenting complaint and goals; his or her general physical condition (strength, flexibility, endurance); health history (accidents, surgeries, broken bones, illnesses, medical conditions, medications), daily activities such as work situation; fitness activities and other recommended exercises; and previous yoga experience. Based on the assessment, the session is tailored to fit the client's needs using various yoga practices—asanas, pranayama, meditation, and so forth—conducted according to the therapist's approach to yoga. The session ends with recommended home yoga practice or routine. The yoga therapy sessions may continue for a number of weeks, depending on the client's needs. The yoga therapy session is designed to encourage the client to take responsibility for his or her well-being. Yoga therapy can be very empowering to the client. The client may come back at a later date for additional yoga therapy sessions to continue his or her yogic development (Kepner, Zador, Gates, & Criswell, 2006).

THE PSYCHOSPIRITUAL DIMENSION OF YOGA

Yoga is not a religion, but it does have a psychospiritual dimension. Yoga has been associated with Hinduism during its history, but it has been practiced in the context of many world religions. It can be practiced effectively with or without a spiritual context. Yoga complements the psychospiritual dimension of mind-body medicine. As the yoga practitioner moves toward integration with the whole of existence, there is a sharing of the energies available from the environment. The feeling of spiritual connection has been found to be healing.

Many approaches to mind-body medicine also include the spiritual dimension. Spiritual may be distinguished from religious. Herbert Benson's group at the Mind/Body Medical Institute report that when they engage in mind-body experiences, they frequently have spiritual experiences. This has often been observed by biofeedback trainers and mind-body (somatics) practitioners.

YOGA AND MIND-BODY MEDICINE

Mind-body medicine uses both mental and physical practices to foster healing. The word healing comes from an Old English word meaning to make whole or sound. Contemporary mind-body medicine combines a variety of mental, physical, and spiritual disciplines. These disciplines come from different cultural traditions. Contemporary research confirms the validity of many of the practices. The combination of approaches is used to create blended forms of medical and health maintenance protocols. The patient may create an informal treatment team in the community using a variety of healthcare approaches. For example, the client may see practitioners from a variety of disciplines: psychotherapy, medicine, yoga, chiropractic, folk healing, massage therapy, acupuncture, and so forth. In a clinical or hospital setting, the client may experience a variety of mind-body therapies and techniques. Practitioners in the medical setting combine on-site mind-body practices appropriate for the particular presenting complaints. For example, the patient in a mind-body medicine pain program may receive biofeedback training, physical therapy, medical treatment, psychosocial therapy, recreational therapy, body mechanics training, and stress management classes—which may include relaxation techniques, visualization, meditation training, stress assessment and stress management, and yoga.

Yoga, used therapeutically, is frequently found in an educational setting or yoga class. For example, a physician may refer a patient to take a yoga class to help with a particular complaint that has a stress component.

APPROACHES TO YOGA IN MIND-BODY MEDICINE

There are a variety of approaches to the use of yoga in mind-body medicine. Yoga classes are offered in clinics and communities for preventive health and wellness. Yoga classes are found within clinics and hospital programs, such as the Osher Center for Integrative Medicine at the University of California, San Francisco. Yoga therapy in private practice settings is a growing phenomenon.

Asanas, pranayama, and meditation are yoga practices with clear uses in mind-body medicine. Asanas are postures developed by yogis over the years. There are traditional postures and more recently created postures. The yoga practitioner moves into the posture and holds the position for a period of time while breathing in a slow, mindful manner. The postures frequently are named after animals or objects of Indian life. As the posture is achieved, the practitioner clears his or her mind and stays as relaxed as possible in the posture.

> The asanas are a link between the individual and the environment in that they are named after animals, trees, rivers, mountains, etc., to remind the individual of the environment. They also exhibit the specific qualities of nature that they are named after. Thus we find the tree pose, tortoise pose, elephant pose, sun salutation pose, peacock pose, lotus pose, etc. The asanas include the movements and postures of yoga. (Criswell & Patel, 2003, p. 214)

Many postures have been found to have health benefits. For example, Chandra Patel (1975) found savasana (the corpse pose) to benefit high blood pressure.

Some of the health benefits for the traditional poses reported by Rammurti Mishra (1959), an Indian physician and yoga authority, were enhanced thyroid, gastrointestinal system, and cardiac function; decreased blood pressure; and correction of faulty postures.

Pranayama refers to breathing practices. The exercises are not just for the respiratory system but are ways of maximizing the available energy in the body. Biofeedback training has found that a correlation between respiration and cardiac function leads to coherence within the body. Health benefits have been attributed to increased heart rate variability. When a person inhales, there is an increase in heart rate; when the person exhales, there is a decrease in heart rate. Sympathetic nervous system activity is associated with inhalation; parasympathetic nervous system activity is associated with exhalation. Respiratory sinus arrhythmia is a normal process. The coordination of heart rate and respiration has been considered healthy response.

According to Criswell and Patel (2003):

> The pranayamas are of fundamental importance because the control of prana [universal energy] helps an individual to attain an undisturbed body and mind. According to hatha yogins, the fluctuations in consciousness result from the fluctuations of breath. Therefore, if the breath is controlled then the fluctuations in consciousness also will be controlled. (p. 214)

Meditation has been found in many cultures throughout history. There are many approaches to meditation; it basically consists of focusing attention on a target and maintaining attention over a sustained period of time. Remaining in meditation for over 15 minutes frequently results in a shift toward parasympathetic nervous system dominance. Meditation greatly aids in relaxation and stress management. It can be done in a simple nonspiritual way, as with Benson's (1975) relaxation response (repeating *one* with each exhale), with a special mantra or with a Sanskrit word, phrase, or sentence. Incorporating meditation in one's day increases relaxation and well-being. There are many other benefits of meditation. A tremendous amount of research has been conducted on the psychophysiological effects of meditation (Murphy, 1992; Murphy & Donovan, 1988).

FUTURE DIRECTIONS FOR YOGA IN MIND-BODY MEDICINE

Future directions for yoga in mind-body medicine may include yoga as an integral part of preventive medicine and health maintenance. Billions of people use yoga for health maintenance, beginning in childhood. Yoga may become integral to the treatment plan for patients in the medical setting. Yoga will be used to a greater extent as self-care for healthcare professionals and patients. Continued yoga and mind-body medical research will increasingly demonstrate the efficacy and applications of yoga. Biofeedback, psychophysiological monitoring, brain imaging techniques (fMRI and others), and future technological developments will be used to assist in yogic development. The *Journal of the International Association of Yoga Therapists,* a peer-reviewed journal featuring yoga research, and other journals will continue to encourage research into all aspects of yoga.

CONCLUSION

Yoga, an ancient practice increasingly validated by current research, can help humans move toward more healthful and fulfilling lives. Yoga practice is growing in acceptance by the modern world. Yoga research needs to be expanded so that more and more people are aware of the mental and physical health-giving potential of yoga.

Yoga is a way of life and a method for lifelong self-care. As more and more people maintain their health and wellness using their own natural resources, yoga practice is a viable way to conduct healthcare and contribute to the enhanced development of the person. Yoga fosters actualization of potential for the whole person. Health and well-being are fundamental to maximum human development; a healthy environment is essential.

This chapter has explored yoga as it relates to mind-body medicine. The understanding of practices from another culture is filtered through one's experiences and cultural context. This chapter has provided the basic principles and practices of yoga within mind-body medicine. Development of a unified mind-body state is facilitated by maximum knowledge. This can include information from a third-person perspective in conjunction with first-person experiences. Profound personal transformation results from bringing together these two kinds of awareness. How the benefits of yoga contribute to mind-body medicine has also been explored. Yoga, regardless of the practitioner's original goal, will lead to the transformation of the practitioner's life. The experience is empowering for the patient/student and mind-body medicine professional.

TOOL KIT FOR CHANGE

These guidelines are designed to expand the contribution of yoga and yoga therapy to mind-body medicine.

Role and Perspective of the Healthcare Professional

1. Assess the suitability of yoga or yoga therapy for the patient and the presenting complaint(s) of the patient, and, if possible, encourage an appropriate referral to a qualified yoga teacher or yoga therapist.

2. Include the yoga teacher or yoga therapist in the therapy team on a formal or informal basis, while monitoring the progress of the patient in resolving or managing presenting complaints with yoga as part of the treatment plan.

3. Evaluate the results of the yoga or yoga therapy in relationship to the patient's presenting complaint.

Role and Perspective of the Participant

1. Assess the relevance of yoga for physical or psychological needs and select a style of yoga compatible with the nature of the individual and the presenting complaint.

2. Select a yoga class or yoga therapist. The class should be taught by an experienced teacher who is affiliated with International Association of Yoga Therapists or the Yoga Alliance. The yoga therapist also should be affiliated with IAYT.

3. Do not engage in yoga practices recommended by a yoga teacher or yoga therapist that are contraindicated for one's condition.

Interconnection: The Global Perspective

1. Yoga is an ancient practice that provides physical and mental training to further refine the unified mind-body and, as such, is unique in including the perspective of the mind-body as an integrated whole.

2. Yoga also means the reunification of the person—mentally, physically, emotionally, and spiritually. Ultimately, yoga refers to the reunification of humankind with the universe, cosmic consciousness, or Absolute and can be an integral part of the treatment plan or an adjunct to other therapies.

3. Yoga complements the psychospiritual dimension of mind-body medicine. As the yoga practitioner moves toward integration with the whole of existence, there is a sharing of the energies available from the environment. The feeling of spiritual connection has been found to be healing.

REFERENCES

Achterberg, J. (1985). *Imagery in healing: Shamanism and modern science.* New York: Shambhala.

Benson, H. (1975). *The relaxation response.* New York: William and Morrow.

Chaudhuri, H. (1975). Yoga psychology. In C. Tart (Ed.), *Transpersonal psychologies.* New York: Harper & Row.

Childre, D., & Martin, H. (1999) *The heart math solution.* San Francisco: HarperSan Francisco.

Criswell, E. (1989). *How yoga works: An introduction to somatic yoga.* Novato, CA: Freeperson Press.

Criswell, E. (1995). *Biofeedback and somatics: Toward personal evolution.* Novato, CA: Freeperson Press.

Criswell, E., & Patel, K. (2003). The yoga path: Awakening from the dream. In S. G. Mijares (Ed.), *Modern psychology and ancient wisdom: Psychological healing practices from the world's religious traditions.* New York: Haworth Press.

Feuerstein, G. (1997a). *The shambhala encyclopedia of yoga.* Boston: Shambhala.

Feuerstein, G. (1997b). *Teachings of yoga.* Boston: Shambhala.

Feuerstein, G. (1998). *The yoga tradition: Its history, literature, philosophy and practice.* Prescott, AZ: Holm Press.

Feuerstein, G. (1999). *Yoga for dummies.* Foster City, CA: IDG Books.

Funderburk, J. (1977). *Science studies yoga: A review of physiological data.* Honesdale, PA: Himalayan International Institute of Yoga Science and Philosophy.

Kepner, J., Zador, V., Gates, J., & Criswell, E. (2006, November 15). Personal communication.

Lamb, T. (2004). *Psychophysiological effects of yoga.* Prescott, AZ: International Association of Yoga Therapists.

Mishra, R. S. (1959). *Fundamentals of yoga: A handbook of theory, practice, application.* New York: Julian Press.

Murphy, M. (1992). *The future of the body: Explorations into the further evolution of human nature.* Los Angeles: Jeremy Tarcher.

Murphy, M., & Donovan, S. (1988) *The physical and psychological effects of meditation.* San Rafael, CA: Esalen Institute Study of Exceptional Functioning.

Ornish, D. (1990). *Dr. Dean Ornish's program for reversing heart disease.* New York: Random House.

Patel, C. (1975). 12-month follow-up of yoga and bio-feedback in the management of hypertension. *Lancet, 1,* 62–64.

Prabhavananda, S., & Isherwood, C. (1953). *How to know God: The yoga of Patanjali.* New York: Signet Books.

Wood, E. (1962). *Yoga.* Harmondsworth, Middlesex, England: Penguin Books.

Chapter Eleven

QIGONG FOR HEALTH AND WELLNESS

Beverly Rubik, PhD

INTRODUCTION

Qigong (also written Chi Kung, and pronounced chee-gung) literally means working with the vital energy (qi) by using mind and body to improve health and well-being. It is a form of enhanced self-care that is reported to protect the health and assist in healing. In traditional Chinese philosophy—beginning with Taoist philosophy of the *Yi Jing* (also written *I Ching*) or *Book of Changes* introduced, some think, over 3,000 years ago—qi is the energy that flows throughout the universe and animates life (Wilhelm & Baynes, 1980). The practice of qigong originated in China over 2,000 years ago.[1] When the qi is cultivated, it flows in the body more smoothly, working through obstacles and leading to greater health and well-being. Qigong is sometimes called "needleless" acupuncture (Cohen, 2003, p. 85). According to traditional Chinese medicine (TCM), when qi is blocked, stagnant, or deficient, people can get sick. When the acupuncture meridians are open and qi is flowing, this sets the stage for self-healing to occur. It is said that qi moves to the parts of the body that need healing.

In the early morning in parks throughout China, thousands of people may be seen practicing qigong in unison, often led by a master. Qigong is related to tai chi chuan (also tai chi or *taiji*) , a choreographed martial art and movement meditation that is widely taught and practiced in the West. Whereas tai chi is a useful discipline for maintaining flexibility and energy, the practice of qigong has evolved more specifically to promote health and healing. Moreover, many forms of qigong are simpler to perform than tai chi. Along with acupuncture and herbology, qigong is considered one of the three pillars of TCM.

Qigong master Greg Yau says that ordinary physical exercise requires effort and expends energy. He distinguishes qigong as the highest level of the martial arts as well as a special form of exercise that conserves energy in order to gain even more energy. Qigong involves minimal effort and produces maximum results (Yau, 2006). The various forms of qigong involve movement and sometimes stillness, including specific postures, sequences of movements, self-massage, breathing techniques, and meditation. While some forms of qigong are quite vigorous, others are gentle and relaxing. Some forms are completely motionless and inward-directed. Certain forms of qigong can be practiced by all, including the severely ill and those confined to bed or a wheelchair. Qigong deeply integrates physical and mental practice. For optimum effect, it is typically practiced daily for about 20 minutes to one hour.

Everyone knows that an automobile needs regular maintenance to keep it running smoothly and prevent it from breaking down. Similarly, qigong can be considered a type of mind-body maintenance that releases the tensions of mind and body and helps one achieve and maintain mental and physical fitness. For thousands of years, qigong has been practiced by many people throughout China to maintain good health and improve mental and physical performance. Furthermore, qigong is said to bring spiritual wisdom, slow the aging process, and contribute to longevity. In past centuries, qigong practices were often kept secret among an elite few, but in recent times, many types of qigong have been taught worldwide.

For one to gain and retain health and happiness, the ancient Chinese masters believed that one must be in harmony with cosmic forces and especially with the flow of qi. With increasing qigong experience, one's qi becomes more balanced, promoting a sense of greater harmony within oneself and with the world. Life becomes less of a struggle and more of a graceful, joyful dance.

THE HISTORY OF QIGONG

The concept of qigong was originally derived from Taoist philosophy and later enriched by Confucian and Buddhist traditions, as well as the continued evolution of Taoist thought. The term, qigong, however, was not used until the twentieth century. While the roots of Taoism and the theory of qi emerged in pre-Confucian *Yi Jing* writings, the classic expression of Taoism can be found in the *Tao Te Ching,* traditionally believed to be written by Lao Tsu. Lao Tsu was thought to be a teacher of Confucius, although scholars wonder whether Lao Tsu might have been a pen name for a group of writers. Confucius, in turn, was traditionally thought to be the author of the extensive commentaries on the *Yi Jing,* adding a focus on the moral order of society to the *Yi Jing*'s original focus on the "way of nature."[2]

The *Tao Te Ching* includes an account of the life force (qi) and (in modern terms) emphasizes the importance of the integration of mind, body, and spirit. The ancient Taoist masters experienced a singular wholeness in all of existence. They identified five basic categories of qi: mineral, plant, animal, human, and divine. Qi is also divided into yin and yang aspects. Yin is passive, receptive, feminine, cold, dark, and soft. Yang is active, creative, masculine, hot, light, and hard. The symbol of Taoism (see Figure 1) shows that the yin and yang are ideally in dynamic balance; yin gives birth to yang and vice versa.

Taoist teachers developed various types of qigong exercises to balance the flow of qi within the body and between humans, Earth, and cosmos. For example, in the second century C.E., Hua Tuo proposed the Five Animal Frolics, qigong exercises that imitate the behavior of the bear, tiger, deer, monkey, and crane. These forms are still widely practiced today.

The Chinese literature shows that qigong was traditionally expounded in most classics of past Chinese dynasties that covered history, philosophy, and medicine. For over several thousand years, the Chinese accumulated theoretical knowledge and personal and clinical experience with qigong. More than 100 Chinese books that are considered to be the ancient, classical literature on qigong have been published. In addition, there are numerous methods handed down within families for generations that form the legacy of qigong (Guorui, 1990).

Since 1949, the Chinese government has organized and conducted comprehensive scientific research on qigong. Research undertaken at the Shanghai Qigong Research Institute in the 1950s confirmed that qigong had positive effects on health and well-being. This finding contributed to the spread of qigong. For a while, the Chinese Cultural Revolution (1966–1976) forced qigong underground, but it reemerged after 1976. Even after qigong practice came out in the open, however, it remained the subject of attack by many critics. Once more, the Chinese government sponsored studies to evaluate the effects of qigong and, once again, found health benefits. Research has also been conducted elsewhere, with similar findings, some of which will be mentioned later in this chapter.

Figure 1
The Taoist symbol, showing the interpenetrating dynamics of yin and yang

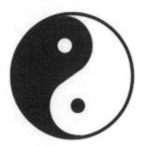

In Beijing, an estimated 1.3 million people practice qigong daily, and in China, 80 million practice it daily (Mayer, 1997). Qigong practice has been growing in the United States, reflected in the fact that the National Qigong Association grew 1,000 percent in six years (Goldberg, 2002). Qigong is regarded worldwide as a beneficial mind-body modality.

MODERN BIOPHYSICS AND THE CONCEPT OF QI

Is there a scientific concept equivalent to the traditional understanding of qi? There is no clear equivalent, although some parallels can be drawn. First, physics has shown that matter and energy are interconvertible, as described by Einstein's famous formula, $E = mc^2$. The transformation of matter into energy, for example, is illustrated by fusion in the sun and also by fission and fusion processes in nuclear reactors. Moreover, all matter vibrates with energy and exchanges energy with other matter whenever it interacts. When positive and negative charges interact through electrical attraction or repulsion, for example, they exchange photons, which are pure energy packets without mass. Even empty space continually produces temporary photons, as well as charged particle pairs such as electrons and positrons (positively charged, antimatter versions of electrons). Called vacuum fluctuations, these temporary—or virtual—particles quickly change into one another; particle pairs annihilate one another to become light or other forms of energy, and photons of light split into charged particle pairs. So, even in so-called empty space, matter becomes energy and energy becomes matter. The relationships among matter, energy, and space explored by contemporary physics may provide keys to the nature of qi and the Tao.

The Taoist Chuang Tze wrote that the Tao (the path, the one, the source) abides only in emptiness (Chang, 1963). The Tao is analogous, in many ways, to the modern physical concept of the quantum vacuum, which gives rise to the buzzing profusion of appearing and disappearing virtual particles described above. Far from being empty, the "vacuum" is paradoxically full. Another way of looking at the vacuum fluctuations described above is in terms of the vast amounts of energy associated with them, which is called the zero-point energy (ZPE). The ZPE constantly interacts with matter, supporting and sustaining it each moment, and may be the closest physical science analogy to the concept of qi. Correspondingly, the qi, which arises from the Tao (emptiness), makes all things move and flourish, from the heavenly bodies to life on Earth, including us. In addition to making us alive, the cosmic qi is believed to revitalize people to the extent that we are "in its flow." When body, mind, and nature become more integrated—if we can interpret Taoist tradition in modern terms—one can experience the qi flowing from the Tao.

Much of contemporary biology is about analyzing the components of life—genes, proteins, and other molecular constituents. This is the dominant Western biomedical paradigm, but it has limitations. It leaves many unanswered questions about what, if anything, animates living things, over and above the organization of their constituents.

Outside of science, there have always been other paradigms that aim to explain the living state. Ancient Taoist masters observed that flowing water never stagnates and concluded, by analogy, that life was associated with flow and energy. There are also many scientists who think that living things are a special kind of system, such as the self-organizing systems studied in far-from-equilibrium thermodynamics (Jantsch, 1980). Such systems are characterized by the ability to change their steady-state patterns in response to extremely small disturbances from within or without. Far-from-equilibrium systems require a continual flow of energy and matter to sustain themselves and enable their self-regulation (Prigogine, 1980). This flow from the outside to the inside of the system is not unlike the Taoist flow of qi.

Many biologists speculate that there must be something more than electrochemical processes that make living things alive and, in particular, make beings such as humans conscious. In biology, there is a long history of a belief in a vital force or life energy, from the philosophical idea of vitalism of the 1600s to the theory of morphogenetic fields that guide development (1890–1950) to the concept of an organizing electromagnetic field within organisms. Most recently, vital energy has been formulated in terms of the biofield.

The human biofield is considered to be an innate energy field that consists of electromagnetic and possibly subtler, higher-order fields, including consciousness. The human biofield is hypothesized to guide development and regulate human physiology and biochemistry (Rubik, 2002a; Rubik et al., 1994). Just as the mental intention (yi) in Taoist philosophy is considered to be a prime mover of the qi, it is proposed that top-down signal transduction, beginning with a shift in consciousness or intention, may interact with and modulate the electromagnetic component of the biofield, which in turn orchestrates changes in the physiology and biochemistry of the body. This then leads to a new dynamic state that may promote healing. This cascade may be key to the foundation of mind-body medicine in general, in which a shift in consciousness is transduced through the biofield to dense levels of the body, ultimately guiding the healing process.

Thus, the biofield, which draws together mind and energy to interact with and regulate the physical body, is another scientific analog of the concept of qi, as both are believed to govern health and wellness. A key premise in traditional Chinese medicine is that where mind (yi) goes, qi flows; and blood follows qi. The biofield, like qi, conveys information throughout the organism and is central to its integration. The biofield is a holistic property of the organism and is proposed to be the super-regulator of the organism, coordinating life functions at multiple levels of organization. The multidimensional biofield is like the conductor of an orchestra whose musicians are found at the various molecular, cellular, and organismic levels of life, all contributing to a special kind of symphony that is responsive to the audience.

Some aspects of the biofield, like qi, may be metaphysical and beyond scientific scrutiny. Although we may not be able to observe qi or life energy directly, we may be able to observe its effects. At the frontiers of science, investigators have used various techniques to observe energy flows believed to correspond to elements of the human biofield. Techniques used include electrodermal testing to measure the flow of electricity at acupuncture points; thermography to map thermal patterns of the body; photodetectors to count biophotons, the ultraweak light emitted from the body; and high-voltage electrophotography that induces light emissions from the human body in order to visualize aspects

Figure 2
Lower, middle, and upper dantians (Johnson, 2000, p. 103). Reprinted with permission from the International Institute of Medical Qigong

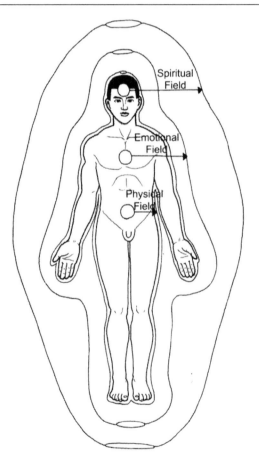

of the human biofield. Discoveries using the latter will be discussed later in this chapter.

In qigong there are three important energy centers within the body, called the dantians, which store and disperse qi from the central core of the body (Johnson, 2000). The region in the lower abdomen just below the navel is called the lower dantian. This is regarded as the major center of qi of the physical body, from which the life force is regulated. The middle dantian, located in the center of the chest, is connected with the qi field of the emotions. The upper dantian is located inside the middle of the head and is associated with the spirit (see Figure 2).

Qi travels along the acupuncture meridians to all organs and tissues of the body. Two key points in the hand that collect and move qi include *lao gong* (the acupuncture point in the center of the palm, the "palace of work") and the *ho gu* (the acupuncture point, also called the "tiger's mouth," near the origin of thumb and forefinger just beyond the metatarsal joint). Scientific research has shown that certain of these energy centers, such as the upper dantian and *lao gong,* emit more visible light energy following certain forms of qigong (Wallace, 1999).

BASIC QIGONG STANCE

Important elements of the ancient self-healing qigongs include proper posture, breathing, relaxation, effortlessness, and tranquility. Qi will not flow properly if one's posture is crooked, muscles are tense, or joints are locked.

There is a basic qigong stance that includes an erect, relaxed upright posture, in which the legs are about shoulder-width apart and the feet planted flat on the ground, slightly turned outward. There is a sense of ease, balance, stability, and rootedness. The knees are slightly bent. All of the joints of the body are relaxed. The buttocks are tucked in and the pelvis is thrust slightly forward. The shoulders are relaxed and hanging down, with the chest muscles relaxed so that the chest is slightly concave. The arms are hanging down at the side of the body in a relaxed manner, suspended a small distance from the sides of the body, with the palms of the hands facing the thighs, lightly touching them. The hands are relaxed with fingers slightly curved, with an inch or so of space between the thumbs and the forefingers. The eyes are open with a soft focus. The face is relaxed with soft smile and slightly parted lips.

Simply holding this qigong stance, often called the *wu ji* posture, will assist in the flow of qi. *Wu ji* is the resting position before any movement begins. This is a state of great emptiness, as in the Tao. This stance has been compared with standing like a tree, rooted deeply in tranquility, power, and vitality. It can be practiced anywhere, often in private. *Wu ji* is considered to be the subtlest qigong.

Breathing is usually regular, relaxed, slow, deep, and easy. In general, the breath should not require attention. However, some forms of qigong involve various types of breathing with certain movements. One is reverse abdominal breathing, in which the abdomen contracts instead of distending during inhalation and relaxes back during exhalation. This form of breathing draws more intensively on the energy of the lower dantian (Alton, 1997).

TYPES OF QIGONG

There are three general categories of qigong. One is medical qigong therapy, whereby a qigong therapist or master treats the qi imbalances of patients with external qi, by passing his or her hands over the patient either directly or at a distance. The second type of qigong includes specific and highly specialized forms of medical qigong that may be prescribed by a doctor of traditional Chinese medicine to treat a specific health condition or disease (such as, for example, breast cancer). The third form of qigong consists of self-exercises. Only the latter will be discussed here.

Qigong is also categorized according to whether it is a still qigong that is meditative, which may be standing or sitting, or an actively moving qigong. Both still and moving forms of qigong are useful to combat the physical and mental tension due to stress, because they both make the qi flow better. According to TCM, the tense exterior of a stressed person masks a sluggish qi inside, which is often associated with symptoms of distress such as pain. As our society becomes increasingly sedentary, some qigong masters believe that active, not meditative, qigong is increasingly what people in modern society most need (Cohen, 1997).

There are many thousands of forms of qigong, and new forms are invented daily. Certain forms of qigong are ancient. A few of the most popular types of qigong that have a long tradition and, moreover, that are considered most useful for prevention and self-healing will be briefly described. For the most part, health-related styles of qigong are more fluid and relaxed than other types of qigong, which can be quite vigorous. Many of the moving forms of qigong are like forms of art that emulate the natural, flowing movements of mammals, birds, and snakes, and they take their names from these animals. The student thus emulates certain characteristic traits of these animals, such as their unique forms of balance, gracefulness, strength, flexibility, and centeredness. There exist many variations of these forms, taught by the many schools and teachers of qigong throughout the world.

The Eight Brocades

First described in an eighth-century Taoist text, the Eight Brocades consist of eight exercises that are considered important for qi cultivation. They are gentle stretching exercises that work on the muscles and tendons as well as stimulating certain acupuncture meridians and key internal organs. Both standing and seated versions of the exercises exist, which are relatively easy and appropriate for everyone. The eight exercises are typically done nine times each, and consist of the following: (1) arms stretching upward; (2) opening the bow; (3) raising each arm; (4) turning the head and looking behind; (5) bending forward; (6) reaching down to the ground; (7) forward punching; (8) bending over and toe touching. Although these movements may seem simple, they have to be coordinated with the breath and mental intent. There are numerous variations of the exercises. The Eight Brocades are sometimes used as warm-ups before another qigong (Cohen, 1997; Guorui, 1990).

Wild Goose Qigong

Dayan qigong, or Wild Goose qigong, can be traced back to about 1100 C.E. as a relatively stable form that was passed down through a lineage of Taoist monks at a monastery on Kunlun Mountain. Master Yang Meijun, a woman and the 27th-generation lineage holder, was the most recent great grandmaster of Dayan qigong; she died in 2002 at 107 years of age. Dayan qigong involves two sets of 64 movements that imitate the movements of the wild goose, a very strong and resilient bird, who migrates thousands of miles each winter. Dayan qigong was designed to boost the qi, combat fatigue, clear negative energy, increase mental clarity, maintain physical fitness, cure and prevent disease, improve health, delay aging, and lengthen life. It leaves one feeling revitalized and refreshed, both mentally and physically. In past centuries, it was kept secret, but, today, Dayan qigong is one of the most highly regarded forms of qigong for health and fitness and is practiced worldwide (Robinson, 2002; Yu, 1998; Zhang, 2000).

Each set of 64 choreographed movements takes about 15 to 20 minutes to perform. Slow, fluid movements and quick movements are involved. The slow movements help massage the internal organs such as the liver and spleen. Gentle movements, such as the hands vibrating over the body, help transmit qi from *lao gong*, in the center of the palm of the hand, to the internal organs. Rapid movements act to stimulate certain acupuncture points with an energy surge to clear out stagnant qi and ensure the flow of fresh qi. The dynamic movements of this form combine strength with grace and gentle stretching of the wild goose. They should be performed softly and smoothly without strain or tension. Dayan qigong is performed with normal breathing.

In Dayan qigong, there are a number of acupuncture points and meridians that one focuses on sequentially to stimulate the energy system. For example, in the beginning of the form, arms are raised forward while visualizing energy moving up the Governing Vessel in the midback and down the Conception

Figure 3
Group practicing Dayan Qigong. Printed with permission from Bett Lujan
Martinez, MEd, Possible Society of CA

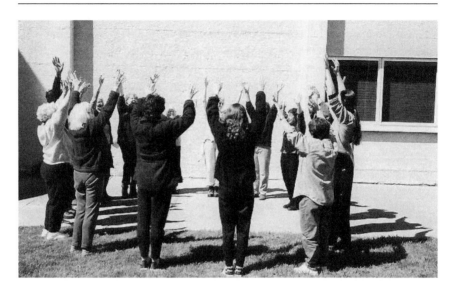

Vessel in the midfront of the body. Then, after collecting qi from the sky, the arms come back down, and the *lao gong* points on the hands are allowed to rest on the lower dantian (about two inches below the naval) to deliver qi. Figure 3 shows a group practicing Dayan qigong.

Dayan qigong stimulates all of the principle meridians and improves the function of the body, as well as strengthens the nerves, regulates the bodily fluids, and balances the organs, including yin and yang aspects. It is said to dispel illnesses of the heart; the nervous, respiratory, digestive, and urinary systems; chronic fatigue; back pain; hypertension; and insomnia.

Five Animal Frolics

Types of qigong whose movements imitate those of animals are among the oldest qigong forms that refer back to ancient Chinese shamanism. There is documentation that some animal forms were practiced as regular exercises in China some 2,300 years ago. Five Animal Frolics (also called Five Animal Play and Five Animal Sports) was developed by Hua Tuo, a famous medical doctor and surgeon in the second century C.E. He taught that, by becoming like and moving like the tiger, monkey, bear, deer, and crane, we balance the Five Elements (according to TCM, the five elements are fire, water, earth, metal, and wood) within us, which promotes health, vibrancy, and longevity. The Five Animal Frolics are a complete qigong system of exercises and one of the oldest healing practices in the world (Cohen, 1997; Fick, 2005; Guorui, 1990; Wu, 2006).

In the Bear Frolic, the heavy, firmly rooted, somewhat clumsy, lumbering movements of the bear warm up and stimulate the body. It is recommended for stimulating and improving functions of the kidneys, adrenals, spleen, and bones and is particularly good to practice in winter. A variety of postures and movements are done, and one main feature of them is on turning the waist while staying centered in the lower dantian. This movement exercises the waist, lower back, hips, and legs.

In the Crane Frolic, one starts with the basic crane stance, which is tall, open, and still and meditative, yet aware. There are six segments in this part of the qigong, which include two-legged standing, forming the beak, flapping the wings, squatting down, standing on one leg, and spreading the wings. The steps are performed lightly and delicately as the movements of a bird. The benefits of the Crane Frolic include relaxation, balance, loosening and opening the joints, strengthening the heart and lungs, cooling the body, diminishing inflammation, and relieving congestion.

Self-Massage Qigong

The practice of self-massage of the acupuncture meridians and key acupuncture points goes back to ancient times. It remains one of the most popular forms of qigong in China and may be practiced from either a standing or sitting position. Qi is enhanced in the hands by vigorous rubbing, and then the fingers or whole hands are placed over key vital centers to stimulate the flow of qi. There are several types of self-massage, from those that focus on the head and face to whole-body qi massage. Certain forms involve light, vigorous slapping of the body at key points as well as rubbing, pressing, pinching, or simply resting a hand on the skin. Self-massage improves circulation, disperses stagnant qi, and invigorates the body (Cohen, 1997; Guorui, 1990).

Other Noteworthy Forms of Qigong for Health and Wellness

Other major forms of qigong for health and wellness are Bone Marrow Washing (Cleansing), Swimming Dragon, Soaring Crane, Coiling Silk, Taiji Ruler, Basic Rock (Cohen, 1997), and Chow qigong (McGee and Chow, 1996).

PRACTICAL CONSIDERATIONS AND PRECAUTIONS

Although there are many books and videos on qigong, it is best to learn qigong from a qualified qigong teacher or master. In choosing a teacher, students and patients should consider the following criteria: whether the teacher has studied directly under a qigong teacher or master in the tradition in which he or she is teaching; number of years of practice; number of years of teaching; recommendations from other students or patients; and recommendations by doctors of TCM.

Because qigong has been shown in numerous studies to enhance health, stimulate self-regulation, and prevent disease, it is offered by some health maintenance organizations and other healthcare organizations as an effective system of self-care that can reduce the high costs of healthcare. Consequently, it is gaining popularity in the United States and is taught increasingly in hospitals, schools, corporate wellness programs, and community centers.

In learning a new practice, one must let go of old habits to form new ones. Here are some tips for beginners:

1. Learning qigong and getting health benefits from it requires time. The Taoists say that a new shoot on a mature tree is delicate and needs time to develop in its own way. Some people will naturally experience the effects and health benefits sooner than others.
2. Excess effort and trying too hard is contrary to what qigong is all about, as it is a relaxed, natural exercise. Moreover, qigong is not a performance. It is more important to practice with relaxation and a quiet mind than perfection. Breathe slowly and deeply, and never strain or force the body or breath. Most active forms of qigong should be done with "soft eyes" (eyes open with a soft, relaxed gaze), normal breathing through the nose, and loose joints (never locked, even in stretching poses).
3. Do not practice immediately after eating. Do not practice if it causes pain or exhaustion. Do not substitute qigong for necessary medical interventions. Do not practice strenuous qigong if pregnant or menstruating.
4. Don't expect too much, too soon. Regular practice over weeks and months is essential to reaping the health benefits of qigong.
5. It is important to perform qigong every day, just as it is healthy to move the bowels at least once a day to prevent stagnation. If you don't do your daily practice, you will not progress rapidly.
6. Do not stop practicing qigong once you have achieved the desired health benefits. Improved regulation along with health benefits are the result of regular practice. These benefits may, in fact, disappear if you stop practicing qigong.
7. Select a form of qigong that appeals to you, and spend between 20 and 40 minutes in daily morning practice. It is best to learn one or two forms of qigong and practice them regularly. Alternate styles of qigong may be practiced on different days. Do not practice more than one form of qigong in any session.
8. Mental intent (or *yi* in Chinese) is one of the most important aspects of qigong practice and also one of the key features that distinguishes qigong from ordinary exercise. One's focus should carry awareness and intent of one's movements, especially with respect to what is being done energetically with one's hands. The gaze of one's eyes should generally follow the movements of one's hands.
9. Always spend some time in a quiescent state (still pose or meditation), a state of inner quietude, after performing an active form of qigong. In this state, be aware of changes in physiological functions inside the body such as the deep relaxation

and increased comfort that follow. There are many ways to do this: by sitting quietly, standing in the qigong stance described earlier, focusing on the lower dantian, counting breaths, or listening to light music. It is important to choose a comfortable and easy posture and to use only one method to induce quiescence (Guorui, 1990).

10. Join a qigong practice group, or start one if a group does not exist in your area. One may also find a qigong partner with whom to practice. Those who practice qigong together often experience a stronger "qi field" that reinforces the benefits of their practice; their mutual commitment may help them to stay on target to improve their practice.

11. It is possible to experience side effects or "qi disturbances" from practicing certain types of qigong. This problem is generally seen in the case of younger people practicing a forceful style of qigong. When taking up any form of qigong, it is wise to discuss possible risks and complications with a qualified instructor (McGee and Chow, 1996).

12. Be advised that there are some forms of qigong that have been invented rather recently and that may not relate directly to ancient teachings. In addition, as with any human system of endeavor, there are always extremists and, moreover, extreme reactions to new thoughts. In relation to this, the Chinese government banned Falun qigong and the book written about it (Li, 2001).

Initially, the beginner may experience no unusual sensations in practicing qigong. However, after some time, one may experience heat and tingling sensations in the hands, and, eventually, that reaction may move slowly through the body. In addition, there may be a sense of tranquility, peace, and increased energy. These are all indicators of the active flow of qi within the body and that the qigong practice is successful (McGee and Chow, 1996).

BASIC SCIENCE STUDIES ON QIGONG

Basic studies on qigong show immediate changes in the biofield after performing qigong, which suggest improved energy regulation. In a study on Wild Goose qigong in 16 middle-aged and elderly adults using electrophotography performed with a gas discharge visualization (GDV) camera (Korotkov, 2002), the light emission of and around the fingertips showed greater density and symmetry immediately following qigong (Rubik, 2002b; Rubik & Brooks, 2005).

Figure 4 shows the electrophotographic data from an elderly man with Parkinson's disease. There is a larger, more intense pattern of light with greater symmetry following qigong. By analogy, consider the blue flame on a gas stovetop. When the gas is flowing irregularly, as when the flame first appears, the flame is irregular and jumpy. When the gas is flowing smoothly, the flame is steady and smooth. Similarly, when qi is flowing smoothly and regularly, the light emission patterns from the fingertips, as observed with the GDV camera, are smoother and more regular. Moreover, for the group of 16 subjects,

Figure 4
GDV-grams (gas discharge visualization camera photos of the light emission patterns) from the two middle fingers of Parkinson's Disease patient, before (left) and after (right) qigong

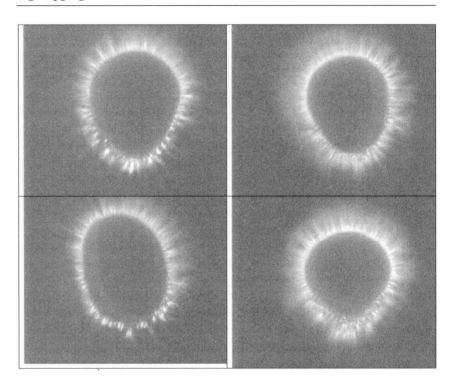

following qigong, the light patterns emitted from the right and left hands become more similar than before qigong, which signifies an improved bilateral energy balance (left-right symmetry). Beginners show the most dramatic changes in the biofield immediately following qigong. By contrast, experienced subjects already have more right-left energy balance initially and, hence, less change overall following qigong (Rubik, 2004a, 2004b).

In another basic science study on qigong, the electrical conductivity of subjects' acupuncture points along the 12 meridians of the acupuncture system was measured before and after qigong using a Ryodoraku device, which is used in Oriental medicine to assess the conductivity of the acupuncture meridians. Results show that the variability (standard deviations) in the measurements decreased following qigong, which suggests fewer fluctuations and improved energy balance (Sancier, 2003).

Numerous basic science studies have been reported in China since the late 1970s, when qigong reemerged. In many of these studies, external qi was projected by qigong masters onto various material systems in laboratories, and various effects have been observed. Some of these effects are quite remarkable from the perspective of mainstream science and include effects such as changes in the rate of decay of radioactive elements, changes in the rate of chemical reactions, and various effects on material systems over extremely large distances. A book summarizing some of the Chinese scientific studies was compiled by Lu Zuyin (1997). The scientific community remains rather skeptical regarding the conclusions of much of the Chinese research in this field and would like to see replication of many of these studies elsewhere under more rigorously controlled conditions. Some studies on the effects of external qi have been conducted in the West, but they show mixed results (Yount et al., 2004).

CLINICAL STUDIES ON QIGONG

Many valuable clinical discoveries regarding the therapeutic benefits of qigong have been made in China and reported in Chinese journals generally not read in the West. Some clinical studies from China that have been translated to English, such as those reviewed by Guorui (1990), show that qigong is particularly effective in treating hypertension, gastric and duodenal ulcer, chronic hepatitis, chronic indigestion, gastroptosis, neurasthenia, tuberculosis, chronic bronchitis, chronic bronchial asthma, senile lumbago, toxemia of pregnancy, and pelvic inflammation.

There remain, however, issues regarding the quality of such studies, including questions about the rigor of research design, the level of detail reported, and the lack of adequate controls, as well as possible issues with the translations. Michael Mayer (2003) has analyzed over 70 studies on the effects of hypertension conducted in China and found that none of the studies were of high enough quality to satisfy Western standards of confirmation in claiming that qigong reduces hypertension. More recently, a Korean pilot study showed a significant reduction in essential hypertension on 36 middle-aged subjects who practiced qigong twice weekly over eight consecutive weeks (Lee, Lim, & Lee, 2004).

Numerous clinical research reports suggest that qigong may contribute to the prevention and treatment of mortality associated with a variety of conditions, such as cancer and cardiovascular disease (Chen & Yeung, 2002; Sancier, 1996). A wide variety of cardiovascular outcomes are reportedly improved by qigong practice, including reduced congestive heart failure and heart attack (Xing & Li, 1993) and reduced incidence of strokes (Kuang, Wang, Xu, & Qian, 1991). In a study on cardiac patients comparing qigong to progressive relaxation, qigong showed greater improvement in psychological measures and reduction in systolic blood pressure (Hui, Wan, Chan, & Yung, 2006).

One of the prime benefits of qigong is stress reduction (Sancier & Holman, 2004). Cohen points out that people in the United States breathe at a rapid rate, on the average, of about17 breaths per minute. Although hyperventilation, with all its medical and psychological consequences, is caused by an excess in the volume of air (and, specifically, carbon dioxide) expired per unit of time rather than a high breathing rate per se (Fried, 1987), hyperventilation has been shown to affect at least 25 percent of the population and indicates a high level of stress and anxiety. An optimal breathing rate of between five and seven breaths per minute, established within three months of qigong practice (Cohen, 2003), will often help to reduce hyperventilation and may indicate other improvements in physiological and psychological self-regulation. In a study done in China, significant improvement was seen in psychological variables such as interpersonal relationships, anxiety, and obsessions after subjects practiced qigong regularly for three months, which was interpreted by the researchers as improved psychological regulation (Hu & Wu, 1989). Qigong has also been shown to help relieve chronic pain (Mayer, 1997).

Considerable evidence suggests that qigong is a useful complementary therapy. For example, it is often used as an adjunct therapy for medical conditions that require drug therapy, such as hypertension, respiratory disease, and cancer. A review of controlled studies was performed to examine the benefits of qigong for these three medical conditions. Taken together, these studies suggest that practicing qigong may favorably affect many functions of the body, permitting reduction of the dosage of drugs required for health maintenance and providing greater health benefits than the use of drug therapy alone. For patients with hypertension, the addition of qigong to their therapeutic program resulted in reduced incidence of stroke, reduced dosage of drugs required for blood pressure maintenance, and reduced mortality. For asthma patients, the combination allowed reductions in drug dosage, the need for sick leave, the duration of hospitalization, and therapy costs. For cancer patients, the combination reduced the side effects of cancer therapy (Sancier, 1999).

Systematic medical observation has shown that qigong is helpful in reducing stress, increasing circulation, improving strength and flexibility, reversing the damage of previous injuries and diseases, improving the immune system, and improving self-regulation processes by decreasing sympathetic nervous system function (the distress response to stressors) (Cohen, 1997). Experimental research from China documents positive effects of qigong on the pulmonary ventilation; invigoration and regulation of digestion; improvements in peripheral blood count of white and red blood cells; improved hormonal secretions related to the adrenal cortex; and improved autonomic nervous system regulation (Guorui, 1990).

Most of the clinical studies in the West thus far have been preliminary or pilot studies conducted on small numbers of subjects. Some have other design limitations such as the lack of randomization, placebo-control group, long-term study, or follow-up. Additional studies that incorporate larger numbers of subjects over longer durations and that use improved study designs are needed to demonstrate more conclusively the efficacy of qigong on improved health and well-being.

Reduction of healthcare costs is also of vital concern, and qigong appears promising. For example, in asthma patients practicing qigong, significant cost decreases were found; patients had fewer sick days out of the work-force, fewer hospitalization days, fewer emergency consultations, fewer respiratory tract infections, fewer drugs taken, and lower drug costs (Reuther & Aldridge, 1998).

QIGONG HEALING ANECDOTES

Scientific and clinical studies are only part of the evidence supporting the efficacy of qigong. Anecdotally, many personal healing stories are revealing. Here are a few stories that show the variety of benefits of qigong, from small positive changes to the dramatic healing of life-threatening diseases when all else had failed. (Note: Names have been changed to protect the privacy of those whose experiences with qigong we report.)

Chronic Pain and Fibromyalgia

Susan was involved in a car accident that resulted in neck and back injury leading to chronic pain and fibromyalgia. She also experienced "devastating fatigue" from her condition and the lack of support that she received from conventional healthcare. Over the next four years, she consulted specialists and tried many forms of Western therapy, including chiropractic and physical therapy, without success. One day she discovered qigong by reading a book and watching a video on the Eight Brocades, and she taught herself the exercises. She practiced the Eight Brocades every day and found that, gradually over time, her level of energy increased while her pain decreased. The more she practiced, the greater were the benefits. She also noticed that when she stopped her practice, her symptoms would return, which motivated her to continue her qigong practice. After a full year of practice, she no longer suffered constant fatigue, felt energetic, and her chronic pain had diminished to the point that it was no longer debilitating. After three and a half years, she claims that she has no symptoms, as long as she practices daily.

Fibrosarcoma Cancer

At age 62, Sandra, who was suffering from a large fibrosarcoma tumor, had a sudden onset of abdominal pain and fever caused by the perforation of her small intestine and peritonitis. Although she was operated on immediately, it was impossible to completely remove the affected portion of her intestine because of the extent of her cancer. Sandra was told that she had, at most, two years to live. Because of the location of her cancer, Sandra was not a candidate for radiation therapy, so she was started on a course of chemotherapy. She experienced the usual side effects of nausea, vomiting, weight loss, and hair loss. Periodic computer tomography (CT) scans did not indicate remission, so her chemotherapy treatment was stopped.

Although her prognosis was seemingly hopeless, Sandra became more hopeful when she learned about qigong. She began to practice Chow qigong, a form of qigong developed by qigong master Effie Poy Yew Chow (McGee & Chow, 1996). When Sandra first started performing qigong, her abdomen was so swollen that she appeared to be six months pregnant. Over the next four months, her abdomen shrank and CT scans showed a steady reduction in the size of her cancer, until it finally disappeared. She also began to feel much better and stepped up her qigong practice to include more intensive training and workshops. Twenty-seven years have now passed since Sandra's recovery. She is cancer free and remains in good health. She continues to practice Chow qigong and leads an active life that includes world travel.

Improved Energy and Well-Being in a Healthy Person

Cynthia has practiced qigong for years for improved energy and vitality. During this time, she experienced several major shifts in her perception of herself and the world that she attributes to qigong. She claims to have achieved greater emotional and physical strength. In the past, she had felt quiet, withdrawn, and in a perpetual fog. After years of qigong, she is more expressive, the fog has lifted, and she feels more like herself. She notes that daily qigong practice increases her energy levels dramatically. She moves more quickly and is rarely sick. At 58 years of age, Cynthia has gained flexibility and can now touch the palms of her hands to the floor while standing. A formerly chronic knee problem has disappeared. Now she can hike five miles in the mountains without hobbling afterward. Cynthia has also noted that qigong has increased her intuition, tuned her senses, and expanded her awareness. Qigong, she writes, has made her a changed person.

Personal Experience of the Author Practicing Qigong

I had actively pursued various forms of Western exercise in my youth, including ballet as a hobby, jogging, and lifting weights. At around 50 years of age, I began to experience frequent pain due to repetitive soft-tissue injuries from these activities and decided to cut down on the rigors of my routine. I began to practice qigong as a recommended gentle exercise for those suffering from chronic injury and in the hope of slowing down the aging process. The first type of qigong I tried was Dayan qigong, which appealed to me because it was like an artistic dance. After a few weeks of practice, a recalcitrant case of tendonitis in my elbow that I had suffered from for years was gone. Moreover, I no longer had cold hands or feet, which had plagued me for many more years. I also felt more relaxed, energized, and centered. This feeling of greater ease had a profound effect on my daily life. Yet when I stopped the practice for about six months, the coldness of my extremities returned, as did my previous stress level. I realized that I needed to practice qigong regularly. Finally, I learned to dance more from a balanced mind-body state that did not strain my aging body, which enabled me to return to my dance hobby without a continuing pattern of injury.

CONCLUSION

Qigong has opened a new window into the human potential for self-healing. Qigong as a self-practice may be used as an adjunct therapy for many disorders and diseases, for the prevention of disease, and to slow the aging process and hopefully contribute to longevity. It may be combined with conventional medicine. It is safe if performed correctly. There are various types of moving and still qigong that may be used for health and healing. Some scientific and clinical evidence of efficacy exists, as well as numerous personal healing stories. There are various scientific analogies to the Taoist concepts underlying qigong, which is an area with potential for future research.

Qigong as a complementary medical modality as well as a form of enhanced self-care shows considerable promise for the reduction of healthcare cost and the improvement of health and well-being around the world. Medical cost containment is an attractive benefit of qigong practice and should be further explored by insurance companies and governments, as well as those considering the practice of qigong. The health benefits of qigong are also attractive, because they are virtually without side effects. As the scientific and clinical databases on qigong continue to grow, qigong is attracting more attention from the scientific and medical communities. There is also a trend toward teaching qigong at mainstream educational, health, and recreational institutions. The public is becoming more aware of qigong, and the practice of qigong is growing. The growth of interest in qigong will be a trend for the foreseeable future.

Roger Jahnke (2002) writes,

> The Chinese realized thousands of years ago that the most profound medicine is produced within the human body for free. Qigong is a power tool that is easy to learn and use for activating this inner medicine. It will play a central role in the emerging new health care system of our country.

Beyond its contribution to health, qigong may do even more; Ken Cohen writes, "Qigong practice can influence every aspect of one's life" (Cohen, 1997,

p. 7). Qigong has the power to foster a clear, calm mind and a strong body and improved confidence and achievement in every realm of human endeavor. In the qigong worldview, Cohen writes,

> We share the breath of life with all of creation. We find the greatest happiness and the deepest health when we are aware of that breath of life—whether it's within your body, or in the sunset, or in the snow outside, or in another person. (Cohen, 2003, p. 87)

Sancier and Holman (2004) conclude,

> From a scientific point of view, the promise of qigong practices provides new avenues for understanding some of the subtle aspects of human life and its natural inclination to strive for balance. For clinicians, it shifts our focus from a battle with disease to a cultivation of health. For practitioners of qigong, it gives us an experiential understanding of greater balance within ourselves and of the cultivation of our individual physical, mental, and spiritual potential. (p. 165)

Additional Resources

The Qigong and Energy Medicine Database is a comprehensive guide to the qigong literature with over 2,000 records of qigong studies, including English abstracts of studies conducted in China. This data base is available from the Qigong Institute (Sancier, 2000). For more information, see www.qigonginstitute.org.

The National Qigong Association (www.nqa.org) provides reliable information and hosts conferences on qigong. Other key organizations include the American Qigong Association (www.eastwestqi.com) and the World Qigong Federation (www.eastwestqi.com).

TOOL KIT FOR CHANGE

Role and Perspective of the Healthcare Professional

1. The professional is the qigong teacher or master, who serves as teacher, guide, and role model to the patient exploring qigong practice. He or she gently corrects the posture and movements of the beginner, ensuring that the patient can obtain maximal benefit from qigong practice without harm.
2. The organization of a practice group for patients learning qigong, led by one or more advanced qigong students, could facilitate the learning of the qigong forms, their regularity of practice, and show patients by example the health benefits they may look forward to.
3. The distribution of instructional videos on the qigong form can help patients to learn and practice qigong with greater efficiency than through infrequent private instructions alone.

Role and Perspective of the Participant

1. Taking responsibility to learn the qigong form(s) correctly and to practice regularly is the key to gaining health benefits from qigong. Working with a qualified teacher and using instructional videos are both recommended.
2. Practicing with a group may provide special benefits from the experience of a group "qi field" that helps to correct the beginner's qi flow patterns.
3. Keeping a diary of practice dates, durations, and any noticed symptoms or results, both mental and physical, is a helpful way to monitor the results of qigong practice and assess any long-term changes.

Interconnection: The Global Perspective

1. Qigong has sometimes been considered arcane by conventional medicine. However, the trend toward increasing globalism has helped to spread qigong. Scientific studies on qigong are also bringing attention to this ancient tradition, although research funding has been scarce in the West.
2. Beyond its benefits for health and wellness, qigong is a time-honored practice for the enhancement of spiritual and psychological development.
3. Disharmony in humans can have its roots in the mind-body system and, beyond it, in the family, environment, and society. With its underlying premise of a circulating cosmic energy called *qi,* qigong offers a worldview that supports healing at multiple levels of being. Just as the Chinese characters that may at once represent a state of person, society, and nature, qi represents the energy that flows in people, society, and nature. Chinese practice, like Chinese philosophy, helps to integrate efforts to find harmony within and harmony without.

ACKNOWLEDGEMENTS

The author is grateful to Dr. Larry Goldberg for his scholarly and detail-oriented editing of the final draft of the manuscript.

NOTES

1. Some historical records, including Shang dynasty oracle bones and Zhou dynasty inscriptions, make reference to aspects of qigong more than 3,000 years ago.
2. For discussions of controversies regarding the history of the *Yi Jing,* see S. Marshall (2001) and R. Rutt (1996).

REFERENCES

Alton, J. (1997). *Living qigong: The Chinese way to good health and long life.* Boston: Shambhala.
Chang, C-Y. (1963). *Creativity and Taoism.* New York: Julian Press.
Chen K., & Yeung, R. (2002). Exploratory studies of qigong therapy for cancer in China. *Integrative Cancer Therapies 1,* 345–370.
Cohen, K. S. (1997). *The way of qigong: The art and science of Chinese energy healing.* New York: Random House.

Cohen, K. S. (2003). Healing through ancient traditions: Qigong and Native American medicine. *Alternative Therapies in Health and Medicine, 9*(3), 83–91.

Fick, F. (2005). *Five animal frolics qigong: Crane and bear frolics.* Shen Long.

Fried, R. (1987). *The hyperventilation syndrome: Research and clinical treatment.* Baltimore: Johns Hopkins University Press.

Goldberg, B. (2002). *Alternative medicine: The definitive guide.* Berkeley, CA: Celestial Arts.

Guorui, J. (1990). *Qigong essentials for health promotion.* Beijing: China Today Press.

Hu, H. C., & Wu, Q. H. (1989). *A collection of scientific articles on qigong.* Beijing: University of Science and Engineering Press.

Hui, P. N., Wan, M., Chan, W. K., & Yung, P.M.B. (2006). An evaluation of two behavioral rehabilitation programs: Qigong vs. progressive relaxation, in improving the quality of life in cardiac patients. *Journal of Alternative and Complementary Medicine, 12*(4), 373–378.

Jahnke, R. (2002). *The healing power of qi: Creating extraordinary wellness through qigong and tai chi.* Chicago: Contemporary Books.

Jantsch, E. (1980). *The self-organizing universe: Scientific and human implications of the emerging paradigm of evolution.* New York: Pergamon Press.

Johnson, J. A. (2000). *Chinese medical qigong therapy: A comprehensive clinical text.* Pacific Grove, CA: International Institute of Medical Qigong.

Korotkov, K. (2002). *Human energy field: Study with GDV bioelectrography.* St. Petersburg, Russia: St. Petersburg State Institute of Fine Mechanics and Optics (Technical University).

Kuang, A., Wang, C., Xu, D., & Qian, Y. (1991). Research on "anti-aging" effect of qigong. *Journal of Traditional Chinese Medicine, 11*(2), 153–158.

Kuang, A., Wang, C., Xu, D., & Qian, Y. (1991). Research on "anti-aging" effect of qigong. *Journal of Traditional Chinese Medicine, 11*(3), 224–227.

Lee, M-S., Lim, H.R.N., & Lee, M. S. (2004). Impact of qigong exercise on self-efficacy and other cognitive perceptual variables in patients with essential hypertension. *Journal of Alternative and Complementary Medicine, 10*(4), 675–680.

Li, H. (2001). *Zhuan Falun: The complete teachings of Falun Gong.* Gloucester, MA: Fair Winds Press.

Lu, Z. (1997). *Scientific qigong exploration: The wonders and mysteries of qi.* Malvern, PA: Amber Leaf Press.

Marshall, S. (2001). *The mandate of heaven: Hidden history in the I Ching.* New York: Columbia University Press.

Mayer, M. (1996–1997). An integrated approach to chronic pain. *Qi: Journal of Traditional Eastern Health and Fitness,* Winter, 22.

Mayer, M. (2003). Qigong clinical studies. In W. B. Jonas & C. C. Crawford (Eds.), *Healing, intention, and energy medicine* (pp. 121–137). New York: Churchill Livingstone.

Mayer, M. (2004). *Secrets to living younger longer: The self-healing path of qigong, standing meditation, and tai chi.* Berkeley, CA: Body Mind Healing Center.

McGee, C. T., & Chow, E.P.Y. (1996). *Miracle healing from China: Qigong.* Coeur d'Alene, ID: Medipress.

Prigogine, I. (1980). *From being to becoming: Time and complexity in the physical sciences.* San Francisco: W. H. Freeman.

Reuther. I., & Aldridge, D. (1998). Treatment of bronchial asthma with qigong yangsheng— A pilot study. *Journal of Alternative and Complementary Medicine, 4,* 173–183.

Robinson, R. (2002). Introduction to Dayan qigong. *Taijiquan and Qigong Journal, 7*(1).

Rubik, B. (2002a). The biofield hypothesis: Its biophysical basis and role in medicine. *Journal of Alternative & Complementary Medicine, 8*(6), 703–717.

Rubik, B. (2002b). Scientific analysis of the human aura. In R. I. Heinze (Ed.), *Proceedings of the 19th Annual International Conference on the Study of Shamanism and Alternative Modes of Healing* (pp. 104–125). Berkeley, CA: Independent Scholars of Asia.

Rubik, B. (2004a). The human biofield and a pilot study on qigong. In J. Fernandes (Ed.), *Proceedings of the International Forum on Science, Religion, and Consciousness* Universidade Fernando Pessoa: Porto, Portugal.

Rubik, B. (2004b). Changes in biofield emission parameters of chronically ill subjects following qigong. In R. I. Heinze (Ed.), *Proceedings of the 20th International Conference on the Study of Shamanism and Alternative Modes of Healing, Santa Sabina Center, Dominican University, San Raphael, CA, September 1–3, 2002* (pp. 235–257). Berkeley, CA: Independent Scholars of Asia.

Rubik, B., & Brooks, A. J. (2005). Digital electrophotographic assessment of the fingertips of subjects practicing qigong. *Evidence-Based Integrative Medicine Journal, 2*(4), 245–252.

Rubik B., Pavek, R., Ward, R., Greene, E., Upledger, J., Lawrence, D., et al. (1994). Manual healing methods. In *Alternative medicine: Expanding medical horizons* (NIH Publication No. 94–066; pp. 134–157). Washington, DC: U.S. Government Printing Office.

Rutt, R. (1996). *Thouyi: The book of changes.* London: Curzon Press.

Sancier, K. M. (1996). Medical applications of qigong. *Alternative Therapies in Health and Medicine, 2,* 40–46.

Sancier, K. M. (1999). Therapeutic benefits of qigong exercises in combination with drugs. *Journal of Alternative and Complementary Medicine, 5*(4), 383–389.

Sancier, K. M. (2000). Qigong database. *Advances in Mind Body Medicine 16,* 159.

Sancier, K. M. (2003). Electrodermal measurements for monitoring the effects of a qigong workshop. *Journal of Alternative and Complementary Medicine, 9*(2), 235–241.

Sancier, K. M., & Holman, D. (2004). Multifaceted health benefits of medical qigong. *Journal of Alternative and Complementary Medicine, 10*(1), 163–165.

Wallace, E. (1999). *Acute alteration of biophoton emission by intention.* PhD dissertation. California Institute of Human Science, Encinitas, CA.

Wilhelm, R., & Baynes, C. F. (Trans.) (1967, 1980). *The I Ching or Book of Changes.* Princeton, NJ: Princeton University Press.

Wu, Z. (2006). *Vital breath of the Dao: Chinese shamanic tiger qigong.* Little Canada, MN: Dragon Door.

Xing Z. H., & Li, W. (1993). Effect of qigong on blood pressure and life quality of essential hypertensive patients. In K. Sancier, *Qigong and energy medicine database.* Retrieved January 2007, from http://www.qigonginstitute.org.

Yount, G., Solfvin, J., Moore, D., Schlitz, M., Aldape, K., & Qian, Y. (2004). In vitro test of external qigong. *Biomed Central Complementary and Alternative Medicine., 4,* 5.

Yu, W-M. (1998). *Chi Kung: Taoist secrets of fitness and longevity.* Burbank, CA: Unique.

Zhang, H-C. (2000). *Wild Goose qigong: Natural movement for healthy living.* Boston: YMAA Publication Center.

Chapter Twelve

THE PSYCHOLOGICAL AND SPIRITUAL CHALLENGES INHERENT IN DYING WELL

David Feinstein, PhD

The individual dying in an ancient or pre-industrial culture is equipped with a religious or philosophical system that transcends death, and is likely to have had considerable experiential training in altered states of consciousness, including symbolic confrontations with death. The approach of death is faced in the nourishing context of the extended family, clan, or tribe, and with its support—sometimes even with specific and expert guidance through the successive stages of dying....The situation of an average Westerner facing death is in sharp contrast to the above in every respect.

—Stanislav and Christina Grof, *Beyond Death*

When death approaches, the healthcare professional is—ready or not—often the default manager of complex psychological, interpersonal, and spiritual challenges. As the Grofs suggest above, however, our culture has not been particularly adept in cultivating the high art of supporting a person through life's final passage. And, as a product of that culture, the attending professional often lacks the perspective and training for ministering to the opportunities and completing the tasks that beckon at the close of a life. The opportunities are significant, often casting into new light the life that has been lived.

This chapter offers healthcare professionals, as well as anyone confronted with these challenges, perspectives and techniques for navigating their way through end-of-life issues in a manner that completes what needs to be completed; seizes the profound and precious opportunities that inevitably present themselves; and meets fear, pain, and uncertainty with love and acceptance. A series of structured exercises throughout the chapter may be used by the professional or the client for exploring various issues involved in coming to a "good death." "A good death," counseled the fourteenth-century founder of humanism, Francesco Petrarca, "does honor to a whole life" (cited in Groves & Klauser, 2005, p. 13).

Many cultures have "books of the dead"—texts that teach about the journey into the afterlife and how to assist another with the process of dying. Scholars find these to be among the most profound spiritual literature generated by the culture. Based on a survey of these texts, Groves and Klauser (2005) provide a summary of the principles that show up consistently. "The common ground of our collective human experience at the end of life" (pp. 35–36) includes, in their analysis, that:

1. The passage through the stages of dying can be enriched profoundly by ordinary people trained to assist in this process.
2. Certain universal patterns or stages in the life-to-death transition process are predictable.
3. There is a clear relationship between physical and spiritual pain.
4. It is necessary to accurately assess spiritual pain before it is likely to be responded to effectively.
5. A "good death" involves maintaining a sense of clear knowing or consciousness at the end of life.
6. Some form of consciousness survives the death of the physical body.
7. The way one lives sets the stage for the way one will die.

This seventh principle underlies a core observation about life and death found in a myriad of cultures: "The sacred art of dying is the sacred art of living" (cited in Groves & Klauser, 2005, p. 16). These words (*Ars sacra moriendi, ars sacra vivendi*) have been inscribed in the rafters of one of the oldest standing hospices, in the medieval town of Beaune in southeastern France, for more than 500 years. Built with a glass floor over a river so patients and caregivers were continually serenaded with the soothing sound of water, the building is a stunning relic from Europe's original hospice movement. Its founder, Nicholas of Rolin, believed "the only measure of a society's greatness depends on how it cares for the poorest of its poor at the end of life" (Groves & Klauser, 2005, p. 14). The European hospice movement has its roots in ancient Celtic practices for relieving both physical and spiritual pain at the end of a person's life, which were exported throughout the Mediterranean world between the ninth and eleventh centuries A.D. The Celtic "midwife to the dying" was called the *anamcara* (soul friend) who used "harp music and special prescriptive poetry together with a wide range of complementary healing modalities...addressing everything from regulating a person's breath and diet to the content of their dreams" (Groves & Klauser, 2005, p. 24).

Every culture and every era of human history has had its own beliefs, customs, and rituals regarding death. Because our culture tends to regard death as a failure of the medical system and a defeat in our quest to dominate nature, we often approach death with greater fear and apprehension than many other societies. But no society has trumped death's unequivocal power over human preferences and fears. Nor has any society fully understood death. "Death," as Hamlet famously ruminated, is that "undiscovered country from whose bourn no traveler returns," leaving us to our own speculations about a Larger Story—about, in fact, the spiritual foundations of our existence. Neither science nor medicine has been able to penetrate the mysteries shrouded in the miracle of a human birth or the journey back into the unknown. Yet no questions are more fundamental.

YOUR PERSONAL PHILOSOPHY ABOUT DEATH

What beliefs and assumptions do you hold about death? The topics in this chapter contain vital questions worthy of deep reflection. You can delve more fully and personally into these topics by simply journaling about your underlying thoughts, images, and intuitions—exploring key assumptions, feelings, and beliefs in each area. Journaling instructions will be provided from time to time, for you to at least mentally consider specific questions and, if you wish, to deepen your inquiries with stream-of-consciousness writing. To experiment here, place the heading "My Philosophy of Death" on the top of a page of a journal, notebook, or word processing file. You will be recording your stream-of-consciousness as you reflect upon your beliefs, attitudes, and feelings regarding death. Place the following question under the heading, where you can glance at it easily. Begin to ponder the question:

• What is death?

Then, for 10 uninterrupted minutes (it is best to set an alarm clock or timer so you don't need to look at the clock), write nonstop in your journal or computer, producing an uncensored flow of thoughts and feelings.

In stream-of-consciousness journaling (also sometimes called automatic writing because the conscious mind lets go and more intuitive levels of the mind are freed to express themselves), the only rule is that you *never stop* writing during the suggested time period. You can write gibberish or "I don't know what to write," but you keep writing. After you have completed this process with the question "What is death?" you might read what you have written and underline or highlight or summarize in another section of your journal the points that are most meaningful to you. An alternative approach is to speak, for at least 10 minutes, your stream-of-consciousness regarding these questions to another person or into a tape recorder, and then to summarize your thoughts and feelings in your journal.

If you wish, you may take this further with additional questions, still under the heading of "My Philosophy of Death." Consider the following, or devise questions you would prefer to explore. The list is provided solely to stimulate your thoughts, feelings, and philosophy about death.

- Why do people die?
- How do I feel about my own death?
- What happens after a person dies?

THE CONSEQUENCES OF WHAT WE BELIEVE

Surveys consistently show that more than 70 percent of Americans believe in some form of afterlife. Such beliefs and visions have consequences. They shape a person's core values and many of the key choices people make. If life is a series of tests through which you earn your way into Everlasting Peace, you had better find out what your spiritual mentors have to say about how to pass those tests. If life is a school in which the soul evolves, from one life time to the next, as many Eastern religions teach, the person is prompted to learn well the lessons life presents. If death is the final curtain, the end of the story, all meaning and purpose must be found during this lifetime.

Death not only provides the context for life, it holds at least three fundamental challenges, beyond facing the moment of our own death, that each of us must confront during our lifetimes. First, what do we do with the fact that we are the only creatures on the planet that possess an ability to reflect upon our ultimate demise? Live in denial? In fear? In rage? Find comfort in some spiritual framework? Second, each of us will probably be called upon to be present in the dying process of someone we love, and there are many ways to answer that call. And, third, each of us will almost inevitably carry the grief of losing a loved one. While science and scientific psychology have much to say in each of these areas, some of the issues regarding death extend, by their nature, beyond the reach of science. This chapter explores how to confront these three deep challenges in ways that are informed by science, psychology, and clinical experience from those who work with death and dying, as well as by your own personal spiritual perspective.

A LIFE ENRICHED BY THE INEVITABILITY OF DEATH

> The dark background which death supplies brings out the tender colors of life in all their purity.
>
> —George Santayana

Robert Jay Lifton, a psychiatrist and pioneer in bringing a psychological perspective to the study of history, believes "the quest for symbolic immortality is an aspect of being human" (1983, p. 35). Symbolic immortality refers to the biological, psychological, social, and spiritual strategies people use to transcend the reality of death. Whether you take great comfort in knowing you will spend eternity in Heaven (or hold another idyllic vision of an afterlife), whether you expect to one day return to Earth in another body, or whether you are quite certain that there is no afterlife, the quest for symbolic immortality is a motivating force in most people's lives. While death "does indeed bring about biological and psychic annihilation," Lifton observes that human "life includes symbolic perceptions of connections that precede and outlast that annihilation" (p. 18).

Lifton describes five modes for attempting to transcend death by achieving symbolic immortality. The first is biological immortality, epitomized by family continuity and imagery of an endless biological chain linked to one's sons and daughters, their offspring, and on and on into eternity. A second mode for attaining symbolic immortality is through one's creative contributions, which may live on "through great works of art, literature, or science, or through more humble influences on people around us" (p. 21). Here we take comfort in the knowledge that our best efforts may become part of human continuity. A third mode of symbolic immortality involves an identity with nature, a knowledge that the natural world will survive our physical demise, and that we, from dust to dust, will be returned to that natural world.

A fourth mode of transcending death involves a belief in "a specific concept of life after death, not only as a form of 'survival,' but even as a release from the profane burdens of life into a higher plane of existence" (Lifton, 1983, p. 20). Lifton believes that the

> common thread in all great religions is the spiritual quest and realization of the hero-founder that enables him to confront and transcend death and to provide a model for generations of believers to do the same....One is offered the opportunity to be reborn into a timeless realm of ultimate, death-transcending truths. (p. 20)

Lifton's fifth mode, "experiential transcendence," is based on an inner experience that is "so intense and all-encompassing that time and space disappear [and there is] a sense of extraordinary psychic unity, and perceptual intensity, and of ineffable illumination and insight" (pp. 24–25). In his classic, *The Varieties of Religious Experience*, William James examined the impact of such experiences and reported that "mystical states of a well-pronounced and emphatic sort *are* usually authoritative over those who have them....Mystical experiences are as direct perceptions of fact for those who have them as any sensations ever were for us" (James, 1902/1961, p. 332).

Write as a second major heading in your journal "My Experiences with 'Symbolic Immortality.'" Write five subheadings corresponding with Lifton's list and record your thoughts and feelings about your relationship to each:

1. Do you have sons or daughters who will carry your biological inheritance from your parents into the future?

2. What will live on in the world in terms of your accomplishments or influence on others?
3. In what ways are you able to take comfort in your connection with the natural world and your knowledge that the natural world will continue after your physical being has reunited with it?
4. What beliefs or concepts, religious or otherwise, do you hold that give comfort or meaning regarding death and what follows death?
5. Have you had experiences that suddenly elevated your understanding and acceptance regarding your limited time here on Earth?

After reflecting on these five questions, consider another uninterrupted 10-minute stream-of-consciousness session on the core question regarding symbolic immortality:

• What gives me peace regarding my eventual inevitable death?

Again, it is best to use a timer or alarm clock so you don't need to keep checking the time, and the only rule is still that you do not stop writing for the entire 10 minutes. When you have completed your stream-of-consciousness writing, go back and underline, highlight, or summarize the most meaningful ideas.

EMBRACING THE PRECIOUSNESS OF THE MOMENT

Elisabeth Kübler-Ross, the physician who in the 1970s did much to dignify death as a topic for public and professional discourse, said the central message she hoped to convey is that death does not have to be feared as a catastrophic, destructive force; that it can, in fact, "be viewed as one of the most constructive, positive, and creative elements of culture and life" (Kübler-Ross, 1975, p. 2). This is not how most Westerners are raised. Even if we accept a vision of an afterlife based on religious or other teachings, more fundamental in our psyches is our culture's scientific/materialistic worldview, which does not provide a framework for understanding death in any terms but annihilation (Templer, 1972).

One of life's ironies, however, is that people who have a close encounter with death often begin to participate more fully in living. A shift in attention occurs as the preciousness of each moment is recognized and savored. Often the change is no less than a spiritual transformation. There is both an opening to one's deeper nature and to qualities of existence that transcend one's individual identity. Regardless of whether traditional religious concepts are used to explain the experience, a deepened sense of purpose and a more profound sense of connection with other people and with the universe are often reported. Higher passions are stimulated; love, beauty, truth, and justice are savored anew.

Two years after a near-fatal heart attack, Abraham Maslow, one of the twentieth century's most innovative psychologists, spoke of the intervening period as "the postmortem life" (Hoffman, 1988, p. 325). Reflecting on how these years were a kind of bonus, an extra gift, he noted that,

> if you're reconciled with death or even if you are pretty well assured that you will have a good death, a dignified one, then every single moment of every single day is transformed because the pervasive undercurrent—the fear of death—is removed.

In the postmortem life:

> Everything gets doubly precious, gets piercingly important. You get stabbed by things, by flowers and by babies and by beautiful things—just the very act of living, of walking and breathing and eating and having friends and chatting. Everything seems to look more beautiful rather than less, and one gets the much-intensified sense of miracles.…The confrontation with death—and the reprieve from it— makes everything look so precious, so sacred, so beautiful that I feel more strongly than ever the impulse to love it, to embrace it, and to let myself be overwhelmed by it. (p. 325)

Those who have seen someone come into such peace and enhanced perception after a near-death encounter may wonder why we must wait until the final season to attain such grace. Perhaps we do not.

We will be exploring ways of intentionally shifting consciousness to find natural sources of inner wisdom and grace, but we can also *do* things that add meaning and richness to our lives. In your journal, write a heading: "If Today Were My Last Day." With 10 minutes of uninterrupted stream-of-consciousness writing, unleash your pen or keyboard to find out what you would do if you knew you were to die tomorrow. Often, people identify actions that could immediately enhance their lives but that they don't seem to get around to doing. Circle the actions you commit to carrying out this week.

SHIFTING CONSCIOUSNESS, SHIFTING PERSPECTIVES

People in every culture throughout time have sought altered states of consciousness. Technologies for inducing these states range from religious rituals to ecstatic drumming, from meditative states to trance dances, from shamanic journeys to elaborate rites of passage, from rhythmic chants to the ingestion of sacred plants. These interventions change brain chemistry in highly specific ways (Austin, 1999). They tend to open what William Blake called the "doors of perception," sometimes sensory perception, sometimes the perception of inner realities (Huxley, 1970). People often emerge from powerful altered states with their perceptions expanded regarding life, nature, and their place in it all. "If the doors of perception were cleansed, every thing would appear," according to Blake, "as it is, infinite." From this expanded perspective, the terror of impending death often dissolves into peaceful acceptance.

Although major shifts of consciousness can be induced, they also can be spontaneous. Known variously as religious experiences, mystical experiences, peak experiences, and ecstatic states, people who go deeply into these states often return with a richer understanding about their life. Some of these experiences also have a direct and lasting influence on their relationship to death. Near-death experiences (NDEs) are particularly powerful in this regard. Best known for the "white light" and "life review" that are widely reported, these are often profound, ecstatic, life-changing events.

Like many men born in the first quarter of the 20th century, Fred was a stern, hard working husband and father. Having grown up desperate for work in the rural South during the Depression, he treated life as serious business. He believed "you get what you earn and you earn what you get. It is best not to be too positive lest you set up expectations that will result in disappointment." For Fred, there was little room for emotion because "feelings keep you from what is important and make you look weak." Unlike many of his peers, he had no use for religion. He was bitter about his early church experiences, and he found no assurance in promises of an afterlife.

At age 55, Fred had a heart attack and was hospitalized. In the hospital, he had another massive coronary. His vital signs indicated that he was clinically dead, but he was revived. Fred had never heard of strange or poignant "near-death" experiences, and he was about the last person on the planet likely to invent one. Yet he reported:

"First I was up near the ceiling and I could see the medical team trying to resuscitate me. I heard a doctor say, 'He's had it!' I yelled back, 'Whatever it is, I don't want it!' but nobody heard me. Suddenly, I was walking over a bridge with a dry wash underneath. On the other side was an open green field. Walking to greet me was Bart [a childhood friend who had died in his early twenties]. I was overjoyed to see Bart. He greeted me warmly and told me to observe everything. But he said that I had to go back. 'Why?' I asked. 'Because you haven't learned a damned thing, Fred. You haven't learned how to love.'"

As Fred became aware of being back in the hospital room, he opened his eyes and met the gaze of a shocked nurse who was putting a sheet over his head. The words "I love you" came out of his mouth. He said "I love you" to each nurse and doctor from the resuscitation team, who were still in the room. One doctor, according to family legend, uncomfortably replied, "That really isn't necessary." His family was amazed. His daughter explained that Fred did not find it easy to say "I love you" to anyone. He would sometimes walk out of the room with a disgusted look on his face when a song on the radio or a program on television got "too mushy."

For the remaining 16 years of Fred's life, he seemed to be making up for lost time—cultivating an ability to listen, taking an intense interest in the lives of others, traveling extensively to various parts of the world to try to understand people from different cultures, making amends for the past with his intimates, and enjoying the company of his grandchildren. At his memorial service, the theme most dwelt upon was the loving spirit Fred brought into his life. (Feinstein & Krippner, 2006, pp. 11–12)

Is this an isolated case? A study published in *Lancet* of 344 cardiac patients who were resuscitated after clinical death showed that 18 percent reported having had NDEs (von Lommel, van Wees, Meyers, & Elfferich, 2001), and thousands of people have been systematically interviewed following such experiences (Moody, 2001). They report—and observations from friends and family confirm—changes in their values, their behavior, and sometimes their personalities. Kenneth Ring, who has been one of the most ardent researchers of this surprising finding, summarizes that, after returning from a near-death experience, "individuals tend to show greater appreciation for life and more concern and love for their fellow humans while their interest in personal status and material possessions wanes. Most NDErs also state that they live afterward with a heightened sense of spiritual purpose and...these self-reports tend to be corroborated by others in a position to observe the behaviors of NDErs" (Ring, 1985, p. 141). In addition to these radical changes in a person's values, in some cases, the NDE is followed by the individual making radical life changes, as if the person has "come into a new and more authentic sense of self" and is able to develop newly appreciated potentials, sometimes to an "astonishing degree" (p. 120).

INNER JOURNEYS

In addition to spontaneous experiences such as NDEs, profound inner experiences that impact one's personality, values, and behavior can be generated with specific interventions. Work with cancer patients at the Chicago Medical School in the early 1960s, using LSD to help control pain, led to the unexpected finding that the treatment also resulted in a range of psychological benefits. A series of clinical trials at the Maryland Psychiatric Research Center confirmed these observations (Grof, 2006) and was apparently leading to new dimensions in end-of-life care until the political climate put an end to such exploration. In one extreme, dramatic, eminently humane program, 31 terminal cancer patients who were experiencing substantial physical and psychological suffering were administered a single session using LSD (Grof, Goodman, Richards, & Kurland, 1973). Twenty-two of the patients showed substantial to dramatic improvements in the alleviation of various emotional symptoms, including depression, anxiety, general tension, sleep disturbances, and psychological withdrawal; a pronounced reduction of physical pain in the weeks or months following the session; and a marked increase in the sense of peace about dying. No significant adverse reactions resulted from the treatment, including in the nine patients who did not show substantial improvement.

Are there pathways to such experience that do not wait for them to occur spontaneously, as in NDEs, and that do not utilize drugs? There are. Stanislav Grof, for instance, one of the investigators in the study just described, surveyed the ways altered states have been induced throughout history. With his wife, Christina, he developed a nondrug approach called holotropic breath work, which utilizes sustained dynamic breathing for evoking powerful internal experiences in a manner that impacts one's sense of self. He claims, in fact, that this method yields positive psychological changes that are similar in scope and impact to those produced by his earlier use of LSD-assisted therapy (Grof, 1990), including the "ego deaths" that lead to self-transcendence. In many cultural traditions, experiences that bring an experiential death to one's ego and identity are seen as preparation and training for dying well.

The embrace by modern psychotherapy of ancient meditation practices (Walsh & Shapiro, 2006) should be of interest to anyone concerned with issues involving healthy living and conscious dying. Meditation has been shown to cultivate positive emotions such as love, joy, and a sense of peace. It helps reduce problematic emotions such as anxiety, fear, depression, and anger. It measurably strengthens desirable personality traits, such as emotional stability, agreeableness, and openness to experience. It improves relationships. Meditators score higher on measures of empathy, interpersonal functioning, and marital satisfaction. Meditation also seems to enhance overall maturation, with meditators scoring higher on measures of ego development, moral development, cognitive development, coping skills, and stage of consciousness (Walsh & Shapiro, 2006).

The practice of meditation seems to produce some outcomes that are similar to those of a spontaneous near-death experience. In a way, meditation training offers practice in dying. One of the phenomena associated with meditation is a "death of the ego" and an awakening into a larger sense of self. According to Ken Wilber,

> If one progresses fairly well in *any* meditation system, one eventually comes to a point of having so exhaustively "witnessed" the mind and body that one actually rises above or transcends the mind and body, thus "dying" to them, and to the ego. (Wilber, 1990, p. 188)

This ego death may be frightening, but what ultimately dies is the sense of being a separate self, and what is born is a higher identity, an experiential identification with the larger forces of nature and of creation. The death of the ego may seem a far cry from physical death, but it is a death that people nonetheless struggle valiantly in their busy outward-directed lives to avoid. Some meditators, however, open themselves to the interior death and rebirth inherent in an ego death. Certain forms of meditation, in fact, serve as an active rehearsal of death. These practices, Wilber elaborates, "contain very precise meditations that mimic or induce the various stages of the dying process very closely—including stopping the breath, the body becoming cold, the heart slowing" (p. 189). Kenneth Kramer (1988), in an examination of "the three faces of death" (biological, psychological, and spiritual) in both Western and Eastern spiritual traditions, observed that practices that result in a spiritual death lead to "self-transcendence," where awareness moves beyond the "prior confines of the self" (p. 24).

Is it necessary to go to these extremes—to seek faux death encounters—in order to live more fully and in a right relationship with death's inevitable call? Meditation, the time-honored approach for transforming consciousness and cultivating a more wholesome relationship with life and death, can be done in many ways and many places. It is available to everyone. And it is free. Some forms of meditation involve focused concentration on an object, on the breath, or on an inner sound. Others cultivate a more open awareness, aiming for "fluid attention to multiple or successively chosen objects" (Walsh & Shapiro, 2006, p. 229). Some forms of meditation simply observe the thoughts and images that arise while others attempt to modify them. Some practices seek to develop general well-being and consciousness expansion while others "focus primarily on developing specific mental qualities, such as concentration, love, or wisdom" (p. 229). Some forms require that the meditator maintain a rigid posture, others are more lax; some involve stretching, and there are even eyes-open "walking meditations."

Meditation may focus on the body, the breath, a sound, an image, or on products of the mind. Some cultures and spiritual disciplines place meditation in about the same relationship to the mind as bathing is to the body. Western culture has not, but as Western psychotherapy is discovering the value and power of meditation for overcoming psychological problems and enhancing mental health, meditation practice is being elevated from a quaint New Age pastime to a viable form of personal development. It is a technology for following the teachings of many wisdom traditions for the person who is in the last stages of dying: "simply, rest in the power of the present" (Groves & Klauser, 2005, p. 27).

DEDICATED TIME AND SACRED SPACE

Dedicated time and sacred space are terms borrowed from Peg Elliott Mayo, the author's first clinical supervisor circa 1968; they are a way of taking a pause from one's daily routines and responsibilities to engage in quiet, uplifting experiences. Setting aside dedicated time in sacred space is a way to attain, in Peg's words, "relief from ordinariness." The term *dedicated time* emphasizes that this is a choice. We have the option of devoting committed time and attention to knowing, enjoying, and cultivating our inner life. *Sacred space* supports the process. It need not be an elaborate temple or altar. A woman who lived in a tiny apartment with her husband and three young sons claimed a dresser drawer and put into it things she treasured and that had strong positive associations for her (drawings she had made in her late teens of her mother and her father, photos of her sons in infancy and at various stages since, a seashell from her honeymoon, a few favorite poems, Gibran's *The Prophet*, a candle, and a walkman with spiritually uplifting CDs). After the boys were in bed and her husband was watching sports on TV, she regularly took the drawer from the dresser, set it on a table, spread the contents, lit the candle, put on the headphones, and browsed the treasures or went within. She looked forward to these makeshift ceremonies, which took her outside her ordinary routines, refreshed her, and provided a route to simple contemplative reveries.

Whether journaling, meditating, engaging in breath work, reveling in nature, creating art, performing personal spiritual rituals, conducting dresser-drawer ceremonies, or doing other forms of inner work, activities that bring us to the edge of our ordinary consciousness and daily routines enhance our appreciation of life. Peg recommends finding or creating a sacred space that you *want* to enter and visiting regularly. In a new area of your journal, place the heading "Dedicated Time, Sacred Space," and write for 10 uninterrupted stream-of-consciousness minutes. When finished, go back and underline, highlight, or summarize the most meaningful ideas.

HELPING A LOVED ONE PASS THROUGH THE FINAL GATEWAY

> There is no greater gift of charity you can give than helping a person to die well.
> —Sogyal Rinpoche, *The Tibetan Book of Living and Dying*

The social context of dying with an incurable disease in the United States today not only fails to support the psychological tasks and spiritual opportunities that arise at the end of a life, it breeds unnecessary suffering in the patient and the patient's family (Byock, 1997). Healthcare providers have rarely had more than a few hours of coursework in caring for persons as they die. Realistic fears hover about untreated pain, abandonment, loss of dignity, and financial hardship. Physical comfort, psychological needs, and quality of life are secondary to aggressive medical strategies involving "ever more toxic regimens and all-out efforts to forestall death" (Byock, 1997, p. 243). Attention stays focused on heroically prolonging life even after circumstances dictate a shift to the challenges of providing effective, enlightened end-of-life care. Meanwhile, the attendant costs are increasingly placed on the patient's family. Nearly a third of families caring for a loved one with a prolonged illness lose most or all of their savings. Tragically,

> a dying father who feels that he is a drain on his family, physically and financially, will experience being a burden every moment of every day; that will be what his life has come to mean. Though his wife and children may affectionately acknowledge

his years of love and selfless devotion, he will fret, feel worthless, and suffer. (Byock, 1997, p. 242)

Ira Byock, a physician and former president of the American Academy of Hospice and Palliative Medicine, after vividly describing the untenable situations faced by many people who are dying, observes:

> The root cause underlying the mistreatment and needless misery of the dying is that America has no positive vision and no sense of direction with regard to life's end. Without a position on the compass pointing the way, the health care profession's and society's approach to care for the dying has been confused, inconsistent, and frequently ill-considered. (Byock, 1997, p. 244)

Byock calls for communities to, as in earlier times, assume coordinated responsibility to see that the physical, social, and spiritual needs of dying persons are met.

> Of the fundamental needs of persons as they die, only the need to control physical symptoms is uniquely medical. Their more basic needs are broader than the scope of medicine....In recognizing these needs, we can say to the dying person with our words and, more importantly with our actions: "We will keep you warm and we will keep you dry. We will keep you clean. We will help you with elimination, with your bowels and your bladder function. We will always offer you food and fluid. We will be with you. We will bear witness to your pain and your sorrows, your disappointment and your triumphs; we will listen to the stories of your life and will remember the story of your passing." (Byock, 1997, p. 247)

COMMUNICATING WITH PEOPLE WHO ARE DYING

The physical, legal, and medical needs involved in caring for a person who is dying have been identified, studied, and ably described (Tobin, 1998). Effective protocols exist even for the most overwhelming physical pain and distress.

> Pain and other symptoms causing physical distress can be alleviated, even when they are severe. It is not always easy, but by being careful and comprehensive, and by being absolutely committed to do whatever is necessary to control physical distress, it can *always* be done. (Byock, 1997, p. 245)

Less tangible or predictable are the unique psychological, interpersonal, and spiritual needs that emerge during the final phase of life.

Maggie Callanan and Patricia Kelley are hospice nurses who, after many years of working with people who are dying, identified the recurring themes in the communications that are of special significance during the final phase of life. They observe that these communications fall into two categories: "attempts to describe what someone is experiencing while dying and requests for something that a person needs for a peaceful death" (Callanan & Kelley, 1997, p. 14). Accurately discerning such messages can be the difference between knowing or not knowing how to alleviate anxiety and suffering, how to provide the most effective care at any moment, how to elevate good intentions into empathy and rapport, and how to join the dying person on a journey that reviews a life that is ending, completes what is emotionally unfinished, and moves peacefully into the unfamiliar and unknown.

While it is almost too obvious to say that communication is important, a depth and quality of listening may be required that goes far beyond normal discourse. Callanan and Kelley (1997) observe that

> many dying people are lonely, not only because people don't visit, but also because of what happens when people do visit. Visitors may spend their time with the person wrapped up in idle talk about the weather, sports, or politics....A dying person's world shrinks, narrowing to a few important relationships and the progress of [the] illness. When dying people aren't allowed to talk about what's happening to them, they become lonely, even amid loving concerned people. (p. 59)

People who are dying often have experiences unlike any they have ever previously encountered, and they may not have the language, or even the concepts, for communicating about them. Caregivers frequently discount the attempts to express these unfamiliar experiences as stemming from confusion, physical deterioration, or medication, missing the nuance and symbolic language being presented. Callanan and Kelley (1997) observe that "bewilderment or disorientation may stem from the unfamiliar, unexpected experiences of dying [and] too often, the responses of those caring for dying people only add to that bewilderment" (p. 17). Yet a dying person's attempts to describe uncommon phenomena "offer unique opportunities to enter that landscape, to participate by responding to their needs and wishes, and to learn what death is like for them—and, perhaps, what it will be like for us" (p. 16).

TERRITORY DYING PEOPLE ARE LIKELY TO ENCOUNTER

Researchers have noted remarkable similarities of deathbed visions in radically different cultures (Osis & Haraldsson, 1977). Dying people often have the sense of being two places at once: in the room and in another realm. They may have glimpses or lucid visions of another world with deceased relatives waiting to greet them, of spiritual beings, or of religious figures. These may include precise communications about "the other side" that bring feelings of peace and understanding. In fact, most of the elements associated with near-death experiences—such as seeing a bright light, sensing the presence of a greater intelligence, visits with loved ones who have died, or experiencing a life review that brings profound insight and meaning—are frequently reported during the last days of life. People who have such encounters may not, however, have the words to describe them, and if the caregiver lacks a framework for making sense of the attempts, they may easily be missed or dismissed. The dying person's most subjectively meaningful experiences may become a source of isolation.

Beyond the need of the dying person to speak about unexpected experiences that may emerge as a natural part of the dying process, Callanan and Kelley's second category of communication involves requests about the dying person's emerging sense of what needs to be completed before a peaceful death can occur. This may include a desire to reconcile personal relationships or to remove other barriers to achieving peace. Because this is delicate, emotionally laden psychological terrain, these requests may be vague or indirect, and, again, they may easily be missed or ignored if the caregiver is not alert.

The five stages of dying elaborated by Elisabeth Kübler-Ross (1975) provide a map for some of the psychological territory a dying person will traverse. Although clinical experience has shown that dying people do not necessarily experience each phase or progress through the phases in an orderly sequence—and may in fact shift back and forth among these phases (Callanan & Kelley, 1997)—familiarity with Kübler-Ross's observations about denial, anger, bargaining, depression, and acceptance helps prepare the caregiver for understanding the deeper dynamics of a dying person's experience.

Denial, a refusal to accept reality, is sometimes a healthy coping mechanism that gives people time to integrate difficult news. The fine line for the caregiver is that, while it is not useful or appropriate to try to dismantle a coping mechanism such as denial, neither is it helpful to encourage a refusal to face reality or enter into a *conspiracy* of denial where the patient, the family, and the caregivers all pretend a terminal patient is going to recover. Callanan and Kelley (1997) discuss this dilemma:

> If you should neither challenge nor encourage denial, what should you do? You should recognize the wish or desire behind it. When your dying friend talks about getting better and going camping again, you could say, "Wouldn't that be fun!" or "I bet you'd like that!" These responses acknowledge your friend's hopes and wishes without reinforcing denial. (p. 40)

Most dying people move beyond denial about their medical situation. Some do not. Gentle exploration and unfaltering support rather than a direct assault on any coping mechanism is part of the challenge facing the caregiver.

Anger is generally oriented toward a real or supposed grievance. When people realize that an illness that seems arbitrary and unfair is probably going to take their lives, anger is one of the strong emotions likely to follow. The anger may be at God, at society and its carcinogens, at others who get to go on living oblivious to the dying person's suffering, at the medical system and caregivers that are treating the patient, or at other parts of the patient's physical and interpersonal surroundings. Wherever it may be focused, it is in the safety of the patient's closest relationships that the anger is most likely to be expressed, and often the vehemence is directed toward family, friends, or caring professionals. At such times it is difficult to avoid feeling hurt or defensive. The least useful responses are to attempt to talk the patient out of the anger or to strike back with your own unprocessed anger. Rather, Callanan and Kelley (1997) suggest: "Look for the cause. Think of anger as a feeling that develops from another emotion. In people who are terminally ill, the roots of anger often are frustration, resentment, or fear" (p. 42). Add loss, helplessness, humiliation, and the inability to care for one's most basic needs.

When these emotions can be raised and explored within the container of a caring and knowledgeable relationship, the energy bound in anger can be directed to addressing its causes more effectively. Frustration does not have to create isolation. Resentments can be expressed, dealt with, and discharged. Losses can be discussed and mourned. Examining the sense of helplessness, humiliation, and the inability to care for oneself can lead to more effective strategies for keeping the patient in control and for accepting that the patient's situation is a natural and inevitable part of the life cycle. Fear can be particularly challenging, because the dying person's fears may intersect with the caregiver's fears and anxieties.

Fear may arise around the progressive symptoms of the illness. Fear may permeate thoughts about the process of dying, or, as Woody Allen quipped, "I'm not afraid of dying, I just don't want to be there when it happens." Fears about what occurs after death are also common. One of the best ways to help a person deal with and counter fear is with accurate information. Consultations with doctors, nurses, hospice workers, or clergy that focus specifically on the fears and concerns that have emerged can be extremely helpful in curbing escalating fear.

Nonetheless, the prospect of death brings us to the edge of everything we know and know how to control. Engaging one's fears is not just a psychological challenge; it can push us into an encounter with the foundations of our spiritual beliefs. One of the most effective tools for engaging this territory is mindfulness meditation, discussed below. Stephen Levine, a meditation instructor and one of the modern pioneers in teaching people to die consciously and well, once advised a woman who was going through the agony of watching her daughter die, "Let her death be surrounded by your care for her and a willingness to go beyond your fear" (Levine, 1989, p. 5). Procedures such as mindfulness meditation and acupressure for the emotions (also discussed below) can be invaluable resources for dealing with fear and anxiety.

The *bargaining* phase of coping with a terminal diagnosis involves attempts to postpone the inevitable. Whether with God, through heroic but unlikely medical interventions, an embrace of a healthy diet, or a promise to be a better person if given more time, these "deals" are typically not discussed and often go unnoticed. They have been likened to the way a child at bedtime may bargain for another goodnight kiss, another song, another drink of water. But they should not be discounted. Callanan and Kelley (1997) describe how

> people with AIDS often make deals to spend the time they have left working to stop the epidemic. "I'll get involved," they may think. "I'll take care of others. I'll teach people how not to get infected. But, God, if I do this you have to let me live longer." Amazingly, such bargains often seem to work. (p. 50)

Depression is a natural reaction to loss and a fundamental emotional component of grief. For a dying person, loss has many faces. The illness may already have extracted the ability to hold a job, to continue roles in the family and community that had always been taken for granted, to care for oneself, or a thousand other insults to one's sense of self. Meanwhile, even greater losses approach: further physical debilitation, never again seeing loved ones, and, finally, the loss of life itself. Mourning is the process of emotionally working through such losses, and depression keeps the mind from focusing on much else. In this way, it serves an adaptive function. Reactive depression helps the person cope with losses that have already occurred; preparatory depression helps the person emotionally prepare for coming losses. For the caregiver, the dying person's depression may be extremely difficult to encounter. As adaptive as grief and depression may be in theory, they usually do not appear to be serving a constructive purpose. Yet you cannot talk a person out of depression, and the depression itself can be contagious. Asking the person to cheer up in one way or another (e.g., "Hey, it's been a good life") discounts the emotional pain and further isolates the individual. Callanan and Kelley (1997) counsel that, presented with a dying person's expressions of sadness and depression, "All you can do when they voice these feelings is listen. Often, no answer is needed—only the attempt to understand" (p. 50). Describing work with the father of two small children who was dying of cancer, they conclude:

> He didn't need cheering up. He didn't need someone to say, "I'll help raise your children," or "I'll try to be there for Joyce after you're gone."…What Mark needed was to have someone listen to his pain, empathize with his sadness, and share his tears. (p. 51)

Acceptance, according to Callanan and Kelley (1997),

> is a feeling of peaceful resignation that usually doesn't come to stay until death is very close. It's common for patients to experience interludes of acceptance and then, in one day, in one conversation, on one sentence, slip into another emotional stage. But eventually death nears, at which time permanent acceptance may arrive. When

this occurs—provided a dying person is comfortable—she needs little except the presence of one or two important people....If you are one of these people, you may experience mixed emotions. The peace of another's acceptance of death can be comforting, but with acceptance comes detachment, a drawing away from others no matter how close they have been. This can be painful for those being left behind. (pp. 51–52)

Interlaced with these five emotional states that people regularly encounter during the dying process—denial, anger and the feelings that underlie it, bargaining, depression, and acceptance—is the need to complete or abandon various *unfinished physical and emotional tasks*. Books and screenplays have been completed in the last days of life, sometimes with a feeble body prolonging life beyond what seems imaginable in order to get to the final word. Sometimes life extends itself to allow the person to attend an event, such as the marriage of a son or daughter, or experience the arrival of a loved one from far away. Other times, projects that had been central in a person's existence have been abandoned as no longer possible or as having never really been worthy of the person's life force. Such decisions may be met with grief or relief. In many instances, the unfinished business seems to be more about core life lessons, such as how to live more fully or with a more open heart, than about completing specific projects. Not infrequently, when a major long-standing issue is resolved or a core life lesson is learned—even if it is not until the person's last few weeks, or even days—the entire life may take on "retrospective meaning," accompanied by a greater sense of peace about dying. A literary depiction of this process is Tolstoy's Ivan Ilych, who, after an existential crisis in the last days of his life, "transformed himself and was able to flood, retrospectively, his entire life with meaning" (Yalom, 1980, p. 208).

The area of unfinished business that frequently becomes the most complex involves other individuals. Sometimes this can be expressing an intimate feeling that has never been stated. Sometimes it involves a long-held resentment or unresolved conflict. Often it entails asking for or rendering forgiveness. The issue of forgiveness may be complicated by confusion between forgiving and condoning an intolerable action. Complex family dynamics may emerge. When the caregiver is able to maintain and model an open heart, the interpersonal atmosphere can change in beautiful ways, a process gracefully described in a classic series of books by Stephen Levine (1982, 1987, 1989) and in an enlightening audio program, *Being with Dying*, by Joan Halifax (1997).

Although a quick, unexpected death may relieve a person of having to face frightening trials, dying with an illness over time provides opportunity for being able to complete what has not been completed. Byock (1997) observes that, when Americans have been asked how they want to die, they sometimes respond with flippant quips about wishing for a sudden death, such as "I want to be struck by lightening after sinking a birdie on the eighteenth hole" or

"I want to be a hundred and be shot in the back by a jealous husband." But he notes that,

> while sudden deaths are attractive among the healthy, in reality, they leave many things undone, and they are often the hardest deaths for families to accept. In contrast to an abrupt, easy death, dying of a progressive illness offers precious opportunities to complete the most important of life's relationships. This includes the chance to reconcile strained relationships, perhaps between previous spouses, or between a parent and an estranged adult child. When the story of two people ends well, a warm light is shone on all that has preceded. Even at the very end of life, healing a relationship can transform the history of a family....When a dying person and a loved one come to feel complete between themselves, time together tends to be as full of joy and loving affection as sadness. (p. 53)

MINDFULNESS MEDITATION AND ACUPRESSURE FOR THE EMOTIONS

Skills in deep, open-hearted listening and responsiveness are the first pillar for assisting a person who is dying to more effectively confront the psychological and spiritual challenges that will emerge, and skills in meeting emotions in ways that open awareness and provide a sense of command form a second pillar. Two procedures from Eastern spiritual and healing traditions that are being adopted increasingly by Western psychotherapists can be invaluable for helping the dying person as well as the caregiver. Each can be self-administered outside the clinical context. Each may be enormously empowering, giving a person a measure of control and a sense of mastery over the ebb and flow of feelings that may run wild in the face of a terminal diagnosis for oneself or a loved one. Each teaches a person to encounter and manage difficult emotions in ways that are generally unfamiliar to individuals brought up in our culture.

Mindfulness Meditation

The stream-of-consciousness writing exercises in the previous section can be training wheels for mindfulness meditation. They can be used for any of the issues discussed in this section as well. You might experiment with this now, using headings such as "My Sadness about Jim's Illness," "My Terror of Losing Jim," "My Helplessness," "Jim's Pain," "My Anger with Jim," "Not Knowing What to Say to Jim," "The Unfairness." Again, focusing on a single topic, write without pausing for 10 uninterrupted minutes, and then review.

Like stream-of-consciousness writing, mindfulness meditation involves turning inward and keeping one's attention on the present moment. Mindfulness meditation, however, is a more subtle art that offers an alternative way of being with pain, anxiety, depression, and stress (Segal, Williams, & Teasdale,

2002). In mindfulness meditation, one pays attention, nonjudgmentally, to the unfolding of experience, moment by moment. You learn to witness the emergence of your inner landscape as an ongoing process rather than a fixed state. The result is that you become less attached to your thoughts and emotions, recognizing how they rise and fall, and this starts to free you from the tyranny of your thoughts (a bumper sticker instructs that "Meditation is not what you think"). You learn how your thoughts change with your mood and discover that *thoughts* are not *facts*. You become a witness of rather than a slave to habitual, automatic thought patterns. And by *turning toward* rather than *turning away from* difficult feelings, you are able to notice and identify negative thought patterns that keep you trapped (Lau & McMain, 2005).

Mindfulness involves a "deep, penetrative non-conceptual seeing into the nature of mind and world" (Kabat-Zinn, 2003, p. 146) that can be cultivated through the types of attention and concentration that are developed in the practice of meditation. Mindfulness and other forms of meditation were originally "nested within a larger conceptual and practice-based ethical framework" (p. 146). The management of one's emotions may be a more modest aspiration than Buddha-like compassion or the liberation from "the wheel of life and death," but it is still a practice that can lead to a skillful understanding of how unexamined thoughts, emotions, and behaviors "contribute directly to human suffering, one's own and that of others" (p. 146). Meditation is far more than a mind game. Because "mind" and "heart" are conveyed by the same word in Asian languages, mindfulness implies attending to the moment with "an affectionate, compassionate quality...a sense of openhearted, friendly presence and interest" (p. 145).

Books such as Jon Kabat-Zinn's *Wherever You Go, There You Are* (1994) and classes (eight two-hour weekly sessions are typical when mindfulness meditation is introduced into a person's psychotherapy) can teach the basic principles. But there is no way around regular practice to keep the principles alive and active in one's awareness. A daily practice of mindful meditation for a person who is faced with a life-threatening illness can significantly enhance the quality of the final days. To experiment, one of the most immediate ways to move into a space of mindfulness, as taught by Stephen Levine, is to simply, one breath at a time, "Soften belly. Notice breath. Open heart." Over and over. Try it.

Acupressure for Emotions

Reviewing a major text in the field of energy psychology for the prestigious online book review journal of the American Psychological Association, Ilene Serlin notes: "Energy psychology is a new discipline that has been receiving attention due to its speed and effectiveness with difficult cases"

(Serlin, 2005). Energy psychology, also sometimes called "acupressure for the emotions," is an approach for emotional self-management and therapeutic change that draws from both Traditional Chinese Medicine and modern cognitive-behavioral therapies. It combines the stimulation of specified manner that seems to quickly change the way the brain organizes specific emotional response patterns (Feinstein, 2006a). Among the emotions that seem to readily respond are excessive anxiety, fear, anger, guilt, jealousy, and shame, as well as mild depression.

Although the psychotherapy establishment has been slow to embrace the methods of and explanations about moving energy, an e-newsletter that provides instruction on how to utilize energy psychology techniques on a professional as well as self-help basis had 318,000 active subscribers at the time of this writing, and this number was increasing at a rate of 5,000 to 10,000 per month. People seem to find the approach effective for emotional self-management. Growing numbers of psychotherapists are incorporating it into their practices. Reports of its effectiveness in the extreme challenge of treating postdisaster trauma have come out of more than a dozen countries (Feinstein, 2006b). Most relevant for the context of a person dying at home is that the method can be readily learned and self-applied (Feinstein, Eden, & Craig, 2005).

Tools that can help a person place difficult feelings into a larger context, or even subdue intense and sometimes extreme emotional reactions, would have obvious value in helping a person move through the psychological challenges as life's final passage draws near. Such tools are readily available. Family members and caregivers must, however, remain very sensitive to not badgering the dying person with the availability of such aids. Fear, anger, depression, and grief all have constructive purposes within the economy of the psyche. Although an onlooker might be tempted to encourage a person to transcend such feelings, it is for each individual to navigate his or her way through complex internal landscapes. Still, experience among energy psychology practitioners suggests that reducing overwhelming emotional intensity does not rob the person of the lesson life is trying to provide. Rather, it allows the entire situation to be received, evaluated, and traversed with greater clarity and equanimity.

INDIVIDUALLY TAILORED RITUALS THAT BRING A FULLNESS OF MEANING

If deep, compassionate listening and responsiveness comprise the first pillar of being a presence in helping a person die well and introducing emotional self-management techniques the second, the third pillar involves introducing rituals that move a person forward on the journey with greater resolution, peace, and awareness. Groves and Klauser (2005) note that, "Death is a mystery so deep that sometimes only sacred ritual can express the fullness of its meaning for both the dying person and the caregivers" (p. 268).

Rituals, according to Megory Anderson (2003), "transform one state of being into another. They carry us from childhood into adulthood, or from membership in our family of birth to the creation of a new family through marriage" (p. 33). They have

> the ability to bring people an experience of something greater. They create a safe space and time in which we can touch the deeper issues of our existence. They have the power to bring to the surface and resolve very deep feelings and unnamed blocks that have been buried in our unconscious. (p. 35)

Rituals may be highly elaborate or exquisitely simple, planned or spontaneous. Anderson, a specialist in creating rituals for people who are about to cross over and their families, tells the story of walking by a hospital room where a man was being taken off of life support. A situation had arisen with the man's adult daughter, and Anderson, who was known to the hospital staff, stepped in to help:

> The woman, who was witnessing her father's death, was weeping uncontrollably. She was so distraught that one of the nurses had to hold her back. She was the only family member there, and I was sure she felt horribly guilty about making the decision to stop his life support.
>
> I asked the nurses to hold everything for just a few minutes while I took the woman into the hallway. I took her by the shoulders and spoke to her very firmly.
>
> "I know this is a horrible experience for you, but let's think for a moment about your father. He's hearing everything going on around him. Do you really want the last thing he hears to be a hysterical daughter? Why don't you talk to him as this is happening? Tell him how much you love him. You might even sing to him!"
>
> Her eyes grew round in amazement.
>
> "I never thought about it that way," she said through tears and hiccups.
>
> The woman took a deep breath and marched back in. She took his hand and said, "Daddy, I'm sorry I behaved that way. I was thinking about me more than I was thinking about you."
>
> She sniffled, wiped her eyes with the back of her hand, and then began singing in the most extraordinary voice.
>
> Amazing Grace! How sweet the sound
> That saved a wretch like me!
> I once was lost, but now am found
> Was blind, but now I see.
>
> I stared at the woman. Five minutes before, she was hysterical, almost having to be restrained, and now she was sitting here with a beautiful glow on her face. Her

voice was pure and exquisite. The nurses were transformed as they listened to her sing. I watched people from the hallway stop and then come to the door of the room, listening.

The nurse at the machines had tears in her eyes as she sang softly with the daughter. Then, quiet. We let the echoes stay with us a bit longer, and the nurse came over to the bed and unhooked tubes and monitors. She looked at the daughter and nodded, without saying anything. We both left the room allowing privacy for father and daughter. (pp. 217–218)

Ritual provides structure for helping what *wants* to happen at the deepest levels to *be able* to happen. They may or may not be rooted in religious or spiritual symbolism. Many rituals are highly attuned to the psychological needs of the dying person and the family. The themes of the rituals Anderson performs most frequently involve (1) letting go of the body, of loved ones, of life; (2) rituals for unresolved issues such as anger, remorse, sadness, fear, and relationships; (3) rituals for physical, emotional, and spiritual purification; and (4) rituals of transition from the state of living to the state of existence in the afterlife. She usually begins by creating "sacred space": devoid of clutter, contained for privacy and intimacy, and adorned with objects of beauty, candles, music, incense, or other devices that shift awareness through the senses. Symbols of personal, spiritual, or religious significance are brought, each ritualistically imbued with sacred intention. Sacred space can be created anywhere, from the person's bedroom to an antiseptic, machine-strewn room in a critical care unit. The rituals Anderson creates are based on an astute assessment of the emotional and spiritual needs the situation presents. She listens intently to all involved and pays close attention to the deep desires of the dying person in particular. She learns about the person's religious and cultural background and builds upon symbols and rituals that were meaningful to the person in their past.

While Anderson's *Sacred Dying: Creating Rituals for Embracing the End of Life* (2003) is perhaps the best practical overview of the subject, Groves and Klauser's *The American Book of Dying* (2005) provides a toolkit that also can be enormously useful. It includes rituals for the bedside, rituals for release, vigil rituals, rituals for remembering, meditation practices, religious rites, journaling and sacred writing exercises, life review exercises, forgiveness exercises, breath work, dream work, guided visualizations, the use of artistic expression, the use of music, the use of prayer, the use of energy therapies, ways of working with people in a coma, and ways of invoking the help and spiritual guidance of one's ancestors. A beautiful and poignant account of the way rituals can be created and can evolve to illuminate the journey of each family member during the illness and death of a young father is also highly instructive (Mayo, 1990a).

Through these three pillars—the power of deep listening, techniques for emotional self-management, and wisely crafted rituals—the process of dying can be transformed. Byock (1997) summarizes:

> Without adequate medical care, dying can be horrible. With skillful medical care and attention to the personal experience of the patient and the patient's family, dying can be made bearable. When the human dimension of dying is nurtured, for many the transition from life can become as profound, intimate, and precious as the miracle of birth. (p. 57)

EXPRESSIVE GRIEF WORK

Death is that curse that makes sweet love our anguish.

—The Buddha

"The terrible fire of grief," writes Peg Elliott Mayo, "is an energetic furnace, refining character, personality, intellect, and soul. It is a catalyst for creation. What is created may be dreadful—a distorted, unapproachable monument to despair—or a distillation of experience that is wholesome, useful, bright, and even wise" (Mayo, 1990b, p. 121). Mayo coined the term *expressive grief work* to describe the importance of emotional expression, psychological discharge, ventilation, and catharsis in the process of "conscious, ritualized grieving" (p. 128). Most cultures have memorials, services, and other practices that allow time where the family and other bereaved "are supported, expected, and encouraged to experience and express their anguish" (p. 128). She guides the reader through a series of internal "rituals for transmuting grief to creativity," including visualization, meditation, movement, sounding, auditory drawing, internal dialogues, reframing, and rituals for saying good-bye (Mayo, 1990b, 2001). One ritual for saying good-bye, after appropriate preparation, involves invoking the one being grieved, making the person present in one's imagination, placing the person in an "empty chair," and very consciously working through (perhaps in numerous sessions) the four stages associated "with the final phase of transmuting grief to creativity in expressive grief work" (Mayo, 1990b, p. 168):

> First, we express the resentment and anger associated with the loss.
> Second, we dredge our memories and recall the person we've lost and our associations about the person. Making a long list of "I remembers" is very useful and often primes the pump for the last two stages.
> Third, we do well to express our appreciations. Speaking or listing these brings balance and gives a sense of legacy from our absent loved one.
> Finally, and with much resolution, we give a benediction and say good-bye.

The presentation of Mayo's rituals for expressive grief work is imbued with enormously moving and instructive accounts of her personal struggles and steps toward resolution following the suicide of her son Patrick not long after his graduation from Yale. In addition to the deeply personal rituals Mayo describes, the essential principles of heartfelt listening discussed in the previous section apply to grief as well. In another moving account about losing a child, Bachu (1997) notes how important it was to talk, in a bereavement support group, with other grieving parents:

> I think it was the sharing of stories that saved my life. There were stories of confession, of regrets, of laments, of fury....We let it all spill out into the collective pool of tears. Compassion filled our hearts. We held each other, remembered other times, and eventually we dared to begin to dream new dreams. (p. 208)

The same three pillars for helping a person die well (deep expression and witnessing, internal and shared rituals, and emotional self-management tools) can also help transform the anguish of grief into the wisdom, compassion, and treasured memories of a life well lived. Each can be useful with the emotional issues that are part of grieving, including sorrow, anger, depression, anxiety, denial, emptiness, longing, loneliness, loss of meaning and identity, withdrawal, thoughts of suicide, and pessimism about the future. Any of these topics can, in fact, be a focus for stream-of-consciousness journaling or mindfulness meditation. For journaling, again, put the topic at the top of the page, write without pausing for 10 minutes, and reflect. In mindfulness meditation, one turns toward rather than away from difficult feelings, going deeper and deeper into the feeling of, say, inconsolable sorrow. Watching its ebb and flow, watching the thoughts one's mind creates around it, can itself be healing.

The elements of effective therapeutic approaches to grief are also instructive. In the first phase of a promising method called *traumatic grief therapy* (Shear, Frank, Houck, & Reynolds 2005), the therapist provides information about normal grief and unresolved, protracted, complicated grief. A model of coping is introduced in which focus alternates between *adjusting to the loss* and *restoring a satisfying life*. The process addresses both the loss and goals for the future. One way of focusing on the loss is through memories. For instance, the person's death may be revisited, told as a story, with eyes closed, and tape recorded. At various points, the person may be asked to describe the amount of distress being experienced. At the moments of greatest distress, techniques to promote a sense of connection with the deceased are used, such as imaginal conversations, concentrating on both positive and negative memories. The person might be asked to imagine that the one who has died is able to hear and respond and is then encouraged to engage in a dialogue with the deceased. A technique that focuses on restoring a satisfying life is to have the person consider what would be desirable at this time if the grief were not so intense. These desirable visions become goals. Other goals might also be identified, such as finding ways of stepping into one's new role in life without the loved one, resolving existing interpersonal difficulties that interfere with moving forward, and reengaging in meaningful relationships. Concrete plans for putting envisioned goals into action are discussed, along with ways of identifying progress toward them.

CONCLUSION

In each of the areas discussed in this chapter—using an awareness of the inevitability of death to enhance one's life, being the "soul friend" with someone who is dying, and moving forward creatively after losing a loved one—the three pillars of deep listening and responsiveness, emotional self-management, and transformative rituals can help guide the way. Although U.S. culture is known for its denial of death, caregivers can draw from the rich traditions and rituals from societies throughout recorded history. Such a multicultural perspective on death is not only enormously empowering, culturally sensitive practices regarding death have, with the increased mobility of the world's population, become essential training for healthcare professionals.

TOOL KIT FOR CHANGE

Perspective of the Healthcare Professional

1. The patient will provide the cues about the care that is needed.
2. Denial, anger, fear, bargaining, and depression all have important psychological functions. Listen well.
3. The dying process includes unusual internal experiences and the need to complete unfinished business. Powerful palliative care methods for reducing pain and increasing physical comfort are available, as are methods for effectively engaging difficult emotions. Ensure that they are used.
4. Rituals bring structure that helps what wants and needs—psychologically and spiritually—to occur.

Perspective of the Participant

1. This is a time to express what you feel and what you need and come to resolution about what is not completed.
2. This is a time to accept where you are on the wheel of life. Do not waste your energies or quality time with loved ones mired in shame or guilt.
3. You will go through a myriad of emotions—engage them in a "soften belly, notice breath, open heart" manner.
4. Spiritual and religious questions, and questions about what happens after death, will occur to you. Request visits from people with whom you would like to discuss them.

Interconnection: The Global Perspective

1. While every culture has its own beliefs and practices regarding death and dying, universal principles found in all cultures help us map what is required in caring for a dying person.

2. The spiritual dimensions of the dying process frequently become important even for people who have not considered themselves religious or spiritual.

REFERENCES

Anderson, M. (2003). *Sacred dying: Rituals for embracing the end of life* (Rev. ed.). New York: Marlowe.

Austin, J. H. (1999). *Zen and the brain: Toward an understanding of meditation and consciousness.* Cambridge, MA: MIT Press.

Bachu, L. (1997). A scent of grace: Surviving the death of a child. In Starhawk et al., *The pagan book of living and dying: Practical rituals, prayers, blessings, and meditations on crossing over* (pp. 205–209). San Francisco: HarperCollins.

Byock, I. (1997). *Dying well: Peace and possibilities at the end of life.* New York: Riverhead Books.

Callanan, M., & Kelley, P. (1997). *Final gifts: Understanding the special awareness, needs, and communications of the dying.* New York: Bantam.

Feinstein, D. (2006a). *Energy psychology: Background, methods, evidence.* Unpublished manuscript. Available from http://www.innersource.net/energy_psych/epi_research.htm.

Feinstein, D. (2006b). Energy psychology in the treatment of post-disaster trauma. Unpublished manuscript. Available from http://www.innersource.net/energy_psych/articles/ep_energy-trauma-treatment.htm.

Feinstein, D., Eden, D., & Craig, G. (2005). *The promise of energy psychology.* New York: Tarcher/Penguin.

Feinstein, D., & Krippner, S. (2006). *The mythic path: Discovering the guiding stories of your past—Creating a vision for your future* (3rd ed.). Santa Rosa, CA: Elite.

Grof, S. (1990). *The holotropic mind: The three levels of human consciousness and how they shape our lives.* San Francisco: HarperCollins.

Grof, S. (2006). *The ultimate journey: Consciousness and the mystery of death.* Ben Lomond, CA: Multidisciplinary Association for Psychedelic Studies.

Grof, S., Goodman, L. E., Richards, W. A., & Kurland, A. A. (1973). LSD-assisted psychotherapy in patients with terminal cancer. *International Pharmacopsychiatry, 8,* 129–144.

Groves, R. F., & Klauser, H. A. (2005). *The American book of dying: Lessons in healing spiritual pain.* Berkeley, CA: Celestial Arts.

Halifax, J. (Presenter). (1997). *Being with dying* [audio cassettes]. Louisville, CO: Sounds True.

Hoffman, E. (1988). *The right to be human: A biography of Abraham Maslow.* Los Angeles: Tarcher.

Huxley, A. (1970). *The doors of perception.* New York: Harper & Row.

James, W. (1961). *Varieties of religious experience.* New York: Crowell-Collier (original work published 1902).

Kabat-Zinn, J. (1994). *Wherever you go, there you are: Mindfulness meditation in everyday life.* New York: Hyperion.

Kabat-Zinn, J. (2003). Mindfulness-based interventions in context: Past, present, and future. *Clinical Psychology: Science and Practice, 10,* 144–156.

Kramer, K. (1988). *The sacred art of dying: How world religions understand death.* New York: Paulist Press.

Kübler-Ross, E. (Ed.). (1975). *Death: The final stage of growth.* [Upper Saddle River, NJ: Prentice-Hall.

Lau, M. A., & McMain, S. F. (2005). Integrating mindfulness meditation with cognitive and behavioural therapies: The challenge of combining acceptance- and change-based strategies. *Canadian Journal of Psychiatry, 50,* 863–869.

Levine, S. (1982). *Who dies? An investigation of conscious living and dying.* Garden City, NY: Anchor.

Levine, S. (1987). *Healing into life and death.* Garden City, NY: Anchor.

Levine, S. (1989). *Meetings at the edge: Dialogues with the grieving and the dying, the healing and the healed.* Garden City, NY: Anchor.

Lifton, R. J. (1983). *The broken connection: On death and the continuity of life.* New York: Basic Books.

Mayo, P. E. (1990a). Rituals for living and dying: One family's experience. In D. Feinstein & P. E. Mayo (Eds.), *Rituals for living and dying: From life's wounds to spiritual awakening* (pp. 1–34). San Francisco: HarperCollins.

Mayo, P. E. (1990b). The alchemy of transmuting grief to creativity. In D. Feinstein & P. E. Mayo (Eds.), *Rituals for living and dying: From life's wounds to spiritual awakening* (pp. 121–172). San Francisco: HarperCollins.

Mayo, P. E. (2001). *The healing sorrow workbook: Rituals of transforming grief and loss.* Oakland, CA: New Harbinger.

Moody, R. (2001). *Life after life: The investigation of a phenomenon—survival of bodily death* (2nd ed.). San Francisco: HarperCollins.

Osis, K., & Haraldsson, E. (1977). *At the hour of death.* New York: Avon.

Ring, K. (1985). *Heading toward Omega: In search of the meaning of the near-death experience.* New York: William Morrow.

Santayana, G. (1972). *Realms of being.* New York: Cooper Square Publishers

Segal, Z. V., Williams, J.M.G., & Teasdale, J. D. (2002). *Mindfulness-based cognitive therapy for depression: A new approach to preventing relapse.* New York: Guilford Press.

Serlin, I. (2005, March 2). Energy psychology—An emerging form of integrative psychology [Review of the book/CD *Energy psychology interactive: Rapid interventions for lasting change*]. *PsychCritiques* [On-line serial]. 50(9), Article 12.

Shear, K., Frank, E., Houck, P. R., & Reynolds, C. F. (2005). Treatment of complicated grief: A randomized controlled trial. *Journal of the American Medical Association, 293,* 2601–2608.

Templer, D. I. (1972). Death anxiety in religiously very involved persons. *Psychological Reports, 31,* 361–362.

Tobin, D. R. (1998). *Peaceful dying: The step-by-step guide to preserving your dignity, your choice, and your inner peace at the end of life.* Reading, MA: Perseus.

von Lommel, P., van Wees, R., Meyers, V., & Elfferich, I. (2001). Near-death experience in survivors of cardiac arrest: A prospective study in The Netherlands. *Lancet, 358,* 2039–2045.

Walsh, R., & Shapiro, S. L. (2006). The meeting of meditative disciplines and Western psychology: A mutually enriching dialogue. *American Psychologist, 61,* 227–339.

Wilber, K. (1990). Death, rebirth, and meditation. In G. Doore (Ed.), *What survives? Contemporary explorations of life after death.* Los Angeles: Tarcher.

Yalom, I. D. (1980). *Existential psychotherapy.* New York: Basic Books.

Chapter Thirteen

THE ROLE OF RITUALS
IN PSYCHOTHERAPY

*Jeanne Achterberg, PhD, Christian Dombrowe, PhD,
and Stanley Krippner, PhD*

The Blood of the Ancients Runs through Our Veins The Forms Pass But the Circle
Remains
                          —Healing chant, Charlie Murphy and Betsy Rose

Since the dawn of history, human societies have used a multitude of healing
practices to deal with illness and disease and to resolve interpersonal and
intrapersonal conflicts. Typically, these practices involved alleged spiritual
forces, and rituals were designed to evoke the aid of deities, spirits, and allies
from "other worlds" (Eliade, 1972; Levi-Strauss, 1967).

Several of these traditional healing practices, as well as the rituals that
accompany them, are still used in various parts of the world. Many people
from immigrant and refugee communities consult traditional healers in developed North American and European countries. Furthermore, increasing numbers of people of the dominant or mainstream culture seek out traditional
healing methods as well (Field, 1990). The interest in traditional healing practices and their accompanying rituals has forced mainstream psychology and
psychiatry to examine this topic and to realize that ritual may play a hitherto
unacknowledged role in Western psychotherapy (West, 2000). Therefore, psychotherapists in the twenty-first century would benefit from learning about
the relevance and possible efficacy of traditional healing modalities and the
rituals that accompany them.

Knowledge of the therapeutic dimension of ritual is especially important
for psychotherapists working in multicultural contexts with culturally diverse clients who rely on traditional forms of healing. For example, thera-

pists working with North American aboriginal peoples will be more effective if they establish working relationships with traditional healers who serve their clients through the performance of healing rituals and ceremonies. Many Native American health and treatment centers not only provide medical and psychotherapeutic services, but also offer culturally integrated treatment modalities such as healing rituals and ceremonies through collaboration with traditional healers. One of the authors (Dombrowe) is personally familiar with a Native American residential treatment center for alcoholism in Manteca, California, that regularly offers sweat lodge ceremonies to its clients.

Although knowledge of the functions and the healing potential of rituals is a crucial aspect of cultural sensitivity for psychotherapists who work with clients from indigenous or immigrant communities and who want to build collaborative relationships with traditional healers based on understanding and respect, it is equally capable of enhancing the effectiveness of conventional therapeutic practice with clients of the mainstream culture. Knowledge about rituals and their functions can help contemporary psychotherapists clearly recognize ritual aspects of their work as well as to consciously integrate rituals into their treatment approach.

Rituals are effective interventions founded on patterned interactions between the client/patient and the therapist/healer within the framework of a culturally shared belief system. Rituals maintain and improve the bond between the therapist and the client. Rituals supply the client with a conceptual framework that provides a sense of direction, mastery, and self-worth. Rituals help clients to overcome despair and to combat demoralization (Frank & Frank, 1991). The emotional intensity of rituals awakens confidence, hope, and a healing expectation and thereby builds the client's morale—an ingredient that is necessary for staying engaged in the sometimes painful process of personal change.

The term *ritual* can be conceptualized as a prescribed, stylized, step-by-step, goal-directed performance of a mythological theme. It is prescribed by such practitioners as shamans, religious functionaries, and family or community elders. It is stylized in a form that symbolizes deeper meaning to the participants. It is mythological in the sense that myths are imaginative narratives concerning vital, existential human concerns that have behavioral consequences. It is goal-directed in that its performance is expected to lead to practical, observable results (Krippner, 2000).

Nothing is as timeless or as universal as the ritualistic circle. For millennia, various circle rituals have been the vehicle for transpersonal medicine; that is, medicine (in the broadest sense of the word) that seems to emanate from beyond the self, from others, and even from sources that a culture considers to be divine in nature (Achterberg, Dossey, & Kolkmeier, 1994). Power is imparted from the circle to its components—the symbols and metaphors that represent various dimensions of healing—and the reverse is also true (Krippner, 1997a).

The coming together of people in a ritual is linked through these symbols and metaphors whether they have concrete referents in everyday reality or are spun by imagination. For example, Native American medicine wheels are examples of the healing circle; the symbols (such as power animals and power objects) placed at different points on the wheel and the metaphors (such as the stories told during the utilization of the wheel) are potent healing agents (Halifax, 1991).

What contemporary practitioners refer to as therapy typically involves a relationship between a healer (practitioner or therapist) and a healee (patient or client). Psychotherapy relies on the healer's ability to mobilize the healee's restorative resources by psychological means (Frank & Frank, 1991). A study of how humans help themselves and each other in times of distress is sobering and humbling and shreds any mantle of arrogance that holds effective treatment to be a modern invention.

From the beginning of recorded history, the search for substances and procedures to cure or relieve suffering has been a convoluted and mutating path. Methods for healing the mind and body come and go. Drugs come and go. Technologies come and go. If there is a thread of common experience running through the past and present of medicine and psychotherapy, it is the ritual that accompanies the medicaments, ministrations, and various gadgets that humans have used to treat each other over the years. Indeed, external ministrations may be regarded more as symbols of healing than as the active ingredient of healing—or the restorative ability of the mind and body. Therefore, it is necessary to focus on the potential of rituals as well as on the practices that accompany them (Achterberg, 1996).

THE POTENTIAL OF RITUALS

For many years, the study of rituals has been the province of ethnologists and cultural anthropologists (e.g., Eliade, 1972; Heinze, 2000; Lévi-Strauss, 1967; Turner, 1986). As a result, the term *ritual* took on overtones of something foreign and exotic, even primitive in nature, something based on ignorance and superstition. In recent years, however, a number of psychologists and psychiatrists (e.g., Achterberg & Lawlis, 1981, 1985, 1996, 1997; Dombrowe, 2005; Frank & Frank, 1991; Krippner, 1982; Torrey, 1986) have observed that the study of indigenous healing practices can be instructive for Western health-care practitioners. Even in technologically advanced societies, rituals hold an unacknowledged potential to fulfill important physical, psychological, social, and spiritual needs.

Krippner (2000) remarked that modern technological societies have lost touch with the sacred aspects of ritual and that most remaining rituals—such as birthdays, marriages, or graduations—have become secularized and thereby lost their magic. What this loss may signify comes more into focus when we consider that the disappearance of ritual among indigenous communities of Australia has been linked to increased violence, despair, and mental confusion (Bond, 2006). The problem is not so much that modern societies lack rituals, but that these modern practices often fail to honor deep human feelings, the need for sacred connections, and the ultimate power of the conscious mind. Whenever humans faced challenges alone, or when they came together in groups or societies, they developed rituals. Without rituals, they had no map for behavior, and no occasions during which they could share their common experiences (Achterberg et al., 1994).

Historically, rituals have been closely associated with the sacred dimension of life. They were frequently used to establish contact with whatever sources the culture ascribed to the divine. Generally, a ritual involves an activity apart from ordinary life—spatially, temporally, and psychologically (Lyon, 2000). Rituals create meanings, maintain or transform social roles and identities, establish contact with transpersonal sources, and mediate healing. Rituals communicate meanings in a multidimensional way, using multisensory involvement, focused attention, and aroused emotionality. They involve symbols, metaphors, objects, and actions that converge around a mythological theme. The skillful manipulation of culturally sanctioned symbols and metaphors seems to be of considerable importance in a ritual's efficacy (Jilek, 1989).

Moore and Myerhoff (1977) observed that rituals can either reinforce existing values, beliefs, and behaviors or can help change them, both individually and collectively. For example, a ritual that is intended to be a rite of passage can change the social roles of an individual from a child to an adult. A ritual can introduce a cultural innovation, such as adding a new deity to the theological panoply. One of the reasons for its efficacy in facilitating individual or social change is that a ritual occurs at the intersection of the private and public worlds. The ritual participants reorganize their inner world and psychological identity in the presence of others who witness and validate those transformations. A ritual regulates the interaction between group members by defining roles, rules, and boundaries. A ritual helps people to identify with their group and to connect with each other. Rituals prevent social isolation, communalize emotional burdens, and help people to bond through shared experience.

A culturally shared belief system—a culture's worldview or mythology—gives meaning to ritual activities, ritual objects, and ritualistic metaphors and symbols (Chapple & Coon, 1978). Conversely, ritual activities enact the belief system or mythology of the community (Bourguignon, 1979; Moore,

1983). This mythology defines the actions, objects, and roles enacted in the ritual.

Because a ritual is a step-by-step process, its performance is carried out with precision. The required behavior is prescribed, yet there is usually some space for improvisation and creativity. Repetition of ritual acts serves to familiarize people with appropriate ritual behavior and to establish a shared sense of meaning and a sense of authenticity (Moore & Myerhoff, 1977). Ritual performances typically are highly stylized, and it is these activities, gestures, and movements that transmit meaning. Heightened emotionality is regularly evoked and regulated by theatrical presentation, music and dance, charismatic leadership, reinforcement from others, and expectations from past experiences. Participants may become highly absorbed in the ritual proceedings and transcend their usual conceptual boundaries (Gilligan, 1997).

TRANSITION RITUALS AND HEALING RITUALS

Scholars have identified several different kinds of rituals (e.g., Wallace, 1966). For example, Krippner (2000) defines "rites" as "mini-rituals," because they are usually simple and straightforward (as in "rites of passage"); "ceremonies" can be termed "maxi-rituals," because they tend to be long and complicated (as in "coronation ceremonies"). There are two primary types of ritual that hold special relevance to psychotherapy: healing rituals and transition rituals (Hart, 1983). Both are prescribed, stylized, and goal-directed, and are characterized by a step-by-step performance.

Transition rituals recreate and transform identity; they facilitate structural changes of the group (e.g., new leadership) as well as status changes of individuals (e.g., from unmarried to married status). In so doing, they provide social cohesion, unite people with their environment, and serve the well-being of the whole society. Van Gennep (1960) described the basic structure that underlies most transition rituals: (a) separation—setting the ritual space apart from ordinary reality; temporary separation from the customary group or activities; (b) liminality—altering one's customary social status, normative behavior, or identity; placing the participant or participants in a state of limbo or on a threshold for change; and (c) integration—the return to ordinary life, but in a transformed fashion. Transition rituals allow individuals and groups to return to ordinary life after the balance in their relationship with their environment, their community, or transpersonal agencies has been disturbed and then restored. These disturbances are seen as a natural part of life transitions that groups and individuals go through in the service of a developmental process.

When discussing transition rituals, vision quests are common examples. Quests in search of a vision that will yield wisdom, power, or insight have been carefully crafted. Some vision quests have been designed to mark transitions from one state of being to another. For example, in preparation for adulthood, adolescents may be temporarily separated from their community. The initiates leave their customary habitat and go to the forest, desert, mountain, or other place that is regarded as having sacred qualities. Once the vision has been received, they return and share their experience with the community. If their vision is deemed authentic and worthy, the initiates become adult members of the tribe.

Healing rituals can be regarded as a special type of transition ritual (van Gennep, 1960). The purpose of transition rituals is to steer individuals and groups safely through life transitions (childhood to adulthood, marriage, death, etc.). Healing rituals serve the same purpose, but in an intrapersonal rather than an interpersonal fashion. The situations that demand the performance of healing rituals have more of a crisis character than regular life transitions, as in cases of sickness, accidents, and disruptive behaviors. Healing rituals derive their power from a shared worldview that informs the client, the healing practitioner, and the community. They sanction and define the healer's role, help the client make sense of a specific symptom or problem, and prescribe a certain course of action to solve the issue at hand. To regain health and wholeness, healing rituals often utilize symbols (for example, the figures on a Navaho sand painting) and metaphors (the *chant way* story that accompanies the use of a Navaho sand painting). The symbols and metaphors of a healing ritual cement the healer-healee bond and engender faith and hope that suffering will be relieved by one's passage into the realm of wholeness and harmony (Torrey, 1986). Healing images are typically evoked through ritual procedures (Achterberg et al., 1994).

The dual function of a healing ritual is that all members of the participating community benefit by receiving and by giving. They surrender to the power of the ritual, and they become empowered to care for those who need assistance. In general, traditional societies regard sickness as due to fragmentation or alienation or as a loss of one's soul. Healing, accordingly, is seen as becoming whole, regaining balance, and restoring one's soul and other missing pieces of one's being. This wholeness is understood in an ecological fashion as regained harmony with oneself as well as a reunion with one's family, society, nature, and the spiritual forces of the cosmos.

For example, the traditional Navaho (or *Diné*) healing ritual comprises six steps: purification of the client, presentation of the client to the healing spirits, calling the spirits to the *Hogan* where the ritual is taking place, selecting the appropriate *chant way* for the client, focusing the client's attention on the images in the sand painting and the story of the *chant way* (i.e., the healing symbols and metaphors), and returning the client to the everyday world (Sandner, 1979).

Achterberg (1985) delineated the following functions of both traditional and contemporary healing rituals:

1. Friends and family members can express their concern by engaging in preparations required for the ritual.
2. Ritual preparations and participation are a way for both the patient and the community to feel in control of what appeared to be a hopeless situation. The ritual enhances group solidarity, and the features of the ritual cement the ties between the patient and a community from which he or she may have felt alienated.
3. The ritual both soothes and distracts a client.
4. The relationship between the healee and the community is strengthened by the ritual.
5. There is a sense of relief through belief in a restored harmony with the spiritual dimensions of the cosmos.
6. The rituals and symbols serve to interpret the meaning of disease as well as the patient's role in sickness and health, all within a cultural context.
7. The emotional intensity of the ritual increases hope or expectant trust that something important will happen.
8. Most rituals are costly in terms of time, money, and resources, and this can serve to enhance the healee's pride and self-esteem.
9. When psychoactive substances are used, community singing and dancing occur, or altered states of consciousness are employed as a consequence of the ritual, the power of the healer and the healer's belief system is strengthened and validated (pp. 157–158).

THE PATTERN OF RITUALS

Both transition and healing rituals, and traditional rituals in general, appear to follow basic patterns (Heinze, 2000; Somé, 1993). This procedure is of special interest to psychotherapists contemplating the incorporation of rituals into their clinical practice. Anthropologist Ruth Inge Heinze (2000) has outlined the following basic ritual structure:

1. Marking and purifying the sacred space and the ritual's participants.
2. Ritually entering the sacred space.
3. Evoking spiritual sources.
4. Encountering these sources.
5. Celebrating the presence of these sources.
6. Thanking these sources, leaving the sacred space, and allowing for closure.

Contemporary psychotherapists who intend to draw on the power of ritual in their clinical practice may be assisted by knowing the structure of traditional rituals. They might want to reframe such terms as *sacred* and *spiritual* in ways that reflect their clients' belief systems and make other adaptations as circumstances make necessary.

RITUALS AND ALTERED STATES OF CONSCIOUSNESS

Rituals (especially shamanic rituals) frequently aim at instigating alterations, shifts, and changes in the attention, cognition, and awareness of participants (see Eliade, 1972; Lévi-Strauss, 1967). These alterations range from focused attention to profound changes in the perception of oneself, space, and time. Rituals have been used not only to induce altered states of consciousness (ASCs), but also to structure what happens during ASCs and to utilize the resulting experiences positively (Wallace, 1959).

The central characteristic of ASCs is a clearly felt qualitative shift in one's patterns of mental functioning (Tart, 1969). Ludwig (1966) mentions the following defining features of ASCs: alterations in thinking, sense of time, emotional expression, and body image, as well as perceptual shifts, changes in meaning or significance, a sense of ineffability, and feelings of rejuvenation and hyper-suggestibility.

Tart (1980) pointed out that ordinary consciousness is often perceived as normal or even optimal and ASCs as odd, inferior, or pathological. This common misperception has been corrected by cross-cultural investigations and by scholars who have pointed out that ASCs actually fulfill important adaptive, hygienic functions (e.g., Dittrich & Scharfetter, 1987; Wittkover, 1970).

From an evolutionary perspective, participation in rituals that induce ASCs and thereby enable participants to overcome their sense of separateness and to experience transpersonal bonding has adaptive values. Rappaport (1978) pointed out that this bonding enhances social integration and solidarity, both of which are essential for the survival of human communities. Krippner (1997b) noted that the ubiquity of ASCs suggests that they were instrumental in helping individuals and communities solve problems that customary procedures failed to address. Other authors have argued that humans have an innate drive to seek ASCs (Kremer, 2003; Samorini, 2000; Siegel, 1990, Weil, 1998, Winkelman, 1996).

Certainly there exist pathological ASCs, but ASCs are not necessarily pathological. Over the centuries, the cultivation of ASCs has been vitally important to indigenous cultures that devoted considerable attention to their systematic induction (Eliade, 1972). Extensive study of the social and cultural patterning of ASCs has demonstrated that in about 90 percent of the world's traditional cultures one can find institutionalized use of ASCs (Bourguignon, 1973).

Rituals have induced ASCs through a variety of techniques, such as fasting, sleep deprivation, suggestion, sensory deprivation or overload, rhythmic stimulation, dancing or chanting, hyperventilation, and psychoactive substances. Dobkin de Rios (1984) reported that each society interprets and structures the ASC experience through its own lens, through its own patterning of visionary experience.

Ritually induced ASCs can effect cognitive and behavioral changes by suspending the individual's defenses and opening the individual to experiences that have the potential to challenge that person's assumptive world. During an ASC, the cognitive filters that structure the way an individual perceives reality (often in maladaptive ways) become temporarily disrupted, and the individual consequently is open to new corrective perceptions and experiences. The experiences available through ASCs, in turn, may also be fully accommodated by the individual's cognitive maps, in which case the individual's belief system is reinforced. At times, the individual's habitual cognitive maps may fail to explain those experiences, in which case the power of that belief system is weakened. This process affords the individual with the opportunity to gain insight, grow in self-awareness, and behave in new ways. The emotional intensity of ritually induced ASCs makes it unlikely for them to be denied later on.

Yet it is important to point out that the experience of an ASC does not guarantee therapeutic change. The experiences may be negative. Learning that occurs in ASC may be state-specific and may not be recalled when the individual returns to an ordinary state of consciousness (Tart, 1975).

In traditional societies, a ritual structures the entry into and exit from an ASC. The ritual provides a sense of security when traversing unfamiliar mental and emotional landscapes. Rituals structure the experience, focus the evoked emotions, and allow the symbolic and mythic elements to provide interpretative cognitive maps that help integrate new insights. The ritual boundaries that separate ritual space and ordinary life help to contain the experience of an ASC and increase the individual's sense of control and safety.

In short, ritual helps to structure and integrate experiences in an ASC (Dobkin de Rios, 1984). This capacity of a ritual to assist in the integration of the experience of an ASC can contribute to the maintenance of long-term positive therapeutic results. For example, the Navaho *chant way* ritual continues for four days, during which time the client follows a regimen to protect members of the tribe from his or her newly acquired powers (Krippner, 1997a). However, Navaho *hatalii* (singing shamans) do not take mind-altering plants before or during the *chant way*, because their memory must be intact and their attention cannot be distracted (Sandner, 1979).

RITUALS IN CONTEMPORARY HEALTHCARE

In 1971, the renowned Native American shaman, Rolling Thunder, had his first prolonged conversation with a Western doctor, Irving Oyle, an osteopathic physician. The two of them were sequestered in the recording studio of their host, Mickey Hart, a rock musician. After several hours, they came out of the studio, arm in arm. Oyle reported,

> We compared our practices. Rolling Thunder said that when a sick person comes to him, he makes a diagnosis, goes through a ritual, and gives that person some

medicine that will restore health. I replied that when a patient comes to me, I make a diagnosis and go through the ritual of writing a prescription that will give the patient some medicine to restore health. (Krippner & Villoldo, 1976, p. 56)

One of the most obvious examples of contemporary healthcare in which ASCs play an important part is hypnotically facilitated psychotherapy. Even though hypnosis, per se, is not a specific ASC, it involves the use of clients' imaginative processes as well as techniques to heighten their motivation and expectation. Most hypnotic procedures involve an induction of some sort, various suggestions that focus a client's attention, and an interaction between the therapist and client in which hoped-for goals are emphasized. Quite often, step-by-step procedures for attaining these goals are outlined; after the hypnotic session ends, these procedures are carried through, either by posthypnotic suggestions or by homework assignments (Krippner, 2005). The effectiveness of hypnosis in facilitating psychotherapy has been demonstrated in several extensive studies (e.g., Kirsch, 1990), and the role of hypnotic ritual plays an important part in enhancing therapeutic outcome.

Dreaming is a naturally occurring ASC, and several studies vouch for the effectiveness of including dream interpretation sessions in psychotherapy (e.g., Hill & Rochlen, 1999). Hill (1996) has developed a three-step ritual for working with dreams. In the exploration stage, the individual parts or elements of a dream are examined, and the client is encouraged to experience the dream as if it were actually happening in the present time. This process helps the client to access the feelings, thoughts, and previous experiences that are represented in the content and emotions of the dream. In the insight stage, the therapist and client collaborate to construct a new understanding of the dream. Together, they try to extend the client's previous understanding of the dream and help the client to learn something new about himself or herself. Finally, in the action stage, the therapist and client determine what life changes the client might make based on what was learned in the dream.

Achterberg described the use of image, symbol, and ritual in modern healthcare in two major life transitions: menopause (Achterberg, 1997) and death and dying (Achterberg & Lawlis, 1981). She pointed out that modern culture is bereft of rituals for the difficult rite of passage associated with the physical, psychological, and spiritual changes of menopause. Women often feel dishonored, confused, and in desperate need of identifying new and different currencies and sources of beauty, passion, and power. Self-generated rituals (i.e., rituals that are designed for a unique purpose) can have powerful therapeutic implications and may be created in a community of women or as meditations in solitude. Conscious engagement in the events and emotions of the menopausal years may require developing a new life story or mythology and identification with images and symbols that are affirmative and life-enhancing.

On the topic of death and dying, Achterberg and Lawlis (1981) pointed out that much of modern culture is devoid of mythological frameworks when it comes to the process of dying. With the exception of rituals embedded in religious traditions, funeral directors reign as mythmakers for death and the path of bereavement. A medical system dedicated to curing interventions largely dictates the experience of dying. Achterberg and Lawlis (1981) suggested that therapists can don some of the activities of the shaman, and, while not shamans themselves, could well apply shamanistic ideas to their therapeutic interactions. "The therapist, therefore, serves as a guide and a collaborator, hoping to remove some uncertainty from the path and to insure that all possible richness can emanate from the event" (p. 210). Memories from a life review might be savored and resolved. A likely focus for the rituals for death and dying is guided imagery, because it bridges ancient healing traditions with an intervention acceptable to modern healthcare. Guided imagery can enable material stored at a preconscious level to emerge as clarification of values and beliefs about dying and the afterlife, and it can help the guide to be able to react and interact sensitively with a patient's dying images (p. 210). Dying imagery is like a pilot's communication as the plane approaches a landing. It can be a dialogue with an unseen entity. Occasionally, a therapist is privileged to be an eavesdropper on one side of the interchange.

When tribal shamans utilize mind-altering substances in their treatments, highly ritualized procedures attempt to guarantee safety as well as positive outcomes. Similar regimens were followed when LSD and other psychoactive substances were introduced into Western psychotherapy (Sherwood, Stolaroff, & Harman, 1962). When legal difficulties hindered these practices, Grof (1985) developed a technique, holotropic breath work, which attempted to mimic many of the effects of LSD-type drugs. An experimental study utilizing holotropic breath work in combination with experiential-oriented psychotherapy found significant reductions in death anxiety and increased self-esteem compared with a group of clients using a conventional therapeutic approach (Holmes, Morris, Clance, & Putney, 2003). The six breath work sessions in this study followed a step-by-step pattern and were highly ritualized.

RITUALISTIC ASPECTS OF PSYCHOTHERAPY

There are many similarities between traditional indigenous healing practices and contemporary psychotherapeutic techniques. Ritual elements that can be found in psychotherapeutic practice are heightened emotionality, the focus on symbols and metaphors, repetition, and enactment (Frank & Frank, 1991). Parallels in terms of process can be found as well. Rituals as well as psychotherapy involve a separation from ordinary life. Optimally, a client is separated from an old way of being and is led into discovering and implementing a new way of living. Specific boundaries separate ritual and therapy from the rest of the client's life (a certain time and place, noninterference, confidentiality, etc.). In psychotherapy as well as in traditional healing rituals, the client has to confront uncertainty and the unknown. Customary social norms are suspended (e.g., expression of intense emotions may be encouraged).

Contemporary psychotherapy and traditional healing practices also share related functions. Both attempt to reconcile self and society and to manage change processes (such as role transitions). Both engender hope and attempt to decrease demoralization. Both counteract feelings of alienation, especially through the sharing of intense emotions and the experience of meaningful interpersonal contact. Both attempt to increase the self-esteem of the client (Frank & Frank, 1991; Serlin, 1993; Torrey, 1986).

The multisensory nature of the Navaho *chant way,* for example, is designed to make the client feel special and privileged. The sand painting's visual images, the audible recitation of the narrative, the touch of the prayer sticks, the taste of the herbal medicines, and the smell of the incense combine to convey the power of the chant to the client (Sandner, 1979).

By contrast, modern psychotherapy is aligned with a scientific orientation that, for the most part, minimizes such an appeal to the senses. Its orientation values rationality and logic, avoiding spiritual and metaphysical perspectives in the pursuit of objectivity. Ritual, however, is inseparably intertwined with spiritual dimensions of the cosmos. The Navaho Big Star Way *chant way* was designed to protect clients against the dangers of the night, and the Hail Way *chant way* tells the story of a young man's battle against attacks from entities living in a non-Earthly realm. These types of rituals allow a departure from rational thought and encourage nonordinary experiences, even ASCs.

In traditional societies, rituals have been used to influence the belief system of large groups of people, thereby molding the social order. Psychotherapy, on the other hand, is concerned with a different type of social control—a normative way of being to which the client needs to be restored. However, several contemporary psychotherapists have understood the importance of reconnecting clients with families and communities, especially when working with young people at risk for suicide and substance abuse (Hendrin et al., 2005). Bossard and Boll (1950) applied ritual to family life; family therapists may break dysfunctional patterns by arranging role-playing exercises, prescribing communal tasks, creating a family discussion circle, and enhancing family integration through other rituals.

RITUAL SPACE AND ORCHESTRATION

Anthropological accounts identify ritual sites that are literally and symbolically bounded (Turner, 1969). Ritual space, such as the Navaho *Hogan* and the sand painting on its floor, is recognizable as such, because it differs from the space that surrounds it. Ritual sites are carefully planned and created with precise arrangements of necessary objects and paraphernalia. Ritual space is marked by special symbols (e.g., clothes worn, words expressed, enacted behaviors) that set it apart from ordinary life. This separation from ordinary life contributes to the heightened emotionality and the healing expectation that make ritual work so effective (Gilligan, 1997).

The psychotherapist's office can be viewed in terms of ritual space. Psychotherapists can create the desired ambience of their offices by choosing the type of furniture and their spatial arrangement, as well as carefully selecting the wall color and artwork. The deliberate design of these environmental factors creates the liminal space in which healing transformation can occur, shielded from intrusions of daily life and its obligations and responsibilities. Some psychotherapists take great care in decorating their offices, in choosing art for the walls and arranging the furniture. Freud is said to have put his clients on a couch because he did not want to become too intimate with them; for whatever reason, this arrangement served to ritualize the psychoanalytic session. Contemporary psychotherapists rarely use couches, but many have found other ways to ensure that their contact with a client differs from anything else that occurs in the client's everyday life.

Until recently, medicine has been intertwined with the sacred, and patients were treated in what was considered sacred space. Hospitals were (and some still are) affiliated with religious institutions. There has been some movement to reinstitute the role of spirituality in terms of architecture and practice. Woodwinds Hospital in St. Paul, Minnesota, and North Hawaii Community Hospital in Waimea, Hawaii, are both examples of a deliberate design to create liminal and ceremonial space, coupled with the best treatments available in modern healthcare.

North Hawaii Community Hospital, for example, invited a *kahuna* to consult on the buildings, grounds, and artwork during construction. Ti plants are appropriately placed according to Hawaiian healing beliefs. A labyrinth modeled after the one at Chartres Cathedral is available to the whole community. Blessing ceremonies at the hospital are conducted by various types of healers.

Psychotherapists and shamans are ritual specialists who orchestrate the process of change; they are the central figures who lead the ritual. Shamans are consulted for any kind of physical, psychological, social, or spiritual problem (Eliade, 1972; Halifax, 1991; Myerhoff, 1974); their role is to restore health and well-being to individuals and communities. Professional practices that shamans have in common with contemporary psychotherapists are listening, empathizing, advising, and instructing . Both types of practitioners must be skilled to observe both verbal and nonverbal nuances and shifts and to take advantage of them in their practice.

Psychiatrist Milton Erickson (Erickson & Rossi, 1980) was well known for his mirroring of clients' subtle behaviors in order to evoke therapeutic effects. He used both direct and indirect suggestions, many of them as part of "teaching stories" replete with paradoxes, parables, and metaphors. Erickson's use of ritual in psychotherapy can be compared to the three stages of a magician's trick: the pledge displays something ordinary, the turn produces something extraordinary from the ordinary, and the prestige displays a surprise twist. Erickson often began his therapeutic sessions by telling the client a simple story, but, by the time the session was finished, that story had evoked an insight, an attitudinal shift, or a behavior change. In a similar fashion, the Navaho *chant ways* begin by recounting ordinary events, but then meander through strange worlds and times, with a surprise ending that is designed to mobilize the healee's inner resources for positive change.

It would be simplistic to describe Erickson and other psychotherapists as modern-day shamans, because significant differences exist between the roles of shamans and psychotherapists. Shamanic practices involve metaphysical elements (such as the invocations of spiritual entities), whereas modern psychotherapy tends, for the most part, to follow the Western scientific paradigm and to avoid sacred domains.

Additionally, shamans typically rely on directive and persuasive techniques to effect desired changes; they can be openly manipulative, and their ritual procedures may encourage submission and obedience. This aspect of the ritual leader's role is fundamentally alien to modern psychotherapy, because most psychotherapists are trained to encourage independence in their clients and to abstain from undue persuasive influence. This is especially true of person-centered therapists (Rogers, 1957), but this stance has permeated many other schools of therapy to some extent.

Another crucial difference is the use of hallucinogenic substances that is often part of many shamanic ritual practices (Dombrowe, 2005). The ethical guidelines of most psychotherapeutic licensing bodies in the United States and most other countries do not condone the use of hallucinogens as part of psychotherapeutic treatment unless they are part of a federally approved research program. Therefore, if a psychotherapist decides to incorporate ritual work into the therapeutic process, he or she may function as ritual specialist but certainly not as shaman.

PSYCHOTHERAPEUTIC RITUALS

Whenever the psychological balance of a person is disturbed (e.g., by the death of or separation from a loved one), a new balance must be found. Contemporary society possesses fewer rituals that assist individuals in unsettling life transitions than traditional societies (Krippner, 2000). Modern psychotherapy tends to function as a substitute for traditional rituals in providing the means to navigate safely the many transitions in modern life. This functional equivalence becomes more apparent whenever psychotherapists prescribe rituals for their clients.

When psychotherapists consider the integration of a traditional healing practice in their approach, they have to consider that many traditional healing practices cannot easily be transferred from one culture to another. However, certain basic elements and principles can be identified and integrated (e.g., a social support group). Malidoma Somé (1993), an African scholar and initiated shaman of the Dagara tribe, argues that modern culture cannot, in the pursuit of spiritual goals, expect to reproduce the original indigenous way of existence and transplant indigenous rituals. However, according to Somé, contemporary groups can draw inspiration from indigenous rituals. Because rituals both reflect and create the values of a culture, it is important to keep in mind that, for many people, effective modern healing rituals affirm the knowledge and wisdom of the current time and place, including advanced technology.

Whenever psychotherapists decide to deliberately apply rituals in the therapeutic process, they should probably create client-specific and problem-specific therapeutic procedures (Hart, 1983). The role of the psychotherapist, then, is to provide expertise on ritual structure, to prepare the clients, and to secure their commitment. Therapeutic rituals should be constructed by the psychotherapist in consultation with the clients, to make sure that the symbols and metaphors are relevant to the clients and their cultural background and belief system (Hart, 1983). Transition rituals would be appropriate for grief therapy, separation, and divorce. Healing rituals could be helpful during couples therapy, family therapy, and in the treatment of addictive and compulsive behaviors. The use of photographs, letters, dance, and artwork may enhance the ritualistic elements of these psychotherapeutic interventions.

Clients can help develop the symbols and choose the basic ritual acts, as well as the specifics of time and place. These are referred to as self-generated rituals. Whereas traditional healing procedures constitute a complete treatment, psychotherapeutic rituals are part of a longer-lasting treatment plan. This is especially apparent in the use of narrative in psychoanalysis and other forms of psychotherapy, a procedure especially suitable for work with children (Brooks, 1994). The crucial test of a psychotherapeutic story is the kind of person it shapes; the use of narrative for this purpose can be a collaborative effort between therapist and client, between healer and healee. There can never be a correct or objective reading of these types of texts, only one that is more "energetic, interesting, and pleasurable" (Vizenor, 1989, p. 5). The use of narrative in psychotherapy is one way of convincing clients that their psychotherapist understands, cares, and has their best interest at heart (Torrey, 1986).

A healer or psychotherapist playing the role of ritual specialist empowers the client by helping to stay in touch with inner imaginative and somatic processes. Topper (1987) found that Navaho healers raised their healees' expectations by setting examples of stability and competence. This established their value as "transference figures" representing nurturance and wisdom (p. 221).

As noted above, a transition ritual is characterized by a symbolic separation from the rest of the society of an individual or group for whom the ritual is being enacted. An important part of the ritual in the psychotherapeutic setting is a sufficient separation from the client's ordinary world in order to assure confidentiality. Should ritual be used outside the office or other therapeutic setting, it is important to select an appropriate site that is free from external intrusions and to establish boundaries for the ritual space. The temporal space should be equally demarcated with a clear beginning and ending.

During the ritual enactment, the psychotherapist remains a witness and only occasionally directs the process. At the end of the ritual, the client needs to return to ordinary consciousness. The psychotherapist is responsible for making sure that the client leaves the ritual space grounded and fully oriented. The client's attention should be reoriented toward practical responsibilities. The involvement of other persons (especially from the client's milieu) can be especially helpful to witness the changes and to provide an opportunity for continued interaction to maintain the changes (Gilligan, 1997; Hart, 1983).

EXAMPLES OF THE USE OF RITUAL IN PSYCHOTHERAPY

Therapeutic rituals are indicated whenever a client has to deal with loss, has to part with a person or life circumstance. These therapeutic rituals are based on performing acts with symbols that represent a relation to a person or situation in question, or they may consist of writing one or several farewell letters. In the case of a divorce that a client has not properly resolved, the therapist can suggest a parting ritual in which the client has the opportunity to work through feelings of grief and depression or anger. The ritual can consist of disposing of the wedding ring in a prescribed fashion at a specified time (e.g., melting it into something else or burying it). Another ritual could be writing a farewell letter in which everything is expressed that the client still wants to say to the former partner. Then the letter is ceremoniously destroyed. Another variation could be the ritual disposal of objects that belonged to the divorced partner (e.g., burning or burying clothes and gifts). Or it may consist of a ritual house-cleaning and rearranging the furniture to ritually mark the beginning of a new stage in life. Since these ritual acts are likely to involve the expression of strong emotions, it is the therapist's responsibility to consider what influence his or her performance might have on the client's milieu (other family members, etc.) and eventually to provide a framework of understanding for those family members who might be indirectly affected by the ritual.

Another life event that can be addressed by rites of separation is the loss of a loved one—one of the most difficult transitions for individuals and families. Mourning rituals can help friends and relatives express the different emotional reactions to the loss. Personal memories of the deceased can be revived and mourning then becomes a process shared by all involved in the ritual. The prescription of therapeutic mourning rituals is indicated whenever a client has not been able to complete the grief process properly (e.g., the client lives too far away to participate in the funeral). In the group therapy setting, a symbolic funeral can take place that can help the client to deal with unresolved feelings about the death. One person may be asked to play the role of the deceased. The therapist may then ask the client questions such as: "What would you say if the deceased were here now?" This gives the client a chance to express all things that were left unspoken. In another version of the ritual, the participants may symbolically bury the deceased by forming a funeral procession, carrying the "deceased" to a designated area in the room, and then covering the person representing the deceased with blankets and flowers. Throughout the ritual drama, the therapist's role consists of encouraging the expression of ambivalent feelings that are involved in the grieving process—hostility, rage, anger, guilt, fear, and despair. At the end of the symbolic funeral, all participants may give their condolences to the bereaved.

Rituals and ritual prescriptions also may be successfully applied in family therapy. Many interactions in family life are, to some degree, ritualized. The stability of family life—the sense of togetherness as a family—is shaped by rites of continuity (Bossard & Boll, 1950), such as shared meals, the execution of communal tasks (e.g., cleaning dishes), and putting the children to bed. Through these rituals, relationships among family members are confirmed and strengthened and the integration of the family is enhanced. Many family problems articulate themselves in poor functioning of these rites of continuity. A family therapist may break dysfunctional interaction patterns by special ritualized assignments. First the therapist needs to identify the rules that guide the ritualized interaction patterns among family members. Then the family therapist may prescribe specific changes in the family rituals. These ritual assignments break the destructive interaction patterns. Hart (1983) gives an example of a family that sought help because of the daughter's compulsive behavior. Every night at bedtime, the 11-year-old girl brushed her teeth four times, opened and shut the door to her room four times, took her clothes off and put them on again four times, and got in and out of bed four times. The mother could not cope with the daughter's behavior any longer. She had no support from her husband, who often worked overtime and believed that it was the mother's duty to raise the children. The therapist suspected tensions between the parents, but the daughter's compulsive rituals were presented as the only problem. The therapist gave the parents the following assignment: Every night, both father and mother were to take the daughter to bed together and allow her to do what she usually did, only instead of four times, the daughter had to repeat everything six times. The next week, the therapist gave the assignment for the daughter to repeat the compulsive acts five times. Each following week, the therapist reduced the number of repetitions prescribed until the behavior disappeared. The parents reported that their relationship also improved. Taking their daughter to bed together every night led them to talk more to each other and to do more together. The daughter's compulsive behavior was a symptom of a dysfunctional family structure, and the prescribed alteration of the existing family ritual not only reduced the symptomatic behavior but also improved the defective relationship between mother and father.

THE HEALING POWER OF RITUALS

Perhaps the most widespread diagnosis on the planet is soul loss (known as *susto* among many Spanish-speaking indigenous practitioners), which usually implies dissociation from vital aspects of oneself or alienation from one's family, friends, and community (Achterberg, 1985). Soul loss, historically, has been treated with the most powerful transpersonal medicine known to the community: social support. Its remediation requires the skills of the shaman, intricate rituals, and the intense involvement of family and friends. The loss of the soul means something far more than imminent demise; it is coping head-on with the meaningless void of life now and in the hereafter and the dissolution of all particulates of self.

In modern times, there is sufficient clinical, anecdotal, and even some empirical evidence that contemporary persons are not immune to soul loss. Although soul loss may not be a necessary precursor to serious illness, it is sufficient to predispose one to danger, threatened suicide, addictions, and clinical depressions, to name most of the serious and visible afflictions. The skilled medical attention demanded by these conditions often obscures the nature of the inner crisis—the substantive loss of meaning that crushes the life or vital force. Soul loss, in its modern incarnation, can be predicated on loss of self-esteem or loved ones. Loss of soul can manifest after a long siege of events, some major traumas, some only the hassles of being alive. How can a practitioner recapture the soul in modern life? Perhaps it can be revitalized through an epiphany of remembrance, gained through connection with the transpersonal forces of community and spirit, or restored through healing rituals that attempt to revive and recapture the soul.

These types of rituals were invariably designed to move the healer, client, and community into ASCs where sacred realities or "places of knowing" were more likely to be reached. The activities included all manner of procedures to alter the senses: drumming, chants, incense, fasting, plant medicines, sensory deprivation, sweats and other temperature extremes, movement, and the power of hope, love, and trust that what was being done was of a healing nature.

Traditional people often describe sickness as disharmony—a synonym for disease (Achterberg et al., 1994). Feeling alone, different, unloved, and rejected or having lost a sense of connection to life all are cofactors, or even primary factors, that play a key role in the etiology and exacerbation of many stress-related killers and cripplers. These include heart disease, cancer, diabetes, stroke, infectious disease, herpes, and psychological disorders and life-style problems such as substance abuse.

Feeling alienated is very stressful—stress impedes the immune system and all aspects of healing, including wound healing. Any ritual that reintegrates a disenfranchised individual or restores harmony will have the outcome of making one whole. Healing rituals in Western culture can be as simple as gift-giving during a time of illness, gatherings associated with religious traditions, or self-generated creative activities.

Storytelling is a valuable aspect of ritual, and listening to or telling stories can reintegrate a person into family and community. The world, as noted by sages and mystics, is made up of stories. Stories, not research data, touch people's hearts and sway their opinions. The elders in one's culture could be asked to tell their stories as part of the tribal lore. When families know the stories of their ancestral or cultural history, they realize that they are not doomed to recapitulate the negative patterns of the past.

Most cultural rituals designed for healing individuals, or for integrating or harmonizing the community as a whole, involve some activity that synchronizes or involves the senses, emotions, or body rhythms. Dancing, drumming, chants, songs, sensory deprivations—such as fasting prior to rites of passage or other celebrations—and laughing together all bring a community into a resonant phase or common plane. This can occur on many levels, including the psychological and emotional, and incorporates the achievement of consensus or group consciousness. Thus, the sense of social alienation, loneliness, dissociation, and being miscast in some aberrant, purposeless human mold is dealt a mighty blow. When rituals provide social integration, connection, or support and reduce feelings of social alienation or loneliness, they may affect biochemistry in ways that facilitate physical well-being.

In a classic review article in the prestigious journal *Science* by House, Landis, and Umberson (1988), 62 studies were cited that provide compelling evidence that (1) a lack of social support constitutes a major risk factor for mortality, and (2) social relationships protect health and enhance healing. Social support networks (defined as marital ties, friends, extended family, group membership, and healthcare professionals and the activities these contacts involved) were found to have a positive effect on such behaviors as surgical recovery time, complications of pregnancy and low birth weight, reported symptoms of chronic diseases, presence of infectious disease (such as tuberculosis), cardiovascular reactivity, ulcers, and stress responses in intensive care units.

Biochemical correlates of social support include increased growth hormone levels (necessary for wound healing), lower cholesterol levels, enhanced immunity (particularly natural killer cell function), and a generally reduced output of the sympathetic nervous system (SNS).

Continuous SNS activity has been implicated in a number of diseases, including heart disease, stroke, cancer, and infectious disease. Encouraging rituals of support in hospital settings not only enhances psychological well-being, but also directly facilitates the healing process. At the least, these studies support the continued presence of family and friends during medical crises, particularly if a person is in intensive care or in a life-threatening condition—the times when they are likely surrounded by machines instead of humans.

Any healing ritual that facilitates the positive emotion of hope and reduces depression and anxiety can have a significant impact on a person's total well-being. The senses of helplessness and hopelessness are well-known companions of depression and have been repeatedly shown to have a negative impact on health, including increased cancer growth. To be told that "there is nothing more that you can do," with no further information, is tantamount to prescribing a poison. There is always something that can be done, and, at some point, that might mean entering into a well thought-through ritual for engaging fully in the dying process.

On the other hand, even in the face of significant pain and crisis, a belief in one's ability to survive, overcome, and even transcend the situation has been a lifeline for people who are victims of abandonment, abuse, or catastrophic disease. Narratives from survivors of the Holocaust often attribute the robust survival of certain women to the fact that they held their communities together by sustained observation of religious and personal rituals (such as birthdays) that marked the passage of time.

The activity of rituals, particularly if they prescribe a series of thoughts or actions, has the critical effect of pacing people through difficult times—such as dying or emotional crises—by providing a roadmap for the unseen, unknown, uncharted territory ahead. Repetitive acts such as chants, songs, or prayers often quiet a troubled mind, making space for mental and spiritual clarity.

Reducing anxiety directly affects the healing process. Prolonged anxiety or stress, as well as helplessness, has long been held to impede healing through sustained chemistry of arousal (such as through the adrenocorticosteroids), causing conditions that foster the development of cardiovascular and other diseases and ultimately act to inhibit components of the immune system (including interleukin 1, natural killer cells, and many others). The body's resistance to disease may even be significantly decreased. Distress has been associated with a decrease in the recovery of damaged cells through an inhibition of the DNA repair mechanism (Kiecolt-Glaser et al., 1988). This information is not new, but the results are not well known, even though the ramifications are extraordinary. The study suggests that anxiety or fear can impede healing or cause disease because of an effect at the basic level of the cell's repair machinery.

To the extent that healing rituals aid in the development of an effective coping strategy, they may successfully ameliorate or prevent physical disease or further deterioration. Coping or belief in self (sometimes called self-efficacy) has been associated with a drop in catecholamines, which are suspected impediments to healing (Kiecolt-Glaser et al., 1988).

Henry (1982), after describing the biochemical effects of coping, suggested that coping preempts the deleterious effects of negative emotions. He reported a rise in adrenal corticoids as an individual moves from an emotional dimension of security to helplessness, a rise in catecholamines as the emotional affect shifts from relaxation to a concern with maintenance of status, and a drop in gonadotropins when a sense of social success changes to social failure. The latter shift may have severe ramifications for sexual responsiveness and parenting activity. In support of healing rituals, one can extrapolate from the information on the biochemistry of hope and positive emotions. Hope, unlike anxiety or helplessness, is correlated with a decrease in corticosteroids, and relaxation and joy have been associated with a decrease in the vasoconstricting catecholamines and therefore an increase in circulation in painful or wounded areas—a necessary condition for adequate tissue repair.

The biochemical effect of transcendent or ecstatic experiences, anecdotally reported for healing rituals from many cultures, is a wasteland of investigation. At best, there is some well-documented evidence that the neuropeptides serve as the biological mediators of emotions, in addition to scattered evidence that a certain category of neuropeptides, the endorphins, is stimulated during the experience and that the neuropeptides have a stimulating effect on the immune system. Despite these deficiencies in the attention of the scientific community, the existing research supports the positive effect on health of decreasing distress; alleviating helplessness, hopelessness, and depression; and encouraging the sustaining power of hope (Kiecolt-Glaser et al., 1988).

Gilligan (1997) noted that the earliest forms of therapy involved ritual because they were intense, structured activities that attempted to recreate or transform one's identity. This transformation can occur at several levels; that is, significant metabolic shifts, changes in electrolyte balances and blood gases, and other neurochemical phenomena can be produced by serious healing rituals and may occasion a major shift in brain activity. Ritual activities also can induce altered perceptions of time and space, a change in sensorium, and a blurring of the boundaries of self and nonself. All of these activities are capable of driving a wedge into consciousness through which light can shine into the dark place of crisis, lifting the veil so the integrity of the client can return or be created.

Lang and Nayer (2000) take a similar perspective to that of Gilligan, pointing out how basic ritual is to all forms of transformation. They have urged people to bring ritual into everyday life, suggesting rituals for family meetings, a preschooler's first day of school, a child's first time at a sleep-away camp, saying goodbye when a friend moves away, an adolescent's first time driving an automobile, going away to college, losing a job, or burying a cherished pet. Feinstein and Mayo (1990) have described rituals for living and dying, while Feinstein and Krippner (2006) have designed many rituals for assisting people to find their mythic path.

Rituals can mark quiet moments, such as enjoying the twilight. In the Jewish tradition, the family sits *shiva* when a loved one dies. The Q'ero Indians of the Andes have a practice of sitting in silence at twilight, "the hour of power" (Wilcox, 1999). Many Eastern traditions use meditation as a way of accessing inner knowing. In other words, ritual need not be confined to indigenous tribal practices or the psychotherapeutic office. These step-by-step procedures can frame people's lives in novel and beneficial ways. Rituals are for everyone.

TOOL KIT FOR CHANGE

Role and Perspective of the Healthcare Professional

1. Rituals can provide structure, meaning, and practical exercises to aid life transitions such as birth, treatment protocols, and death.
2. Rituals help patients and their families cope with these transitions.
3. Rituals are culturally sensitive and can assist interactions between professional and patient.

Role and Perspective of the Participant

1. Rituals and symbols can be useful in interpreting and understanding the deeper meaning of disease and illness.
2. Rituals can help restore balance to the life of the client and his or her family following diagnosis and treatment.
3. Rituals can be done by the client, thus promoting empowerment and self-efficacy.

Interconnection: The Global Perspective

1. Rituals maintain and transform social rites and identities.
2. Rituals create a healing environment, connecting the self to the environment, nature, and spiritual forces.

REFERENCES

Achterberg, J. (1985). *Imagery in healing: Shamanism and modern medicine*. Boston: Shambhala.

Achterberg, J. (1996). What is medicine? *Alternative Therapies in Health and Medicine, 2*(3), 58–61.

Achterberg, J. (1997). Imagery and ceremony for a rite of passage. In B. Horrigan (Ed.), *Red moon passages: The power and wisdom of menopause*. New York: Random House.

Achterberg, J., Dossey, B., & Kolkmeier, L. (1994). *Rituals of healing: Using imagery for health and wellness*. New York: Bantam.

Achterberg, J., & Lawlis, G. F. (1981). Imagery approaches for death and dying. In H. Sobel (Ed.), *Behavioral therapy in terminal care: A humanistic approach*. Cambridge, MA: Ballinger.

Bond, H. (2006). Punishing terrains: The land strikes back. *Shamanism, 19*(2), 26–35.

Bossard, J.H.S., & Boll, E. S. (1950). *Ritual in family living*. Philadelphia: University of Pennsylvania Press.

Bourguignon, E. (1973). Introduction: A framework for the comparative study of altered states of consciousness. In E. Bourguignon, *Religion, altered states of consciousness and social change* (pp. 3–36). Columbus: Ohio State University Press.

Bourguignon, E. (1979). *Psychological anthropology. An introduction to human nature and cultural differences*. New York: Holt, Rinehart and Winston.

Brooks, P. (1994). *Psychoanalysis and storytelling*. Cambridge, MA: Blackwell.

Chapple, E. D., & Coon, C. S. (1978). *Principles of anthropology*. Huntington, NY: Krieger.

Dittrich, A., & Scharfetter, C. (1987). *Ethnopsychotherapie: Psychotherapie mittels aussergewöhnlicher Bewusstseinszustände in westlichen und indigenen Kulturen* [Ethnopsychotherapy: Psychotherapy in the context of unusual states of consciousness in Western and indigenous cultures]. Stuttgart, Germany: Enke.

Dobkin de Rios, M. (1984). *Hallucinogens: Cross-cultural perspectives*. Albuquerque: University of New Mexico Press.

Dombrowe, C. (2005). Touched by spirit. A heuristic study of healing experiences in peyote ceremonies. *DAI-B 66*. Unpublished dissertation, California Institute for Integral Studies, San Francisco, CA. Accession Number AAT 3177318.

Eliade, M. (1972). *Shamanism: Archaic techniques of ecstasy*. Princeton, NJ: Princeton University Press.

Erickson, M. H., & Rossi, E. L. (Eds.). (1980). *The collected papers of Milton H. Erickson on hypnosis*. New York: Irvington.

Feinstein, D., & Krippner, S. (2006). *The mythic path* (3rd ed.). Santa Rosa, CA: Elite Books.

Feinstein, D., & Mayo, P. E. (1990). *Rituals for living and dying*. San Francisco: Harper-Collins.

Field, N. (1990). Healing, exorcism and objects relation theory. *British Journal of Psychotherapy, 6*, 274–284.

Frank, J. D., & Frank, J. B. (1991). *Persuasion and healing* (3rd ed.). Baltimore: Johns Hopkins University Press.

Gilligan, S. (1997). *The courage to love: Principles and practices of self-regulation*. New York: Norton.

Grof, S. (1985). *Beyond the brain: Birth, death, and transcendence in psychotherapy*. Albany: State University of New York Press.

Halifax, J. (1991). *Shamanic voices: A survey of visionary narratives.* New York: Penguin.

Hart, O., van der (1983). *Rituals in psychotherapy. Transition and continuity.* New York: Irvington.

Heinze, R. I. (Ed.). (2000). *The nature and function of rituals: Fire from heaven.* Westport, CT: Bergin & Garvey.

Hendrin, H., Brent, D. A., Cornelius, J. R., Coyne-Beasley, T., et al. (2005). Youth suicide. In D. L. Evans, E. B. Foa, R. E. Gur, H. Hendin, et al. (Eds.), *Treating and preventing adolescent mental health disorders: What we know and what we don't know.* New York: Oxford University Press.

Henry, J. P. (1982). The relation of social to biological processes in disease. *Social Science and Medicine, 16,* 369–380.

Hill, C. E. (1996). *Working with dreams in psychotherapy.* New York: Guilford Press.

Hill, C. E., & Rochlen, A. B. (1999). A cognitive-experiential model for working with dreams in psychotherapy. In L. Vandecreek & T. L. Jackson (Eds.), *Innovations in clinical practice: A source book* (pp. 467–480). Sarasota, FL: Professional Resources Press.

Holmes, S. W., Morris, R., Clance, P. R., & Putney, R. T. (2003). Holotropic breathwork: An experimental approach to psychotherapy. *Subtle Energies & Energy Medicine, 12,* 125–138.

House, J. S., Landis, K. R., & Umberson, D. (1988). Social relationships and health. *Science, 241,* 540–545.

Jilek, W. G. (1989). Therapeutic use of altered states of consciousness in contemporary North American Indian dance ceremonials. In C. A. Ward (Ed.), *Altered states of consciousness and mental health: A cross-cultural perspective* (pp. 167–185). Newbury Park, CA: Sage.

Kiecolt-Glaser, J. K., Kennedy, S., Malkoff, S., Fisher. L., Speicher, C. E., & Glaser, R. (1988). Marital discord and immunity in males. *Psychosomatic Medicine, 50,* 213–229.

Kirsch, I. (1990). *Changing expectations: A key to effective therapy.* Pacific Grove, CA: Brooks/Cole.

Kremer, J. (2003). *Trance als multisensuelle Kreativitätstechnik* [Trance as a multisensory creativity technique]. In P. Luckner (Ed.), *Multisensuelles design: Eine Anthologie* (pp. 591–620). Halle, Germany: University Press of Burg Giebichsteiner—Hochschule für Kunst und Design.

Krippner, S. (1982). The shaman as healer and psychotherapist. *Voices, 28*(4), 12–23.

Krippner, S. (1997a). The role of mandalas in Navajo and Tibetan rituals. *Anthropology of Consciousness, 8,* 22–31.

Krippner, S. (1997b). The varieties of dissociative experience. In S. Krippner & S. M. Powers (Eds.), *Broken images, broken selves: Dissociative narratives in clinical practice* (pp. 336–361). Washington, DC: Brunner/Mazel.

Krippner, S. (2000). Altered states of consciousness and shamanic healing. In R. I. Heinze (Ed.), *The nature and function of rituals: Fire from heaven* (pp. 191–212). Westport, CT: Bergin & Garvey.

Krippner, S. (2005). Trance and the trickster: Hypnosis as a liminal phenomenon. *Journal of Clinical and Experimental Hypnosis, 53,* 97–118.

Krippner, S., & Villoldo, A. (1976). *The realms of healing* (Rev. ed.). Millbrae, CA: Celestial Arts.

Lang, V. E., & Nayer, L. B. (2000). *How to bury a goldfish and 113 other family rituals for everyday life.* New York: Daybreak/Rodale/St. Martin's.

Lévi-Strauss, C. (1967). *Structural anthropology.* New York: Basic Books.

Ludwig, A. M. (1966). Altered states of consciousness. *Archives of General Psychiatry, 15,* 225–234.

Lyon, W. S. (2000). The ritual core of shamanism: Observations on an international gathering of shamans. In R. I. Heinze (Ed.), *The nature and function of rituals: Fire from heaven* (pp. 179–189). Westport, CT: Bergin & Garvey.

Moore, T. (1983). *Rituals of the imagination.* Dallas, TX: Pegasus Foundation.

Moore, S. F., & Myerhoff, B. G. (Eds.). (1977). *Secular ritual.* Assen, The Netherlands: Van Gorcum.

Murphy, C., & Rose, B. (n.d.). The blood of the ancients [Recorded by Betsy Rose]. On *Welcome to the circle* [CD]. Berkeley, CA: Paper Crane Music.

Myerhoff, B. G. (1974). *Peyote hunt: The sacred journey of the Huichol* Indians. Ithaca, NY: Cornell University Press.

Rappaport, R. (1978). Adaptation and the structure of ritual. In N. Burton Jones & V. Reynolds (Eds.), *Human behavior and adaptation* (Vol. 18). New York: Halsted Press.

Rogers, C. R. (1957). The necessary and sufficient conditions of therapeutic personality change. *Journal of Consulting Psychology, 21,* 95–103.

Samorini, G. (2000). *Animals and psychedelics: The natural world and the instinct to alter consciousness.* Rochester, VT: Park Street Press.

Sandner, D. (1979). *Navajo symbols of healing.* New York: Harcourt, Brace, Jovanovich.

Serlin, I. (1993). Root images of healing in dance therapy. *American Dance Therapy Journal, 15*(2), 65–75.

Sherwood, J. N., Stolaroff, M. J., & Harman, W. W. (1962). The psychedelic experience: A new concept in psychotherapy. *Journal of Neuropsychiatry, 4,* 69–80.

Siegel, R. K. (1990). *Intoxication: Life in pursuit of artificial paradise.* New York: Dutton.

Somé, M. P. (1993). *Ritual—Power, healing, and community.* New York: Penguin/Arkana.

Tart, C. (Ed.). (1969). *Altered states of consciousness.* New York: Wiley.

Tart, C. T. (1975). *States of consciousness.* New York: Dutton.

Tart, C. (1980). A systems approach to altered states of consciousness. In J. M. Davidson & R. J. Davidson (Eds.), *The psychobiology of consciousness* (pp. 243–269). New York: Plenum.

Topper, M. D. (1987). The traditional Navajo medicine man: Therapist, counselor, and community leader. *Journal of Psychoanalytic Anthropology, 10,* 217–249.

Torrey, E. F. (1986). *Witchdoctors and psychiatrists: The common roots of psychotherapy and its future.* New York: Harper & Row.

Turner, E. (1986). Encounters with neurobiology: The response of ritual studies. *Zygon: Journal of Religion and Science, 21,* 249–256.

Turner, V. (1969). *The ritual process: Structure and anti-structure.* Chicago: Aldine.

van Gennep, A. (1960). *The rites of passage.* London: Routledge & Kegan Paul.

Vizenor, G. (1989). Introduction. In G. Vizenor (Ed.), *Narrative chance: Postmodern discourse on Native American Indian literature* (pp. 3–16). Norman: University of Oklahoma Press.

Wallace, A.C.F. (1959). Cultural determinants of response to hallucinatory experiences. *Archives of General Psychiatry, 1,* 58–69.

Wallace, A.C.F. (1966). *Religion: An anthropological view.* New York: Random House.

Weil, A. (1998). *The natural mind* (Rev. ed.). New York: Houghton Mifflin.

West, W. (2000). *Psychotherapy and spirituality: Crossing the line between therapy and religion.* London: Sage.

Wilcox, J. P. (1999). *Keepers of the ancient knowledge: The mystical world of the Q'ero Indians of Peru.* Boston: Element.

Winkelman, M. (1996). Psychointegrator plants: Their roles in human culture, consciousness and health. In M. Winkelman & W. Andritzky (Eds.), *Yearbook of cross-cultural medicine and psychotherapy 1995* (pp. 9–53). Berlin: VWB.

Wittkover, E. D. (1970). Trance and possession states. *International Journal of Social Psychiatry, 16,* 153–160.

AFTERWORD

Cynthia D. Belar, PhD

Human beings have a long history of seeking methods to decrease discomfort and to increase comfort; indeed over the millennia, multiple substances, procedures, and practices have been explored to alleviate disease and to promote health, which is a broader construct than simply the absence of disease. A definition of health that includes a sense of well-being also results in a variety of procedures being considered part of healthcare practice that traditionally have not been seen as such. Using this broad definition of health, the chapter authors in this volume provide informative histories of current practices and procedures that have been used to promote health and offer their own views on their relevance to healthcare. This volume's final chapter, "The Role of Rituals in Psychotherapy," provides a cross-cutting framework through which it was most interesting to re-read and reconsider every chapter in this volume.

Some of the practices described in this volume have been researched with respect to their impact on disease status and outcomes, including attempts to identify active and inactive ingredients within the procedures. Other practices are described related to the broader concept of sense of well-being as measured by self-report or as based on either theoretical or spiritual assumptions about human behavior. The work emanates from a variety of disciplines and professions. It is most important for healthcare professionals to be aware of these

The ideas expressed represent the views of the author and do not represent policy of the American Psychological Association.

diverse perspectives on health and well-being, as understanding health belief models and patient values are essential to treatment planning.

A holistic view of health in its broadest sense might also include a focus on the environment, with attention to the behavior of individuals in relationship to their environment. Although humans require a healthy environment in order to survive and prosper, this topic is not often addressed in the education of health professionals. In addressing education for a sustainable future, Anthony Cortese said, "We have known for quite some time that a healthy environment is essential to human existence, health and well-being. Humans can live for about four minutes without air, four days without water, and four weeks without food. Plants, animals, and the habitats they occupy provide the food that sustains human life. The earth and all its living organisms supply all raw materials for human activities" (Cortese, 1997, p. 3). Yet Cortese noted that American medical students received only about one day's training in environmental and occupational medicine.

My purpose in noting the link between the environment and health within the context of a holistic view of healthcare is not to review the well-documented health problems associated with air and water pollution, toxic waste, or the damage to the environment caused by human consumption. Rather, I want to highlight the relationship between human behavior and the environment and the importance of that interface for the health and well-being of humans.

In discussing research needs, Deborah Du Nann Winter reported work by William Bevan who, over 25 years ago, argued that "myopically investigating small questions while the big problem of human survival goes unattended is professionally irresponsible" (Winter, 2000, p. 516). Others might argue that a holistic model of healthcare must include care for the environment among its practices and that patient behavior in this arena should be encouraged as much as self-care.

More mainstream is the view that *all* citizens should receive education for a sustainable future and that all educators are responsible for attending to this need. A resolution for such has been endorsed by over 300 college presidents and organizations in higher education. It has been emphasized that the role of higher education is critical to make the shift in values and actions required to create a sustainable world and that a paradigm shift toward a systemic perspective that "encompasses the complex interdependence of individual, social, cultural, economic and political activities and the biosphere" must be made in order to maintain health (Cortese, 1997, p. 8). These concepts are not new but they are receiving considerable support internationally. For example in December 2002 the United Nations General Assembly adopted resolution 57/254 on the United Nations Decade of Education for Sustainable Development (2005–2014), and named the United Nations Education, Scientific and Cultural Organization (UNESCO) as the agency to promote the Decade.

A special difficulty in using such an all-encompassing definition of health and healthcare practices in these discussions is related to how healthcare services are financed in this country. In general, practices that are deemed medically necessary are the ones covered by health insurance or government programs, although some procedures relevant to disease prevention are covered (e.g., inoculations), and some secondary prevention services have received more support over the last decade (e.g., smoking cessation, weight reduction). Demands for accountability in healthcare have also resulted in an increased focus on practices that are supported by scientific evidence and on evidence-based practice involving the integration of the best research data with clinical expertise and patient preferences. Practices that are primarily associated with a sense of well-being or spiritual health are seen as discretionary and thus outside the scope of insurance designed to cover health problems. It will be interesting to note whether the same level of demand for accountability and scientifically based services will be found in the arena of discretionary services (for want of a better term) and how that will impact related research and the education and credentialing of service providers.

With respect to the discipline of psychology, the scientific basis of practice has been core to its profession. Some of its earliest professional applications to societal problems were in the area of education—in attempts to understand learning and in the measurement of aptitude for learning in children who were experiencing school-related problems. The assessment of intelligence was also important in World War I and II, wars whose sequelae fostered psychology's focus on mental health problems. With the increased sophistication of behavioral research, the decrease in infectious disease, the increased focus on chronic disease, and the inadequate explanatory power of the biomedical model, more psychologists focused on broader aspects of health and behavior and not solely on mental health issues. When I began my work in the early 1970s in what we then called medical psychology, it was certainly not mainstream in organized psychology as it is today. Perhaps environmental psychology will also become more mainstream in education and in health so that we can foster the behavior change required to avoid outstripping our resources for our own future health.

REFERENCES

Cortese, A. D. (1997). *Engineering education for a sustainable future.* Presented at the Conference on Engineering Education and Training for Sustainable Development: Towards Improved Performance, September 24–26, 1997. Paris, France.
Winter, D.D.N. (2000). Some big ideas for some big problems. *American Psychologist, 55*(5), 516–522.

ABOUT THE GENERAL EDITOR

Ilene Ava Serlin, PhD, ADTR, is a recognized leader and has been practicing whole person health care for over 35 years. She is a clinical psychologist and registered dance/movement therapist at Union Street Health Associates in San Francisco and Marin County. She is a fellow of the American Psychological Association (APA), past-president of the APA's Division of Humanistic Psychology, and served on APA's Presidential and Division 42 (Independent Practice) Health Care Task Force. She is the founder of the Arts Medicine program at the Institute of Health and Healing at California Pacific Medical Center and of the movement support group at the Integrative Health Care for Women with Breast Cancer at the University of California, and is on the advisory committee for Sutter Hospital's Integrative Health and Healing Services in Santa Rosa. Her videotape called *Dance Movement Therapy for Women with Breast Cancer* was awarded the Marian Chace Award by the American Dance Therapy Association.

Dr. Serlin has taught at Saybrook Graduate School, UCLA, Lesley University, and abroad. She is on the Editorial Board of *PsycCritiques PsycCRITIQUES—Contemporary Psychology: APA Review of Books*, the *American Journal of Dance Therapy*, and *The Journal of Humanistic Psychology* and is a reviewer for APA's *Professional Psychology: Research and Practice* and *Division 32's The Humanistic Psychologist*. Her writings include the following:

Serlin, I. A. (2000). Symposium: Support groups for women with breast cancer. *The Arts in Psychotherapy, 27*(2), 123–138.

Serlin, I. A. (2004a). Religious and spiritual issues in couples therapy. In M. Harway (Ed.), *Handbook of couples therapy* (pp. 352–369).New York: John Wiley & Sons.

Serlin, I. A. (2004b). Spiritual diversity in clinical practice. In J. Chin (Ed.), *The psychology of prejudice and discrimination* (pp. 27–49). Westport, CT: Praeger.

Serlin, I. A. (2005). Year of the whole person. *Psychotherapy Bulletin: Division 29 (APA),* *40*(1), 34–39.

Serlin, I. A. (2006). Expressive therapies. In M. Micozzi (Ed.), *Complementary and integrative medicine in cancer and prevention: Foundations and evidence-based interventions* (pp. 81–91).

Her Web site is www.ileneserlin.com.

ABOUT THE VOLUME EDITORS

VOL. I

Marie A. DiCowden, PhD, is a nationally known healthcare psychologist and behavioral medicine specialist. Dr. DiCowden joined the University of Miami/Jackson Memorial Hospital staff in the Department of Orthopedics and Rehabilitation in 1981. She maintains her adjunct faculty position at the medical school in addition to faculty affiliations with Nova University and Saybrook Graduate School. In 1988 Dr. DiCowden founded The Biscayne Institutes of Health and Living, Inc. and The Biscayne Foundation in Miami, Florida. This program was an extension of her work on the medical campus and evolved into the HealthCare Community model. This innovative program provides frontline, integrative care for disabled children and adults in addition to integrative health programs for mind and body for the community at large. She serves as the executive director of this program. Dr. DiCowden is a Fellow of the American Psychological Association and a member of the National Academy of Practice. She writes and lectures extensively, both nationally and internationally, on issues of disability, healthcare, and healthcare policy.

VOL. II

Kirwan Rockefeller, PhD, is the director of arts and humanities continuing education at the University of California, Irvine. His expertise includes psychology, visual and performing arts, humanities, and body-mind modalities. He has taught organizational behavior and social psychology at the doctoral level and has consulted with top national and entertainment organizations on the accurate depiction of social and mental health issues, including the Entertainment Industries Council, ABC, CBS, NBC, FOX, Paramount Pictures, Universal Studios, Warner Bros., Centers for Disease Control and Prevention, National Institute on Drug Abuse, The Robert Wood Johnson Foundation, and Ogilvy Public Relations Worldwide. He is the author of *Visualize Confidence: How to Use Guided Imagery to Overcome Self-Doubt.* He has presented at the Susan Samueli Center for Integrative Medicine and is a member of the American Psychological Association and the California Psychological Association.

Stephen S. Brown, MA, is a freelance editor in San Francisco, California. He holds a master's degree in philosophy from San Francisco State University, where he studied with Jacob Needleman and taught philosophy and religion. His interests include contemporary spiritual thought, aesthetics, particularly the philosophy of music, and the philosophy of technology and culture.

VOL. III

Jill Sonke-Henderson, BA, is cofounder and codirector of the Center for the Arts in Healthcare Research and Education (CAHRE) at the University of Florida (UF) and is on the faculty of the School of Theatre and Dance at the University of Florida. She has been an artist in residence in the Shands Arts in Medicine program since 1994, where she founded the Dance for Life program. She has been developing and teaching arts in healthcare coursework and conducting research at UF for over a decade, and is a frequent lecturer throughout the United States and abroad. Jill serves on the board of directors and as a consultant for the Society for the Arts in Healthcare, and is the recipient of a New Forms Florida Award, an Individual Artist Fellowship Award from the State of Florida, and a 2001 Excellence in Teaching Award from the National Institute for Staff and Organizational Development (NISOD).

Ilene Ava Serlin, PhD, ADTR, is a nationally known clinical psychologist and registered dance/movement therapist in private practice in San Francisco and Marin County. She is a Fellow of the American Psychological Association, is past president of the Division of Humanistic Psychology, and served on APA's Presidential Task Force on Whole Person Psychology. She is the founder of the Arts Medicine program at the Institute of Health and Healing at California Pacific Medical Center, and has taught at Saybrook Graduate School, University of California at Los Angeles, Lesley University, and abroad. She is on the editorial board of *PsycCritiques, American Journal of Dance Therapy,* and *The Journal of Humanistic Psychology.*

Rusti Brandman, PhD, is codirector of the Center for the Arts in Healthcare Research and Education (CAHRE) and is coordinator of dance at the University of Florida. Credits include directorships of professional dance companies, international appearances in Holland, receipt of awards from the Florida Fine Arts Council, the National Dance Association, and the American College Dance Festival Association, and service as a national officer for ACDFA. She was a founder of CAHRE and has served as an artist in residence at Shands Hospital at UF and at Alachua General Hospital. She has presented internationally on the arts in healthcare for the American Holistic Medical Association, the Society for the Arts in Healthcare, the International Institute on the Arts in Healing, the Congress on Research in Dance, and the Hawaii International Conference on the Arts and Humanities. She has received five Scholarship Enhancement grants for her arts in health research, producing the Dancing in Hospitals video.

John Graham-Pole, MD, graduated from London University in 1966, and has been on the faculties of London and Case Western Reserve Universities. He is now professor of pediatrics, adjunct professor of clinical and health psychology, medical director of Shands Arts in Medicine, University of Florida, and medical director of Pediatric Hospice of North Central Florida. He has authored or edited five books and made a CD of original poetry and music. He has published about 250 book chapters, articles, and poems in peer-reviewed journals. He has given several hundred presentations across the world on holistic medicine, palliative care, humor, and the healing arts.

ABOUT THE CONTRIBUTORS

Jeanne Achterberg, PhD, is a scientist who has received international recognition for her pioneering research in medicine and psychology. A faculty member for 11 years at Southwestern Medical School, she is currently a professor of psychology at Saybrook Institute, San Francisco. Achterberg co-chaired the mind-body interventions ad hoc advisory panel and the Research Technologies Conference of the Office of Alternative Medicine and was a member of the Advisory Board, Unconventional Cancer Treatments Study Group, Office of Technology Assessment, U.S. Congress. She has authored over 100 articles and five books, including *Imagery in Healing, Woman as Healer, Rituals of Healing,* and *Lightning at the Gate.* In April 2001, she was featured in *Time* magazine as one of the six innovators of alternative and complementary medicine for the coming century. Achterberg is past president of the Association of Transpersonal Psychology and was senior editor for *Alternative Therapies.* Her current research is at North Hawaii Community Hospital in Waimea, Hawaii, studying prayer and healing.

Cynthia D. Belar, PhD, is the executive director of the Education Directorate of the American Psychological Association (APA) and professor emerita in the Department of Clinical and Health Psychology at the University of Florida Health Science Center. From 1984 to 1990 she served as chief psychologist and clinical director of behavioral medicine for the Kaiser Permanente Medical Care Program in Los Angeles. Belar has published numerous articles and chapters on professional practice, including those with a focus on clinical psychology, clinical health psychology, managed healthcare, and primary care. One of her books, *Clinical Health Psychology in Medical Settings,* has served as a primer for practitioners. She has served as president of the American Board of Clinical Health Psychology and APA's Division of Health Psychology, and received the first Timothy B. Jeffrey award for Outstanding Contributions to Clinical Health Psychology.

Jennifer Block, MA, is the director of public education and chaplain at Zen Hospice Project in San Francisco, California. From 1999 to 2003, Block was a supervisory candidate with the Association of Clinical Pastoral Education and chaplain at St. Mary's Medical Center in San Francisco, where she taught spiritual care and professional chaplaincy to year-long residents and summer interns. Since 1998, she has been an active member of the Zen Hospice Project, a sangha (faith community of Buddhist practitioners) who practice Shakya- muni Buddha's teaching of the Four Noble Truths through compassionate service to individuals facing the final weeks of life. She completed end-of-life counselor training with the Zen Hospice Project in November 2002. Block received a BS degree in communications from Boston University in 1985, an MA degree in postmodern theology from Naropa University in 1999, and ordination from the Interfaith Seminary of Santa Cruz, California, in 1998. She also serves as adjunct faculty for the Sati Center for Buddhist Studies and the Chaplaincy Institute for Arts and Interfaith Ministries in Berkeley, California.

Matthew Cowden, MDiv, MFA, is an Episcopal priest serving as associate rector at Christ Church in Alexandria, Virginia. He received his training in clinical pastoral education at Children's National Medical Center in Washington, DC, where he also has served as on-call chaplain. He is the author of a cross-cultural study in theater and liturgical arts, *Drama & Liturgy: Dramatic Methods for Discerning a Methodological Approach to Primary Theology.* For the last two years, Cowden has been invited to present his research in religion and the arts at the regional conference for the American Academy of Religion/ Society of Biblical Literature.

Eleanor Criswell, EdD, is a professor of psychology and former chair of the psychology department, Sonoma State University. She is founding director of the Humanistic Psychology Institute (now Saybrook Graduate School and Research Center). She is the editor of *Somatics Magazine* and director of the Novato Institute for Somatic Research and Training; her books include *Biofeedback and Somatics: Toward Personal Evolution* and *How Yoga Works: An Introduction to Somatic Yoga.* Criswell is past president of Division 32—Humanistic

Psychology of the American Psychological Association and the Association for Humanistic Psychology, and she is currently secretary/treasurer of the International Association of Yoga Therapists.

Christian Dombrowe, PhD, received his MA in clinical psychology from the University of Heidelberg and his PhD in East-West psychology from the California Institute for Integral Studies. He has been actively pursuing training in Zen Buddhist meditation since 1991, Tibetan Buddhist philosophy since 1994, and Native American healing practices since 1995. His special interests are the integration of spirituality and psychology/psychotherapy, eco-psychology, transpersonal psychology, and cross-cultural entheogen-based healing practices.

Betty Ervin-Cox, PhD, received her PhD from United States International University (now Alliant University) and an honorary PsyD from Forest Institute of Professional Psychology. Prior to her doctoral work, she had theological seminary training and received her bachelor's degree from Lewis-National University. Ervin-Cox served for over 25 years as director of student affairs and professor (Forest Institute of Professional Psychology) and dean of students and professor (Colorado School of Professional Psychology). She has worked extensively in the field of religion and psychology, edited and co-edited many publications. She practiced and taught for many years in the field of marriage and family therapy. Ervin-Cox continues to do research and consulting in her retirement years. Her favorite pastime is being a grandmother. She lives with her husband in Chapel Hill, North Carolina.

Steve Fehl, MA, is a student in the doctor of clinical psychology program at the Colorado School of Professional Psychology in Colorado Springs, Colorado. He served Lutheran parishes in Texas, Michigan, California, Minnesota, and Colorado before beginning his doctoral work. Fehl has a masters degree in psychology and has done additional graduate work at San Francisco Theological Seminary in San Anselmo, California.

David Feinstein, PhD, is a clinical psychologist and the national director of the Energy Medicine Institute based in Ashland, Oregon. Author of seven books and more than fifty professional papers, he has taught at the Johns Hopkins University School of Medicine and Antioch College. Among his major works are *The Promise of Energy Psychology, The Mythic Path,* and *Rituals for Living and Dying.* His multimedia *Energy Psychology Interactive* was a recipient of the Outstanding Contribution Award of the Association for Comprehensive Energy Psychology.

Bruce D. Feldstein, MD, after 19 years in emergency medicine, became a hospital chaplain in 2000, completing his clinical pastoral education at Stanford Hospital & Clinics. He is the founding director of the Jewish Chaplaincy at Stanford University Medical Center and a member of the National Association of Jewish Chaplains. He teaches spirituality and meaning in medicine at Stanford University School of Medicine as adjunct clinical professor in family and community medicine and is a recipient of a John Templeton Spirituality in Medicine Curricular Award.

John Fox, CPT, is a poet and certified poetry therapist. He is adjunct associate professor at the California Institute of Integral Studies in San Francisco, California. He teaches in the Graduate School of Holistic Studies at John F. Kennedy University in Berkeley, California, and the Institute for Transpersonal Psychology in Palo Alto, California. He is author of *Poetic Medicine: The Healing Art of Poem-making* and *Finding What You Didn't Lose: Expressing Your Truth and Creativity through Poem-Making* and numerous essays. Fox conducts poetry healing circles in the Bay Area and works throughout the United States. He has taught in Ireland, England, Israel, Kuwait, South Korea, and Canada. John is the past president of the National Association for Poetry Therapy 2003 through 2005. He lives in Mountain View, California.

Tamara McClintock Greenberg, PsyD, MS, is assistant clinical professor at the University of California Langley Porter Psychiatric Institute and the University of California San Francisco Medical School. She teaches and supervises in the San Francisco Bay Area on the topics of health psychology and psychoanalytic psychotherapy and on the integration of these two approaches in working with medical patients. Greenberg is author of *The Psychological Impact of Acute and Chronic Illness.* She is in private practice in San Francisco.

Christopher S. M. Grimes, PsyD, is a licensed psychologist practicing in Independence, a suburb of Kansas City, Missouri. He earned his doctorate in clinical psychology from the Forest Institute of Professional Psychology. In addition to clinical work, he maintains research and writing interest in the area of religious and spiritual issues in psychotherapy.

Janice Gronvold, MS, founder of California-based Spectrec, provides business and marketing development services for spa, medical, and healthcare organizations. She graduated from the Stuart School of Business at the Illinois Institute of Technology and eBusiness Strategy Program at the University of Chicago. She has held executive positions with world-renowned resorts, including the Golden Door in California, Rancho La Puerta in Mexico, and medical spas including Medical Spa at Nova in Ashburn, Virginia, and the Obagi Skin Health Institute in Beverly Hills, California. Gronvold serves as an instructor and advisory board member for the Spa and Hospitality Management Program for the University of California, Irvine, is a consultant for Tai Sophia Institute, and a guest instructor for Bastyr University. She has appeared in national and international publications, with projects featured on CNN, BBC, ABC, NBC, NPR, and Travel News Network.

Margaret Heldring, PhD, is a clinical psychologist whose career spans independent practice to public policy. She has served as a clinical assistant professor in family medicine at the University of Washington and senior health advisors to former U.S. Senators Bill Bradley and Paul Wellstone. In 2000, she founded and is president of a national health policy nonprofit organization, America's Health Together (AHT). Funded by the Robert Wood Johnson Foundation, AHT led a groundbreaking partnership after 9/11 to investigate the mental health effects of that disaster and to build capacity in primary healthcare to respond to natural and manmade disasters. AHT is currently working to strengthen philanthropic activity in mental health, both domestically and globally.

Louis Hoffman, PhD, is a core faculty member at the Colorado School of Professional Psychology. In addition, he is an adjunct professor at Fuller Theological Seminary's Graduate School of Psychology, co-director of the God Image Institute, and director of the Depth Psychotherapy Institute, P.C. He is co-editor of *Spirituality and Psychological Health* and the forthcoming *God Image Handbook: Theory, Research, Practice.* His primary professional interests include existential and other depth psychotherapies, religions, and spiritual issues in therapy and the history and philosophy of psychology.

Stanley Krippner, PhD, is professor of psychology at Saybrook Graduate School in San Francisco, California. In 2002, he was given the American Psychological Association's Award for Distinguished Contributions to the International Advancement of Psychology and also has received lifetime achievement awards from the International Association for the Study of Dreams and the Parapsychological Association. He is co-author of *The Mythic Path* and co-editor of *Broken Images, Broken Selves: Dissociative Narratives in Clinical Practice* and *The Psychological Impact of War Trauma on Civilians: An International Perspective.*

Dean Ornish, M.D., is the founder and president of the non-profit Preventive Medicine Research Institute in Sausalito, California, where he holds the Safeway Chair. He is Clinical Professor of Medicine at the University of

California, San Francisco. Dr. Ornish received his medical training in internal medicine from the Baylor College of Medicine, Harvard Medical School, and the Massachusetts General Hospital. He received a BA in Humanities summa cum laude from the University of Texas in Austin, where he gave the baccalaureate address.

For the past 30 years, Dr. Ornish has directed clinical research demonstrating, for the first time, that comprehensive lifestyle changes may begin to reverse even severe coronary heart disease, without drugs or surgery. Recently, Medicare agreed to provide coverage for this program, the first time that Medicare has covered a program of comprehensive lifestyle changes. He recently directed the first randomized controlled trial demonstrating that comprehensive lifestyle changes may stop or reverse the progression of prostate cancer. His current research is focusing on whether comprehensive lifestyle changes may affect gene expression.

He is the author of five best-selling books, including New York Times' bestsellers *Dr. Dean Ornish's Program for Reversing Heart Disease, Eat More, Weigh Less*, and *Love & Survival*. He writes a monthly column for both *Newsweek* and *Reader's Digest* magazines.

The research that he and his colleagues conducted has been published in the *Journal of the American Medical Association, The Lancet, Circulation, The New England Journal of Medicine*, the *American Journal of Cardiology*, and elsewhere. A one-hour documentary of their work was broadcast on *NOVA*, the PBS science series, and was featured on Bill Moyers' PBS series, Healing & *The Mind*. Their work has been featured in all major media, including cover stories in *Newsweek, Time*, and *U.S. News & World Report*.

Dr. Ornish is a member of the boards of directors of the U.S. United Nations High Commission on Refugees, the Quincy Jones Foundation, and the San Francisco Food Bank, and a member of the Google Health Advisory Council. He was appointed to The White House Commission on Complementary and Alternative Medicine Policy and elected to the California Academy of Medicine. He is Chair of the PepsiCo Blue Ribbon Advisory Board and the Safeway Advisory Council on Health and Nutrition and consults directly with the CEO's of McDonald's and Del Monte Foods to make more healthful foods and to provide health education to their customers in this country and worldwide.

He has received several awards, including the 1994 Outstanding Young Alumnus Award from the University of Texas, Austin, the University of California, Berkeley, "National Public Health Hero" award, the Jan J. Kellermann Memorial Award for distinguished contribution in the field of cardiovascular disease prevention from the International Academy of Cardiology, a Presidential Citation from the American Psychological Association, the Beckmann Medal from the German Society for Prevention and Rehabilitation of

Cardiovascular Diseases, the "Pioneer in Integrative Medicine" award from California Pacific Medical Center, the "Excellence in Integrative Medicine" award from the Heal Breast Cancer Foundation, the Golden Plate Award from the American Academy of Achievement, a U.S. Army Surgeon General Medal, and the Bravewell Collaborative Pioneer of Integrative Medicine award. Dr. Ornish has been a physician consultant to The White House and to several bipartisan members of the U.S. Congress. He is listed in *Who's Who in Healthcare and Medicine*, *Who's Who in America*, and *Who's Who in the World*.

Dr. Ornish was recognized as "one of the most interesting people of 1996" by People magazine, featured in the "TIME 100" issue on integrative medicine, and chosen by LIFE magazine as "one of the 50 most influential members of his generation."

A. Griffin Pollock, BA, received her bachelor in arts degree in psychology from Wake Forest University. The focus of her research has been attention process training as well as neuropsychological concomitants of coronary artery bypass surgery. In addition, she is working on the translation of a Russian neuropsychology textbook, *Localization in Clinical Neuropsychology and Neuroscience*. Pollock works as a technician for a home health agency during her application process for graduate training in neuropsychology.

Antonio E. Puente, PhD, received his doctorate from the University of Georgia. He is professor of psychology at the University of North Carolina, Wilmington, and maintains a private practice in clinical neuropsychology. He has published six books and over 150 articles and has been editor of *Neuropsychology Review*. Puente has been president of several organizations (e.g., the National Academy of Neuropsychology) and has chaired several American Psychological Association (APA) boards and committees as well as representing APA on the AMA's Current Procedural Terminology panel.

Dean Radin, PhD, is senior scientist at the Institute of Noetic Sciences (IONS) in Petaluma, California. He also serves as adjunct faculty at Sonoma State University and as a member of the distinguished consulting faculty at Saybrook Graduate School. Radin earned advanced degrees in electrical engineering from the University of Massachusetts and the University of Illinois, Urbana-Champaign, and a PhD in psychology, also from the University of Illinois. Before joining the IONS research staff, he worked at AT&T Bell Laboratories, GTE Laboratories, Princeton University, University of Edinburgh, University of Nevada, and three Silicon Valley research labs. Author of over 200 scientific and popular articles, Radin is also author of *The Conscious Universe* and *Entangled Minds*.

Kirwan Rockefeller, PhD, is director of continuing education at the University of California, Irvine. His expertise includes psychology, visual and performing arts, humanities, and body-mind modalities. He has taught organizational behavior and social psychology at the doctoral level and has consulted with top national and entertainment organizations on the accurate depiction of social and mental health issues, including the Entertainment Industries Council, Inc., ABC, CBS, NBC, FOX, Paramount Pictures, Universal Studios, Warner Bros., Centers for Disease Control and Prevention, National Institute on Drug Abuse, The Robert Wood Johnson Foundation and Ogilvy Public Relations Worldwide. He is the author of *Visualize Confidence: How To Use Guided Imagery to Overcome Self-Doubt.* He has presented at the Susan Samueli Center for Integrative Medicine and is a member of the American Psychological Association and California Psychological Association.

Ronald H. Rozensky, PhD, ABPP, is board certified in both clinical and clinical health psychology by the American Board of Professional Psychology. He is professor and associate dean for international programs in the College of Public Health and Health Professions at the University of Florida, where he served as chair of the Department of Clinical and Health Psychology for eight years. Rozensky has published five books on the science and practice of psychology in medical settings as well as numerous chapters and journal articles on health psychology and professional practice issues in psychology. He is a member of the board of directors of the American Psychological Association and is the founding editor of the *Journal of Clinical Psychology in Medical Settings.*

Beverly Rubik, PhD, is president and founder of the Institute for Frontier Science, a nonprofit organization for research and education on consciousness, subtle energies, and complementary medicine, in Emeryville, California. She has over 60 publications in these areas, including several on qigong research. She serves on the editorial board of the *Journal of Alternative and Complementary Medicine* and that of *Integrative Medicine Insights.* Rubik is also a core professor at the Graduate College of Union Institute and University in Cincinnati, Ohio. She is professionally listed in *Who's Who in the World.* Rubik received the Scientist of the Year Award at the Eighth World Qigong Congress in 2005 for her research on qigong.

Marilyn Schlitz, PhD, is vice president for research and education at the Institute of Noetic Sciences and senior scientist at the Research Institute of the California Pacific Medical Center. Schlitz completed a bachelor of philosophy degree from Montieth College, Wayne State University; a masters of arts in social and behavioral studies from the University of Texas, San Antonio; a PhD in social anthropology from the University of Texas, Austin; a postdoctoral fellowship in the Cognitive Sciences Laboratory, Science Applications International Corporation; and a postdoctoral fellowship in psychology at Stanford University. She has published over 200 articles in the area of consciousness studies and is the co-editor of *Consciousness and Healing: Integral Approaches to Mind Body Medicine*. Schlitz has conducted research at Stanford University, Science Applications International Corporation, the Institute for Parapsychology, and the Mind Science Foundation; has taught at Trinity University, Stanford University, and Harvard Medical School; and has lectured widely at sites including the United Nations and the Smithsonian Institution. She served as a congressionally appointed advisory member for the National Institutes of Health Center for Complementary and Alternative Medicine and is on the board of trustees for the Esalen Institute and the board of directors for the Institute of Noetic Sciences. She also serves on the Scientific Program Committee for the Tucson Center for Consciousness Studies.

Samuel F. Sears, PhD, is an associate professor at the University of Florida Health Science Center in the College of Public Health and Health Professions in the Department of Clinical and Health Psychology. He holds a joint appointment in the Division of Cardiovascular Medicine. His clinical practice is focused on providing psychological services to cardiac patients. He is a nationally recognized expert in research on the psychological care and quality of life outcomes of patients with arrhythmias and implantable cardioverter defibrillators.

Ilene A. Serlin, PhD, ADTR, is a clinical psychologist and registered dance/movement therapist. She is the founder and director of Union Street Health Associates and the Arts Medicine Program at California Pacific Medical Center. She is a fellow of the American Psychological Association, past president and council representative of the Division of Humanistic Psychology of the American Psychological Association. She is on the editorial boards of *The Arts in Psychotherapy*, the *Journal of Dance Therapy*, and the *Journal of Humanistic Psychology* and has taught and published widely in the United States and abroad. Serlin's approach draws on her extensive background of training and experience in dance and the arts, Gestalt and depth psychotherapy, and behavioral medicine. She has been dancing for 40 years and trained in Labanotation with Irmgard Bartenieff. She studied and taught with Laura Perls at the New York Gestalt Institute, did her predoctoral internship at the Children's Clinic of the C. G. Jung Institute of Los Angeles, and taught at the University of California, Los Angeles, Lesley University, Saybrook Graduate School, and the California School of Professional Psychology.

Shauna L. Shapiro, PhD, is a professor of counseling psychology at Santa Clara University. She has published over three dozen articles and book chapters in the area of meditation and has presented her research nationally and internationally. Shapiro's current work is focused on the mechanisms of meditation, examining the ways through which change and transformation occur.

David Spiegel, MD, is the Jack, Lulu, and Sam Willson Professor in the School of Medicine Professor, associate chair of psychiatry and behavioral sciences, director of the Center on Stress and Health, and medical director of the Center for Integrative Medicine at Stanford University School of Medicine, where he has been a member of the academic faculty since 1975. He is past president of the American College of Psychiatrists, and is past president of the Society for Clinical and Experimental Hypnosis. He has published 10 books, 137 book chapters, and 277 scientific journal articles on hypnosis, psychosocial oncology, stress, trauma, and psychotherapy. His research is supported by the National Institute of Mental Health, the National Cancer Institute, the National Institute on Aging, the John D. and Catherine T. MacArthur Foundation, the Fetzer Institute, the Dana Foundation, and the Nathan S. Cummings Foundation, among others. He is winner of 22 awards, including the 2004 Judd Marmor Award from the American Psychiatric Association for biopsychosocial research and the Hilgard Award from the International Society of Hypnosis. His research on cancer patients was featured in Bill Moyers's Emmy award-winning PBS series, *Healing and the Mind,* and recently on the *Jane Pauley Show.*

Lauren Vazquez, MS, is a doctoral candidate at the University of Florida in the College of Public Health and Health Professions in the Department of Clinical and Health Psychology. She has served as project director for multiple grant-supported research studies focusing on the psychological care of cardiac patients. She is the recipient of a predoctoral fellowship from the National Institutes of Health for her research on women with implantable cardioverter defibrillators.

Roger Walsh MD, PhD, is professor of psychiatry, philosophy, and anthropology and is adjunct professor of religious studies at the University of California at Irvine. His books include *Paths Beyond Ego: The Transpersonal Vision, Essential Spirituality: The Seven Central Practices,* and *The World of Shamanism.*

ABOUT THE ADVISERS

Laura Barbanel, EdD, ABPP, served as professor and program head of the graduate program in the School Psychology at Brooklyn College of the City University of New York for many years. She also served as deputy dean for graduate studies for the School of Education at Brooklyn College. Dr. Barbanel is currently in private practice in Brooklyn, New York. She works with adults and children, couples, and families.

Dr. Barbanel is a fellow of the American Psychological Association (APA) and a diplomate of the American Board of Professional Psychology. She has served in a number of elected and appointed positions in the APA, on its board of directors, and currently on the Committee for the Advancement of Practice. She is president-elect of Division 42, the division of independent practice. In this capacity, she has established a Task Force on Health Care for the Whole Person, which focuses on the collaboration of psychologists with physicians in the delivery of healthcare.

William Benda, MD, FACEP, FAAEM, received his professional training at Duke University, University of Miami School of Medicine, Harbor-UCLA Medical Center, and the Program in Integrative Medicine at the University of Arizona. His research and clinical work has focused on patients with breast cancer, animal-assisted therapy, and physician health and well-being. He was principal investigator on two National Center for Complementary and Alternative Medicine–funded investigations of therapeutic horseback riding in the treatment of children with cerebral palsy and is currently extending this research to the field of pediatric autism. Benda is a co-founder of the National Integrative Medicine Council, a nonprofit organization for which he has served as director of medical and public affairs. He is an editor, contributor, and medical advisory board member for a number of conventional and alternative medicine journals and has lectured extensively on a variety of topics in the integrative arena.

Lillian Comas-Diaz, PhD, is the executive director of the Transcultural Mental Health Institute, a clinical professor at the George Washington University Department of Psychiatry and Behavioral Sciences, and a private practitioner in Washington, DC. The former director of the American Psychological Association's Office of Ethnic Minority Affairs, Comas-Diaz was also the director of the Yale University Department of Psychiatry Hispanic Clinic. She is the senior editor of two textbooks: *Clinical Guidelines in Cross-Cultural Mental Health* and *Women of Color: Integrating Ethnic and Gender Identities in Psychotherapy.* Additionally, Comas-Diaz is the founding editor in chief of the American Psychological Association Division 45 official journal, *Cultural Diversity and Ethnic Minority Psychology.* She is a member of numerous editorial boards and currently is an associate editor of *American Psychologist.*

Rita Dudley-Grant, PhD, MPH, ABPP, is a psychologist currently serving as clinical director of Virgin Islands Behavioral Services, a system of residential services for emotionally disturbed and behaviorally disordered adolescents. She has published and presented extensively on child and adolescent mental health and substance abuse both locally and nationally. A practicing Nichiren SGI Buddhist for the past 26 years, she has presented on Buddhism and psychology as well as spirituality at meetings of the American Psychological Association since 1998. Dudley-Grant is co-editor of *Psychology and Buddhism: From Individual to Global Community.*

Jeffrey E. Evans, PhD, is clinical associate professor in the Department of Physical Medicine and Rehabilitation, Division of Rehabilitation Psychology and Neuropsychology, University of Michigan where he treats patients with brain injuries and other conditions. He also holds an appointment in the Residential College at U of M where he has taught courses on the psychology of creativity, psychology of consciousness, and brain and mind since the 1970s. His dissertation, "The Dancer from the Dance: Meaning and Creating in Modern Dance Choreography" (1980), is a life historical exploration of creative style. Recent research includes executive mental processes involved in task switching.

Joseph S. Geller, JD, has been active in policy-making, government relations, and community service for many years. He was elected mayor of the City of North Bay Village, Florida, in 2004 and was reelected in 2006. He previously served North Bay Village as an interim city attorney in 2003. He was chair of the Dade County Democratic Party from 1989 to December 2000. He also served as a member of the Democratic National Committee. He was an attorney for the Gore campaign during the recount litigation and represented former Attorney General Janet Reno in regard to the gubernatorial primary in 2002 and the John Kerry campaign in 2004. Geller is a partner in the Hollywood, Florida, law firm of Geller, Geller, Fisher & Garfinkel, LLP. The partners specialize in governmental relations, real estate, land use, civil litigation, municipal law, administrative and appellate practice, and corporate practice. Geller is admitted to practice in the Supreme Court of the State of Florida, the United States District Court, Southern District of Florida, and the United States Court of Appeals for the Eleventh Circuit.

Marjorie S. Greenberg, MA, is chief of the Classifications and Public Health Data Standards staff at the National Center for Health Statistics (NCHS), Centers for Disease Control and Prevention, Department of Health and Human Services (DHHS). Greenberg, who has been with NCHS since 1982, also serves as executive secretary to the National Committee on Vital and Health Statistics, which is the external advisory committee to DHHS on health information policy, and as head of the World Health Organization Collaborating Center for the Family of International Classifications for North America. Her areas of interest and expertise include health data standardization, uniform health data sets, health classifications, data policy development, and evaluation policy. She received her bachelor's degree from Wellesley College and a master's degree from Harvard University.

Stanislav Grof, MD, is a psychiatrist with more than fifty years of experience in research of nonordinary states of consciousness. He has served as principal investigator in a psychedelic research program at the Psychiatric Research Institute in Prague, Czechoslovakia; chief of psychiatric research at the Maryland Psychiatric Research Center; assistant professor of psychiatry at the Johns Hopkins University; and scholar-in-residence at the Esalen Institute. He is professor of psychology at the California Institute of Integral Studies and Pacifica Graduate Institute, conducts professional training programs in holotropic breathwork and transpersonal psychology, and gives lectures and seminars worldwide. He is one of the founders and chief theoreticians of transpersonal psychology. He has contributed 18 books and more than 130 papers to the professional literature. Among his books are *Psychology* *of the Future, The Ultimate Journey, When the Impossible Happens, The Cosmic Game,* and *The Stormy Search for the Self* (with Chr istina Grof). His Web site is www.holotropic.com.

Gay Powell Hanna, PhD, MFA, is the executive director of the Society for the Arts in Healthcare. Through faculty positions at Florida State University and the University of South Florida (USF) from 1987 to 2002, Hanna directed VSA arts of Florida, an affiliate of the John F. Kennedy Center for the Performing Arts, providing arts education programs for people with disabilities including people with chronic illness. In 2001, she established the Florida Center for Creative Aging at the Florida Policy Exchange Center on Aging at USF to address quality of life issues. A contributing author to numerous articles and books, including the *Fundamentals of Arts Management,* 4th edition, published by the Arts Extension Service of University of Massachusetts Amherst, Hanna is noted for her expertise in accessibility and universal design. In addition, she is a practicing artist who maintains an active studio with work in private and corporate collections through the southeastern United States.

Margaret Heldring, PhD, is a clinical psychologist whose career spans independent practice to public policy. She has served as a clinical assistant professor in family medicine at the University of Washington and senior health advisors to former U.S. Senators Bill Bradley and Paul Wellstone. In 2000, she founded and is president of a national health policy nonprofit organization, America's Health Together (AHT). Funded by the Robert Wood Johnson Foundation, AHT led a groundbreaking partnership after 9/11 to investigate the mental health effects of that disaster and to build capacity in primary healthcare to respond to natural and manmade disasters. AHT is currently working to strengthen philanthropic activity in mental health, both domestically and globally.

James G. Kahn, MD, MPH, is a professor of health policy and epidemiology at the University of California, San Francisco, in the Institute for Health Policy Studies. Kahn is an expert in policy modeling in healthcare, cost-effectiveness analysis, and evidence-based medicine. His work focuses on the use of cost-effectiveness analysis to inform decision-making in public health and medicine. Kahn and colleagues recently published a study in *Health Affairs* entitled "The Cost of Health Insurance Administration in California: Insurer, Physician, and Hospital Estimates." This is the first study to quantify U.S. healthcare administration costs by setting (i.e., insurer, hospital, and physician groups) and within setting by functional department (e.g., billing). It found that insurance-related administration represents at least 21 percent of physician and hospital care funded through private insurance. The research led to the follow-ing in Harper's Index: "Estimated amount the U.S. would save each year on paperwork if it adopted single-payer healthcare: $161,000,000,000" (http://harpers.org/HarpersIndex2006-02.html). Kahn was the leader of a team of Physicians for a National Health Program physicians who submitted a single-payer proposal for the California Health Care Options project.

Gwendolyn Puryear Keita, PhD, is the executive director of the Public Interest Directorate of the American Psychological Association, where she had previously served as director of the Women's Programs Office for 18 years. She has written extensively and made numerous presentations on women's issues, particularly in the areas of women's health and women and depression, and on topics related to work, stress, and health. She has convened three conferences on psychosocial and behavioral factors in women's health and is coauthor of *Health Care and Women: Psychological, Social and Behavioral Influences.* Keita was instrumental in developing the new field of occupational health psychology, has convened six international conferences on occupational stress and health, and coauthored sev-eral books and journal articles on the subject, including *Work and Well-Being: An Agenda for the 1990s* (1992), *Job Stress in a Changing Workforce: Investigating Gen-der, Diversity, and Family Issues* (1994), and *Job Stress Interventions* (1995). Keita has presented before Congress on depression, violence, and other issues.

Kenneth Kushner, PhD, received his PhD in psychology from the University of Michigan in 1977. He is a professor in the Department of Family Medicine of the University of Wisconsin. He has practiced Zen for over 25 years and is a Zen Master in the Chozen-ji lineage. He is founder of the Chozen-ji Betsuin/International Zen Dojo of Wisconsin and the author of *One Arrow, One Life: Zen, Archery and Enlightenment.*

William Mauk, MBA, has a long history in public service and in the private healthcare and administrative consulting arena. Graduating from the Univer-sity of California, Los Angeles, with an MBA degree in finance, Mauk has worked with the Agency for International Development. He was appointed by President Carter to serve as deputy comptroller of that agency in 1977 and in 1979 by President Carter as deputy administrator of the Small Busi-ness Administration. Beginning in the 1980s, he was senior vice president of administration for the John Alden Life Insurance Company. From 1995 to 2002, he was chief executive officer for the Health Maintenance Organiza-tion, Neighborhood Health Partnership. Since that time he has been active as a business and political consultant. He is currently CEO of VIVA Democracy, providing Internet software consultation for political campaigns.

Susan McDaniel, PhD, is professor of psychiatry and family medicine, associate chair of family medicine, and director of family programs and the Wynne Center for Family Research in Psychiatry at the University of Rochester School of Medicine and Dentistry. Her special areas of interest are behavioral health in primary care and family dynamics and genetic conditions. She is a frequent speaker at meetings of both health and mental health professionals. McDaniel is co-editor of the journal *Families, Systems & Health.* She coauthored or edited the following books: *Systems Consultation* (1986), *Family-Oriented Primary Care* (1990 and 2005), *Medical Family Therapy* (1992), *Integrating Family Therapy* (1995), *Counseling Families with Chronic Illness* (1995), *The Shared Experience of Illness* (1997), *Casebook for Integrating Family Therapy* (2001), *Primary Care Psychology* (2004), *The Biopsychosocial Approach* (2004), and *Individuals, Families, and the New Era of Genetics (2007).* Her books have been translated into seven languages.

Marc Micozzi, MD, is a physician-anthropologist who has worked to create science-based tools for the health professions to be better informed and productively engaged in the new fields of complementary and alternative (CAM) and integrative medicine. He was the founding editor-in-chief of the first U.S. journal in CAM, *Journal of Complementary and Alternative Medicine: Research on Paradigm, Practice and Policy* (1994). He organized and edited the first U.S. textbook, *Fundamentals of Complementary & Alternative Medicine* (1996), now in its third edition. In addition, he has served as series editor for Medical Guides to Complementary and Alternative Medicine with 18 titles in print on a broad range of therapies and therapeutic systems within the scope of CAM. In 1999, he edited *Current Complementary Therapies,* focusing on contemporary innovations and controversies, and *Physician's Guide to Complementary and Alternative Medicine.* In 2002, he became founding director of the Policy Institute for Integrative Medicine in Washington, DC.

Geoffrey M. Reed, PhD, is a clinical and health psychologist who, from 1995 to 2006, was assistant executive director for professional development at the American Psychological Association. He has worked with the World Health Organization (WHO) on the development and implementation of the International Classification of Functioning, Disability, and Health (ICF) since 1995. He continues to lead the development of a multidisciplinary procedural manual and guide for standardized application of the ICF with the official involvement of national professional associations representing psychology, speech-language pathology, occupational therapy, recreational therapy, physical therapy, and social work. He is senior consultant for WHO projects with the International Union of Psychological Sciences and is an international consultant on healthcare issues. He is a member of the WHO

International Advisory Group for the revision of the Chapter V: Mental and Behavioural Disorders of the International Classification of Diseases and Related Health Problems. He lives in Madrid, Spain.

Elaine Sims AB, MA, is the director of the University of Michigan Hospitals and Healthcare Centers Gifts of Art program. She has worked in arts in healthcare since 1990. Her areas of expertise include the visual and performing arts, healing gardens, caring for the caregiver initiatives, as well as the full spectrum of arts in healthcare offerings including art cart programs, bedside music, artists-in-residence, medical school arts curriculum, and running a full medical center orchestra. Sims is serving her third term on the board of the Society for the Arts in Healthcare (SAHCS). She is also a consultant for the SAHCS consulting service. Sims is a member of the Ann Arbor Commission for Art in Public Places. She also serves on the University of Michigan Health System Environment of Care Committee and the Interior Design Standards Committee. She particularly enjoys collaborating with university and community partners in exploring and promoting the world of arts in healthcare.

Louise Sundararajan, PhD, received her doctorate in history of religions from Harvard University and her EdD in counseling psychology from Boston University. Currently a forensic psychologist, she was president of the International Society for the Study of Human Ideas on Ultimate Reality and Meaning. A member of American Psychological Association and the International Society for Research on Emotions, she has authored over forty articles in refereed journals and books, on topics ranging from Chinese poetics to alexithymia.

Tobi Zausner, PhD, who has an interdisciplinary PhD in art and psychology, is also an art historian and an award-winning visual artist with works in major museums and private collections around the world. Zausner writes and lectures widely on the psychology of art and teaches at the C. G. Jung Foundation in New York. She is an officer on the board of ACTS (Arts, Crafts, and Theatre Safety), a nonprofit organization investigating health hazards in the arts, and was chair of art history in the Society for Chaos Theory in Psychology and the Life Sciences. Zausner is writing a book on physical illness and the creative process of visual artists titled *When Walls Become Doorways: Creativity and the Transforming Illness.*

CUMULATIVE INDEX

impairments, **1**:236; participation, **1**:236; participation restrictions, **1**:236; performance, **1**:236–37; religion, **1**:243–44; spirituality, **1**:243–44

Clergy, spiritual caretaking role, **2**:135–38

Client, of healthcare, redefined, **1**:47–50

Clifford, Sally, **3**:55

Clinical pastoral education (CPE), **2**:137–38

Clinical psychology: arts inclusion introduction in, **3**:259–60; assessment in, **3**:262–63; doctoral programs curricula, **3**:261–62; integration of arts, **3**:267; psychotherapy training core, **3**:263–65; role for aesthetics, **3**:275–77; training models, **3**:265–67

Clinical Psychology Programme (Canterbury Christ Church University), **3**:266

Clinton, Bill, **1**:35–36

Clinton Health Security Act, **1**:289

Closure phase, of creative process, **3**:82–83

Clown Care Unit, **3**:48

Coalition for the Advancement of Medical Research (CAMR), **1**:291

Codes: current procedural terminology codes, **2**:1; for health/behavior, **1**:4, 268–70; integrated care, **1**:270–71; prevention, **1**:271–72; of ICF: activity, **1**:236; activity limitations, **1**:236; body functions, **1**:236; capacity, **1**:236–37; environmental factors, **1**:236; human rights, **1**:243–44; impairments, **1**:236; participation, **1**:236; participation restrictions, **1**:236; performance, **1**:236–37; religion, **1**:243–44; spirituality, **1**:243–44

Cognitive control, **3**:93

Cognitive therapy, **3**:204

Cognitive-Analytic Therapy (CAT), **3**:264

Cognitive-behavioral strategies: for anxiety management, **2**:9–10; and guided imagery, **2**:65; and mindfulness, **2**:108; for pain management, **2**:11–12

Cohen, S., **2**:56, 58

Coherence: and euthymia, **3**:94; and relaxation/flow, **3**:102–3

Cold Water Treatments (Hahn), **2**:29

Collaborations, between primary care/ mental health providers, **1**:4

Collaborative Family Health Association, **1**:4

College of Fine Arts (University of Florida), **3**:48

Color research, **1**:57–58

COMBI-assessment, Biscayne Academy, **1**:187, 190–91

Communication technologies, **1**:107

Communications: with dying people, **2**:247–48; in hospital settings, **2**:3; nonverbal communication, **2**:68

Communities: approaches to death/dying, **3**:193; and continuity of care issue, **2**:12–17; empowerment of, **1**:44; influence on families, **1**:46; linking of, **1**:49; and psychological interventions, **2**:3; survival of, **1**:48. *See also* Quipunet virtual community

Community health aide/practitioners (CHA/Ps), Alaska model, **1**:204; exposure to community health aide manual, **1**:227; and public/personal knowledge distinction, **1**:206

Community Stress Prevention Center (Israel), **3**:254

Comorbidity concerns, **1**:3

Complementary and alternative medicine (CAM) practitioner: usage by ethnicity, **1**:163, **2**:64–65; view of integrative medicine, **1**:124–30; homeopathy, **1**:129–30; naturopathy, **1**:129; traditional Chinese medicine, **1**:125–29

Complementary and alternative medicines (CAM), **1**:2–3; defined, **1**:33–34, 249; growing pains of, **1**:35; and health insurance, **1**:265; integration with mainstream healthcare, **1**:5; malpractice/negligence issue, **1**:250–51; rating of healing practices, **2**:178; scope of practice, **1**:251–54; treatment offerings in hospitals, **2**:27

Components of health/well-being, of ICF: conceptual model, **1**:235–36; reciprocity, **1**:235; scope, **1**:235; universality, **1**:235

Compton, W. C., **2**:116